T0204162

BLOOD AND CIRCULATORY DISORDERS

SOURCEBOOK

SIXTH EDITION

Health Reference Series

BLOOD AND CIRCULATORY DISORDERS
SOURCEBOOK

SIXTH EDITION

Provides Basic Consumer Health Information about Blood and Circulatory System Disorders, Such as Anemia, Leukemia, Lymphoma, Hemophilia, Thrombophilia, Bleeding and Clotting Disorders, as well as Artery, Vascular, and Venous Diseases, Including Facts about Blood Types, Blood Donation, Diagnostic Tests and Medications, and Tips for Maintaining Healthy Circulatory System

Along with a Glossary of Terms Related to Blood and Circulatory Disorders and a List of Resources for Additional Help and Information

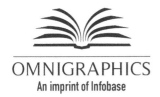

OMNIGRAPHICS
An imprint of Infobase

Bibliographic Note

Because this page cannot legibly accommodate all the copyright notices, the Bibliographic Note portion of the Preface constitutes an extension of the copyright notice.

* * *

OMNIGRAPHICS
An imprint of Infobase
132 W. 31st St.
New York, NY 10001
www.infobase.com
James Chambers, *Editorial Director*

* * *

Copyright © 2023 Infobase
ISBN 978-0-7808-2080-7
E-ISBN 978-0-7808-2081-4

Library of Congress Cataloging-in-Publication Data

Names: Chambers, James (Editor), editor.

Title: Blood and circulatory disorders sourcebook / edited by James Chambers.

Description: Sixth edition. | New York, NY: Omnigraphics, An imprint of Infobase, [2023] | Includes index. | Summary: "Provides basic consumer health information about blood and circulatory system function, various circulatory disorders, and treatment options. Includes index, glossary of related terms, and other resources"-- Provided by publisher.

Identifiers: LCCN 2023024900 (print) | LCCN 2023024901 (ebook) | ISBN 9780780820807 (library binding) | ISBN 9780780820814 (ebook)

Subjects: LCSH: Blood--Diseases--Popular works. | Blood-vessels--Diseases--Popular works.

Classification: LCC RC636.B556 2023 (print) | LCC RC636 (ebook) | DDC 616.1/3--dc23/eng/20230622

LC record available at https://lccn.loc.gov/2023024900
LC ebook record available at https://lccn.loc.gov/2023024901

Table of Contents

Part 4. Bleeding and Clotting Disorders

Part 7. Additional Help and Information

Preface

ABOUT THIS BOOK

Blood plays many important roles in the human body. It carries oxygen and nutrients to the body's cells, helps fight infection, and works to heal wounds. When a disorder inhibits its ability to meet the body's needs or prevents blood from flowing or coagulating properly, a myriad of problems can result. Many blood diseases and disorders are caused by genetic factors. Other risk factors include underlying comorbidities, side effects of medicines, and a lack of certain nutrients in your diet. Notable among these conditions are anemia and bleeding disorders, such as hemophilia.

Blood and Circulatory Disorders Sourcebook, Sixth Edition offers facts about blood function and composition, the maintenance of a healthy circulatory system, and the types of concerns that arise when processes go awry. It discusses the diagnosis and treatment of many common blood cell disorders, bleeding disorders, and circulatory disorders, including anemia, hemochromatosis, leukemia, lymphoma, hemophilia, hypercoagulation, thrombophilia, atherosclerosis, blood pressure irregularities, coronary artery and heart disease, and peripheral vascular disease. Blood donation, cord blood banking, and process of blood transfusions are also discussed. The book concludes with a glossary of terms related to blood and circulatory disorders and a directory of resources for further help and information.

HOW TO USE THIS BOOK

This book is divided into parts and chapters. Parts focus on broad areas of interest. Chapters are devoted to single topics within a part.

Part 1: Understanding the Blood and Circulatory System delves into the composition and functions of blood, covering various types and their roles in the body. It also explores blood donation procedures, cord blood banking, and offers insights for maintaining a healthy circulatory system.

Part 2: Anemia and Related Disorders explores anemia types resulting from inherited or acquired deficiencies in red blood cell production, as well as genetic predisposition-based hemolytic anemias. The part provides comprehensive information on causes, diagnosis, and management of anemia.

Part 3: Cancer and Other Blood Disorders details blood cancers such as leukemia, lymphoma, and plasma cell disorders, as well as white blood cell disorders. The part clarifies causes, diagnosis, and treatment strategies for these conditions.

Part 4: Bleeding and Clotting Disorders examines bleeding disorders from insufficient clotting (e.g., hemophilia, von Willebrand disease) and excess clotting (e.g., DVT, PE). Diagnosis and treatment methods for these conditions are explored, along with comprehensive information on various factors affecting clotting.

Part 5: Circulatory Disorders focuses on disorders of veins, arteries, and the heart, including aneurysms, stroke, blood pressure irregularities, atherosclerosis, and more. The part offers insight into causes, diagnosis, and treatment options for the circulatory disorders.

Part 6: Diagnosing and Treating Blood and Circulatory Disorders provides information about medical tests used for identifying and monitoring blood and circulatory disorders, along with insights into medications and treatment.

Part 7: Additional Help and Information includes a glossary of terms related to blood and circulatory disorders and a directory of resources offering additional help and support.

BIBLIOGRAPHIC NOTE

This volume contains documents and excerpts from publications issued by the following U.S. government agencies: Agency for Healthcare Research and Quality (AHRQ); Centers for Disease Control and Prevention (CDC); Genetic and Rare Diseases Information Center (GARD); Genetics Home Reference (GHR); Health Resources and Services Administration (HRSA); MedlinePlus; National Cancer Institute (NCI); National Heart, Lung, and Blood Institute (NHLBI); National Institute of Arthritis and Musculoskeletal and Skin Diseases (NIAMS); National Institute of Diabetes and Digestive and Kidney Diseases (NIDDK); National Institute of Neurological Disorders and Stroke (NINDS); National Institute on Aging (NIA); National Institutes of Health (NIH); *NIH News in Health*; Office of Dietary Supplements (ODS); Office of Disease Prevention and Health Promotion (ODPHP); Office on Women's Health (OWH); Surveillance, Epidemiology, and End Results (SEER) Program; U.S. Food and Drug Administration (FDA); and U.S. Social Security Administration (SSA).

It also contains original material produced by Infobase and reviewed by medical consultants.

ABOUT THE *HEALTH REFERENCE SERIES*

The *Health Reference Series* is designed to provide basic medical information for patients, families, caregivers, and the general public. Each volume provides comprehensive coverage on a particular topic. This is especially important for people who may be dealing with a newly diagnosed disease or a chronic disorder in themselves or in a family member. People looking for preventive guidance, information about disease warning signs, medical statistics, and risk factors for health problems will also find answers to their questions in the *Health Reference Series*. The *Series*, however, is not intended to serve as a tool for diagnosing illness, in prescribing treatments, or as a substitute for the physician–patient relationship. All people concerned about medical symptoms or the possibility of disease are encouraged to seek professional care from an appropriate health-care provider.

A NOTE ABOUT SPELLING AND STYLE

Health Reference Series editors use *Stedman's Medical Dictionary* as an authority for questions related to the spelling of medical terms and *The Chicago Manual of Style* for questions related to grammatical structures, punctuation, and other editorial concerns. Consistent adherence is not always possible, however, because the individual volumes within the *Series* include many documents from a wide variety of different producers, and the editor's primary goal is to present material from each source as accurately as is possible. This sometimes means that information in different chapters or sections may follow other guidelines and alternate spelling authorities. For example, occasionally a copyright holder may require that eponymous terms be shown in possessive forms (Crohn's disease vs. Crohn disease) or that British spelling norms be retained (leukaemia vs. leukemia).

MEDICAL REVIEW

Infobase contracts with a team of qualified, senior medical professionals who serve as medical consultants for the *Health Reference Series*. As necessary, medical consultants review reprinted and originally written material for currency and accuracy. Citations including the phrase "Reviewed (month, year)" indicate material reviewed by this team. Medical consultation services are provided to the *Health Reference Series* editors by:

Dr. Vijayalakshmi, MBBS, DGO, MD
Dr. Senthil Selvan, MBBS, DCH, MD
Dr. K. Sivanandham, MBBS, DCH, MS (Research), PhD

HEALTH REFERENCE SERIES UPDATE POLICY

The inaugural book in the *Health Reference Series* was the first edition of *Cancer Sourcebook* published in 1989. Since then, the *Series* has been enthusiastically received by librarians and in the medical community. In order to maintain the standard of providing high-quality health information for the layperson, the editorial staff felt it was necessary to implement a policy of updating volumes when warranted.

Medical researchers have been making tremendous strides, and it is the purpose of the *Health Reference Series* to stay current with the most recent advances. Each decision to update a volume is made on an individual basis. Some of the considerations include how much new information is available and the feedback we receive from people who use the books. If there is a topic you would like to see added to the update list, or an area of medical concern you feel has not been adequately addressed, please write to: custserv@infobaselearning.com.

Part 1 | Understanding the Blood and Circulatory System

Chapter 1 | **Blood Function and Composition**

Blood is a connective tissue and, as a connective tissue, it consists of cells and cell fragments (formed elements) that are suspended in an intercellular matrix (plasma). Blood is the only liquid tissue in the body that measures about 5 liters in an adult human and accounts for 8 percent of body weight.

The body consists of metabolically active cells that need a continuous supply of nutrients and oxygen. Metabolic waste products need to be removed from the cells to maintain a stable cellular environment. Blood is the primary transport medium that is responsible for meeting these cellular demands.

Blood cells are formed in the bone marrow, the soft, spongy center of bones. New (immature) blood cells are called "blasts." Some blasts stay in the marrow to mature. Some travel to other parts of the body to mature.

The activities of the blood may be categorized as transportation, regulation, and protection.

These functional categories overlap and interact as the blood carries out its role in providing suitable conditions for cellular functions.

The transport functions include the following:
- carrying oxygen and nutrients to the cells
- transporting carbon dioxide and nitrogenous wastes from the tissues to the lungs and kidneys, where these wastes can be removed from the body
- carrying hormones from the endocrine glands to the target tissues

The regulation functions include the following:
- helping regulate body temperature by removing heat from active areas, such as skeletal muscles, and transporting it to other regions or to the skin where it can be dissipated
- playing a significant role in fluid and electrolyte balance because the salts and plasma proteins contribute to the osmotic pressure
- functioning in pH regulation through the action of buffers in the blood

The protection functions include the following:
- clotting mechanisms to prevent fluid loss through hemorrhage when blood vessels are damaged
- helping (phagocytic white blood cells (WBCs)) to protect the body against microorganisms that cause disease by engulfing and destroying the agent
- protecting (antibodies in the plasma) against disease by their reactions with offending agents

COMPOSITION OF THE BLOOD

When a sample of blood is spun in a centrifuge, the cells and cell fragments are separated from the liquid intercellular matrix. Because the formed elements are heavier than the liquid matrix, they are packed in the bottom of the tube by the centrifugal force. The light-yellow-colored liquid on the top is the plasma, which accounts for about 55 percent of the blood volume and red blood cells (RBCs), also called the "hematocrit" or "packed cell volume" (PCV). The WBCs and platelets form a thin white layer, called the "buffy coat," between the plasma and RBCs. Figure 1.1 shows the different components of the blood.

Plasma

Plasma is the watery fluid portion of blood (90% water) in which the corpuscular elements are suspended. It transports nutrients, as well as waste, throughout the body. Various compounds, including proteins, electrolytes, carbohydrates, minerals, and fats, are dissolved in it.

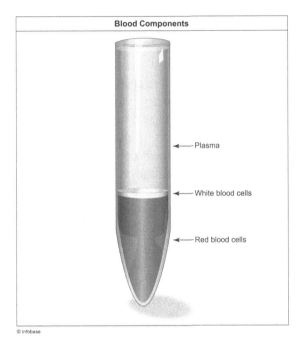

Figure 1.1. Blood Components

Infobase

Formed Elements

The formed elements are cells and cell fragments that are suspended in the plasma. The three classes of formed elements are the erythrocytes (RBCs), leukocytes (WBCs), and thrombocytes (platelets).

ERYTHROCYTES

Erythrocytes, or RBCs, are the most numerous of the formed elements. Erythrocytes are tiny biconcave disks; they are thin in the middle and thicker around the periphery. The shape provides a combination of flexibility for moving through tiny capillaries with a maximum surface area for the diffusion of gases. The primary function of erythrocytes is to transport oxygen and, to a lesser extent, carbon dioxide.

LEUKOCYTES

Leukocytes, or WBCs, are generally larger than erythrocytes, but they are fewer in number. Even though they are considered to be blood cells, leukocytes do most of their work in the tissues. They use the blood as a transport medium. Some are phagocytic, and others produce antibodies; some secrete histamine and heparin, and others neutralize histamine. Leukocytes are able to move through the capillary walls into the tissue spaces, a process called "diapedesis." In the tissue spaces, they provide a defense against organisms that cause disease and either promote or inhibit inflammatory responses.

There are two main groups of leukocytes in the blood. The cells that develop granules in the cytoplasm are called "granulocytes," and those that do not have granules are called "agranulocytes." Neutrophils, eosinophils, and basophils are granulocytes. Monocytes and lymphocytes are agranulocytes.

Neutrophils, the most numerous leukocytes, are phagocytic and have light-colored granules. Eosinophils have granules and help counteract the effects of histamine. Basophils secrete histamine and heparin and have blue granules. In the tissues, they are called "mast cells." Lymphocytes are agranulocytes that have a special role in immune processes. Some attack bacteria directly; others produce antibodies.

THROMBOCYTES

Thrombocytes, or platelets, are not complete cells but are small fragments of very large cells called "megakaryocytes." Megakaryocytes develop from hemocytoblasts in the red bone marrow. Thrombocytes become sticky and clump together to form platelet plugs that close breaks and tears in blood vessels. They also initiate the formation of blood clots.

BLOOD CELL LINEAGE

The production of formed elements, or blood cells, is called "hemopoiesis." Before birth, hemopoiesis occurs primarily in the liver and spleen, but some cells develop in the thymus, lymph nodes, and red bone marrow. After birth, most production is limited to the red bone marrow in specific regions, but some WBCs are produced in lymphoid tissue.

All types of formed elements develop from a single cell type— stem cells (pluripotential cells or hemocytoblasts). Seven different cell lines, each controlled by a specific growth factor, develop from hemocytoblasts. When a stem cell divides, one of the "daughters" remains a stem cell, and the other becomes a precursor cell, either a lymphoid cell or a myeloid cell. These cells continue to mature into various blood cells.

Leukemia can develop at any point in cell differentiation. Figure 1.2 shows the development of the formed elements of the blood.[1]

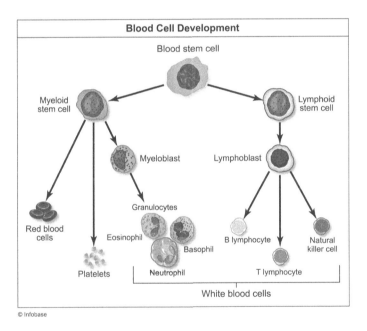

© Infobase

Figure 1.2. Blood Cell Development

Infobase

---

[1] Surveillance, Epidemiology, and End Results (SEER) Program, "Anatomy," National Cancer Institute (NCI), September 7, 2016. Available online. URL: https://training.seer.cancer.gov/leukemia/anatomy. Accessed May 10, 2023.

Chapter 2 | **Blood Groups and Blood Typing**

Blood typing is a classification system used to sort human blood according to the kinds of antigens (blood proteins) found in red blood cells (RBCs). There are four primary types of blood: A, B, O, and AB. Each blood type is further classified by an Rh-positive or Rh-negative designation. Rh refers to the Rhesus factor and indicates the presence (positive) or absence (negative) of a specific protein found on the surface of red blood cells. Blood type is an inherited trait.

Blood typing is important because not all blood types are compatible with each other. Giving the wrong blood type to a person through a blood transfusion can result in serious complications and even death. It is important for pregnant women to know their blood type. If the expectant mother is Rh-negative and the expectant father is Rh-positive, the mother will need to receive treatment to help protect the fetus from complications that could arise from a mix of incompatible blood types.

TESTING BLOOD TYPE

Blood type tests are performed for a variety of reasons. Some of the most common reasons include the following:
- classification of donated blood
- preparation for a blood transfusion or any surgery
- preparation for an organ transplant
- when a woman is pregnant or plans to become pregnant
- identification of individuals (e.g., determining blood relations)

The two most common blood typing tests are the ABO and Rh tests.

The ABO test examines RBCs in order to classify the blood as A, B, AB, or O. Blood that is type A contains the A antigen, and type B contains the B antigen. These two blood types are incompatible. Each type contains antibodies that will attack and destroy the cells of the other. Blood type AB contains both A and B antigens, meaning that it is compatible with both A and B blood types. People with blood type AB can receive blood from anyone of any blood type, making type AB the "universal recipient." Type O blood contains no antigens and can be given to anyone of any blood type. For this reason, type O blood is known as the "universal donor." Figure 2.1 shows which blood types are compatible.

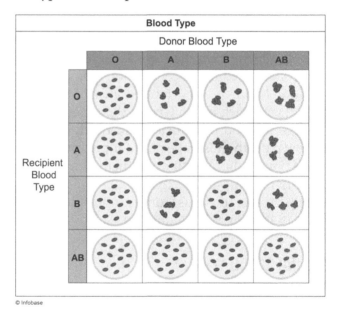

© Infobase

Figure 2.1. Blood Type

Infobase

To test for blood type, a small amount of blood is mixed with serum containing blood antibodies and observed to see if the sample blood cells agglutinate (stick together). Blood cells that stick together when mixed with anti-A serum are classified as type A.

Type B blood cells stick together when mixed with anti-B serum. Type AB blood cells stick together when mixed with both anti-A and anti-B serums. Blood cells that do not stick together when mixed with anti-A or anti-B serums are classified as type O.

A second blood type test is performed to verify the results of the first test. In the second test, known as "back typing," a small amount of the blood being tested is mixed with a small amount of blood that has already been classified as type A or type B and observed for agglutination (sticking together). If the sample blood cells stick together when mixed with type B blood, the sample is identified as type A. Conversely, if the sample blood cells stick together when mixed with type A blood, the sample is identified as type B. If the sample blood cells stick together when mixed with either type A or type B blood, the sample is identified as type O. If the sample blood cells do not stick together when mixed with type A or type B blood, the sample is identified as type AB.

The Rh test is performed by mixing a small blood sample with a serum that contains anti-Rh serum. If the sample blood cells stick together when mixed with anti-Rh serum, the blood is Rh-positive. If the sample blood cells do not stick together when mixed with anti-Rh serum, the blood is Rh-negative. People with Rh-negative blood can only receive Rh-negative blood; people with Rh-positive blood can receive either Rh-positive or Rh-negative blood.

The results of both kinds of blood type testing are used for complete identification of blood type. For example, type A blood that is Rh-positive is A-positive, type B blood that is Rh-negative is B-negative, and so on.

BLOOD TYPE COMPATIBILITY

- A person with A-negative blood can receive A-negative and O-negative blood.
- A person with A-positive blood can receive A-negative, A-positive, O-negative, and O-positive blood.
- A person with B-negative blood can receive B-negative and O-negative blood.
- A person with B-positive blood can receive B-negative, B-positive, O-negative, and O-positive blood.

- A person with AB-negative blood can receive AB-negative and O-negative blood.
- A person with AB-positive blood can receive any type of blood.
- A person with O-negative blood can only receive O-negative blood.
- A person with O-positive blood can receive O-negative or O-positive blood.

References

"Blood Type Test," *WebMD*, September 9, 2014. Available online. URL: www.webmd.com/a-to-z-guides/blood-type-test. Accessed June 1, 2023.

Todd Gersten, MedlinePlus, "Blood Typing," National Institutes of Health (NIH), February 24, 2014. Available online. URL: www.nlm.nih.gov/medlineplus/ency/article/003345.htm. Accessed June 1, 2023.

Chapter 3 | **Blood Donation and Preservation**

Chapter Contents

Section 3.1 | An Overview of Blood Donation

Blood donation is a voluntary procedure in which one person gives some of their blood to help another person. People need to receive blood donations if they are having surgery, if they lost blood from an injury, or if they have certain illnesses such as hemophilia, sickle cell disease (SCD), anemia, or some types of cancer.

BLOOD DONORS

A blood donor is a person who volunteers to give some of their blood through blood donation. Certain requirements must be met in order to become a blood donor. Blood donors must be healthy adults between the ages of 17 and 70 who weigh at least 110 pounds and have normal blood pressure and body temperature. Donors are eligible to give blood once every 56 days.

Certain restrictions exist to protect both blood donors and blood donation recipients. People who are not able to donate blood include pregnant women, people who have recently had a tattoo or piercing, people who are ill, and those taking specific medications. People who have recently traveled to certain countries may also be disqualified from donating blood.

BLOOD DONATION PROCESS

Blood donations are typically collected at blood drives, blood banks, or medical facilities. The process usually begins with a donor screening interview, which is conducted in private. During this interview, a health professional asks a series of questions to determine whether a person is able to donate blood. Questions may focus on past and present health conditions and personal behaviors such as drug use or sexually transmitted diseases (STDs). These questions are asked every time a person donates blood so that any changes in the donor's health can be identified.

After the initial screening interview, the blood donation process takes about 10 minutes. About 1 pint (480 ml) of blood is collected from each blood donor. This amount is equal to about 8 percent of the average adult's total blood volume. The donor's body will replace the volume of donated blood within 24–48 hours. The amount of red blood cells (RBCs) in that volume of blood will be replaced by the donor's body in 10–12 weeks.

Blood donations are tested and screened to ensure the blood is safe to give to another person. These tests usually screen for blood-borne diseases such as hepatitis, human immunodeficiency virus (HIV), West Nile virus (WNV), and other viruses. Blood that tests positive for any of the screened diseases is discarded as medical waste, and the donor is notified of the test results so that they may seek treatment if needed. Donated blood is also checked to identify the blood type (A, B, AB, or O).

TYPES OF DONATED BLOOD

Most donated blood is processed to separate the whole blood into the different components that make up human blood, such as platelets, plasma, and RBCs. This is done because most blood donation recipients only need to receive a certain component of blood.

The following are the different types of blood donation:

- Whole blood contains RBCs, white blood cells (WBCs), plasma, platelets, antibodies, and other components. This type of blood donation is called "homologous."
- Plasma is extracted from donated blood with a centrifuge, which is a machine that spins at a high rate of speed to separate the blood into its components. The plasma is then drawn out of the blood, and the RBCs are returned to the donor. This type of blood donation is called "apheresis."
- Platelets are extracted from blood using a different centrifuge process, and both RBCs and the plasma are returned to the donor. This type of blood donation is called "pheresis."
- Autologous donation refers to blood that is donated by a person for their own use. This type of blood donation is rare and is usually done in special cases.
- Directed or designated donation refers to blood that is donated for use by a specific person. This type of blood donation is also rare and done only in special cases.

RISKS OF DONATING BLOOD

The blood donation process is safe, and there are no health risks associated with donating blood. Sterile, prepackaged equipment is used to collect blood donations, and new equipment is used for each donor. The blood donor may develop a small bruise on their arm at the site from which blood was drawn. Some blood donors feel light-headed or slightly dizzy after giving blood. For this reason, most blood donors are given water, fruit juice, and a small snack and asked to sit for a few minutes after their blood is collected. For the first few hours after donating blood, it is recommended that blood donors refrain from physical activity and drink plenty of fluids.

References

"Blood Donation," Better Health, March 2013. Available online. URL: www.betterhealth.vic.gov.au/health/conditionsandtreatments/blood-donation. Accessed June 1, 2023.

"Donating Blood: Topic Overview," *WebMD*, March 12, 2014. Available online. URL: www.webmd.com/a-to-z-guides/donating-blood-topic-overview. Accessed June 1, 2023.

Section 3.2 | Apheresis

Apheresis, or therapeutic apheresis, is a process in which blood is drawn from the body, then separated, and a selected constituent of the blood, such as plasma or platelets, is removed from the whole blood, and the remaining blood components are returned to the body through reinfusion. This process is carried out using an apheresis machine.

Apheresis is intended to treat a disease by removing unwanted components from whole blood or donating specific blood components from healthy individuals to patients with conditions that can be treated. The procedure for apheresis is similar to blood donation, except that apheresis takes one to two hours and blood donation takes only 20 minutes.

TYPES OF THERAPEUTIC APHERESIS

The types of apheresis are as follows:

- **Plasmapheresis.** During this process, the plasma (the liquid part of the blood) separated from the blood is treated and then reinfused into the body.
- **Cytapheresis.** This is the process of removing specific cellular components, such as red blood cells (RBCs), white blood cells (WBCs), platelets, and sickle cells, from the whole blood.
- **Lipid apheresis.** This is the process of removing low-density lipoprotein cholesterol in patients who have inherited hypercholesterolemia.
- **Photopheresis.** This is the process of removing disease-causing WBCs and exposing them to a medication (8-methoxypsoralen), followed by ultraviolet radiation. The treated WBCs are then returned to the body. This process is also known as "extracorporeal photopheresis" (ECP). It is used in treating graft versus host disease (GVHD), cutaneous T cell lymphoma, psoriasis, Crohn's disease, scleroderma, organ transplant rejection, and many more.

PROCEDURE FOR APHERESIS

The procedure involves the following basic methods:

- **Manual apheresis.** The manual method is similar to the process of blood donation. This method is used when the patient undergoing transfusion has a low RBC count.
- **Automated apheresis.** The automated method uses a cell separator machine to separate the blood components and return the remaining blood to the body. This method is applicable only to healthy donors above the age of 17 and 110 pounds or patients with sufficient RBC count.

APPLICATIONS OF APHERESIS

Apheresis is used clinically to treat various blood disorders and cancer. A few of the applications are as follows:

- **RBC exchange**. The abnormal cells are removed and replaced with healthy RBCs. RBC exchange is widely used for treating sickle cell disease (SCD) and other infectious diseases, such as malaria, caused by mosquitoes, or babesiosis, caused by ticks.
- **Plasma exchange**. This is done to treat conditions such as Guillain-Barré syndrome (GBS), hyperviscosity syndrome, myasthenia gravis, and other severe autoimmune neuron disorders.
- **Autologous stem cell collection**. This is the collection of healthy cells from the patient, which are taken from the bone marrow or the blood before high-dose chemotherapy and returned after completion. Chemotherapy destroys healthy cells and bone marrow. Returning these collected cells helps the damaged cells recover. This autologous stem cell collection treats diseases such as Hodgkin lymphoma, non-Hodgkin lymphoma (NHL), germ cell tumors, symptomatic myeloma, amyloidosis, and sarcoma.
- **Volunteer donor collection**. Blood components are collected from healthy donors for stem cells, which replenish healthy cells; granulocytes, which fight infections; and lymphocytes, which help immune defense. The collected cells are used to treat other patients as needed.
- **Therapies and clinical trials**. Apheresis is used to collect cells for novel therapies that include the treatment of cancers with dendritic cells and chimeric antigen receptor T (CAR-T) cells. They are also used for clinical trials, which are programs to develop new cellular therapies.

COMPLICATIONS IN APHERESIS

The procedure may be risky for individuals who are weak or anemic. Large catheters are inserted for the process, which may lead to heavy bleeding, clotting, and other infections such as pneumothorax (lung collapse). Anticoagulants used to prevent clotting during blood collection may decrease plasma ionized calcium, which is necessary for bone mineralization, secretion of hormones and enzymes, and so on.

References

"Apheresis," Peter MacCallum Cancer Centre, June 22, 2018. Available online. URL: www.petermac.org/services/treatment/haematological-treatments/apheresis/what-apheresis#:~:text=What%20is%20aheresis%20used%20for,range%20of%20other%20blood%20disorders. Accessed July 4, 2023.

"Apheresis in the Office Setting," National Center for Biotechnology Information (NCBI), March 15, 2008. Available online. URL: www.ncbi.nlm.nih.gov/pmc/articles/PMC2793967/#:~:text=Pheresis%20is%20from%20the%20Greek,terms%20often%20are%20used%20interchangeably.&text=Pheresis%20is%20any%20procedure%20in,cells)%20is%20separated%20and%20kept. Accessed July 4, 2023.

"Automated Donations," Community Blood Centre, August 21, 2010. Available online. URL: https://givingblood.org/donate-blood/automated-donations.aspx. Accessed July 4, 2023.

"Bone Marrow Transplant," Mayo Clinic, July 20, 2022. Available online. URL: www.mayoclinic.org/tests-procedures/autologous-stem-cell-transplant/pyc-20384859#. Accessed July 4, 2023.

Brian Castillo and Amer Wahed, "Apheresis," Science Direct, 2018. Available online. URL: www.sciencedirect.com/topics/nursing-and-health-professions/cytapheresis. Accessed July 4, 2023.

Georg Stussi, Andreas Buser, and Andreas Holbro, "Red Blood Cells: Exchange, Transfuse, or Deplete," National Center for Biotechnology Information (NCBI), December 2019. Available online. URL: https://www.ncbi.nlm.nih.gov/pmc/articles/PMC6944943. Accessed July 4, 2023.

Jeffrey L Winters, "Lipid Apheresis, Indications, and Principles," National Center for Biotechnology Information (NCBI), August 10, 2011. Available online. URL: https://pubmed.ncbi.nlm.nih.gov/21834078. Accessed July 4, 2023.

"Photopheresis," Cleveland Clinic, November 14, 2022. Available online. URL: https://my.clevelandclinic.org/health/treatments/10252-photopheresis. Accessed July 4, 2023.

Ravindra Sarode, "Therapeutic Apheresis," MSD Manuals, September 2022. Available online. URL: www.msdmanuals.com/en-in/professional/hematology-and-oncology/transfusion-medicine/therapeutic-apheresis. Accessed July 4, 2023.

Richard T Davey, ClinicalTrials.gov, "Apheresis to Obtain Plasma or White Blood Cells for Laboratory Studies," National Institutes of Health (NIH), June 2, 2023. Available online. URL: https://clinicaltrials.gov/ct2/show/NCT00114647#contacts. Accessed July 4, 2023.

Shane R. Sergent and John V. Ashurst, "Plasmapheresis," National Center for Biotechnology Information (NCBI), July 12, 2022. Available online. URL: www.ncbi.nlm.nih.gov/books/NBK560566. Accessed July 4, 2023.

Section 3.3 | Ensuring Safe Blood Donation

The U.S. Food and Drug Administration (FDA), through the Center for Biologics Evaluation and Research (CBER), is responsible for ensuring the safety of more than approximately 11 million units of whole blood donated each year in the United States. These donations can be further processed into blood components such as red blood cells, platelets, and plasma. In addition, approximately 4 million units of platelets and plasma intended for transfusion are collected annually by apheresis. The FDA's regulations and guidance regarding blood donor eligibility, blood donation, and processing help protect the health of both the donor and the recipient.

FIVE LAYERS OF SAFETY

The FDA's blood safety efforts focus on minimizing the risk of transmitting infectious diseases while maintaining an adequate supply of blood for the nation.

Blood safety is based on five layers of overlapping safeguards:

- **Donor screening**. Donors are provided with educational material and asked to self-defer if they have risk factors that may affect blood safety. Donors are then asked specific questions about their medical history and other risk factors that may affect the safety of their donation. This "up-front" screening identifies ineligible donors.
- **Donor deferral lists**. Blood establishments must keep a current list of deferred donors. They must also check all potential donors against that list to prevent the collection or use of blood from deferred donors.
- **Blood testing**. After donation, blood establishments are required to test each unit of donated blood for the following transfusion-transmitted infections (TTIs):
  - hepatitis B
  - hepatitis C
  - human immunodeficiency virus (HIV) 1 and 2
  - human T-cell lymphotropic virus (HTLV) I and II
  - *Treponema pallidum*, which causes syphilis
  - West Nile virus (WNV)
  - *Trypanosoma cruzi* (Chagas disease)
- **Quarantine**. Donated blood must be quarantined until it is tested and shown to be free of infectious agents.
- **Problems and deficiencies**. Blood establishments must investigate manufacturing problems, correct all deficiencies, and notify the FDA when product deviations occur in distributed products.

If a violation of any one of these safeguards occurs, the blood product is considered unsuitable for transfusion and may be subject to recall.

ARE YOU ELIGIBLE TO DONATE BLOOD?

To meet the basic requirements for donating blood, you must be in good health and:

- have a pulse and blood pressure within acceptable limits
- have a normal temperature
- meet the minimum age requirement per applicable state law
- have an acceptable normal blood hemoglobin level
- be free of infections that can be transmitted through blood transfusion or risk factors closely associated with exposure to these infections
- not have donated blood in the past eight weeks

There are a number of potential reasons that may cause you to be temporarily or permanently deferred from donating blood. These include, but are not limited to:

- not feeling well on the day of the donation
- a history of nonprescription injection drug use
- getting tattooed in the past three months (unless done under sterile conditions and at a state-licensed facility)
- having certain medical conditions or receiving certain medical treatments or medications
- living in or traveling to certain areas for a designated period of time, for example, traveling to an area where malaria is endemic

ONGOING SAFETY EFFORTS

Emerging threats to the blood supply and other potential risks mean that the FDA's blood safety team never stops looking for ways to ensure and preserve the safety of blood and blood products.

The FDA scientists are working to develop sensitive donor screening tests to detect emerging diseases and potential bio-terrorism agents in blood donations. They are also working to improve blood donor screening tests to detect variant strains of HIV, WNV, and hepatitis viruses. In addition, the FDA's Office of

Blood Research and Review addresses donor deferral issues and updates eligibility requirements when appropriate.[1]

Section 3.4 | Storage and Preservation of Blood

Lost blood must be replaced for major surgeries. This is done through transfusion. Blood must be stored and preserved in the right conditions to be used safely.

SAFE STORAGE OF BLOOD

Whole blood and red cells should always be stored between 33.8 °F (1 °C) and 42.8 °F (6 °C), or their oxygen-carrying ability is reduced. The anticoagulant used contains nutrients and prevents the blood from clotting during transport.

Adverse effects may occur if the blood is not transported at the recommended temperatures. Warm temperatures may cause bacterial growth, and freezing temperatures may cause hemolysis or destruction of the blood cells. Cryoprotectants, such as glycerol or hydroxyethyl starch, are used to prevent blood hemolysis. These chemicals protect the blood cells from the damage caused by freezing. Since glycerol is the most popular cryoprotectant, frozen blood is also known as "deglycerolized red blood cells."

Blood should not be frozen in blood collection tubes as it could crack them. Blood samples should be transferred to plastic, pre-screened cryo-vials before freezing since cryo-vials can withstand liquid nitrogen temperatures as low as –320.8 °F (–196 °C). The blood samples in evacuated tubes (sealed, single-use tubes) must be stored at a refrigeration temperature of 39.2 °F (4 °C) and should be shipped in cold packs. Blood samples in cryo-vials should be stored at lower than or equal to –4 °F (–20 °C) and shipped frozen on cold packs or dry ice.

---

[1] "Have You Given Blood Lately?" U.S. Food and Drug Administration (FDA), May 16, 2023. Available online. URL: www.fda.gov/consumers/consumer-updates/have-you-given-blood-lately. Accessed May 31, 2023.

STORAGE CONDITIONS AND SHELF LIFE OF BLOOD COMPONENTS

- Whole blood is stored at 39.2 °F (4 °C) and has a shelf life of 21–35 days. The shelf life of whole blood varies depending on the anticoagulant used.
- Red blood cells or erythrocytes are stored at 39.2 °F (4 °C) and have a shelf life of up to 42 days. The shelf life varies depending on the anticoagulant used.
- Platelets are stored at room temperature and are constantly stirred to prevent clumping and have a shelf life of up to five days.
- Plasma is stored at a temperature of less than or equal to –4 °F (–20 °C) and has a shelf life of one year.
- White blood cells or leukocytes can be risky to donate since they may carry viruses or release toxic substances into the recipient's body. However, granulocytes, a type of white blood cells, that destroy bacteria and viruses can be collected through apheresis and transfused to the patient within 24 hours.

Preservation of Blood

Although blood cells are stored for up to 42 days, the average age of the blood used for transfusion is 18 days. However, depending on the anticoagulant used, the duration of preservation varies. For example, blood preserved in disodium ethylenediamine tetraacetate (Na_2EDTA) can be stored for up to four weeks; in glucose and raffinose at –4 °F (–20 °C), it can last for four to six weeks; and in ethyl-alcohol-saline-sugar solutions, it can last for up to five months.

Shipment of Blood

Sample vials must be stored upright in boxes secured with rubber bands and placed in a biohazard bag with an absorbent material. Containers must be labeled correctly according to sample requirements, such as "Do not freeze," an "up" arrow label in case the box is unlabeled, a dry ice label, an overpack label, and UN3373 Biological Substance, Category B, which must be rotated to a diamond position to be read horizontally.

References

"Blood Components," American Red Cross (ARC), March 16, 2018. Available online. URL: www.redcrossblood.org/donate-blood/how-to-donate/types-of-blood-donations/blood-components.html. Accessed July 4, 2023.

C. Robert Valeri, "Frozen Red Cell Technology," National Library of Medicine (NLM), October 30, 2003. Available online. URL: https://www.ncbi.nlm.nih.gov/books/NBK233117. Accessed July 11, 2023.

"Cryovial Safety," Yale Environmental Health and Safety, September 15, 2020. Available online. URL: https://ehs.yale.edu/sites/default/files/files/cryovial-safety.pdf. Accessed July 4, 2023.

Frederick Proescher and Jean Nolan, "Progress in Blood Preservation," National Center for Biotechnology Information (NCBI), September 1954. Available online. URL: www.ncbi.nlm.nih.gov/pmc/articles/PMC1532116. Accessed July 4, 2023.

"Improving the Collection and Management of Human Samples Used for Biomonitoring," Centers for Disease Control and Prevention (CDC), March 2018. Available online. URL: www.cdc.gov/biomonitoring/pdf/Human_Sample_Collection-508.pdf. Accessed July 4, 2023.

Shokoufeh Aalaei, et al., "Monitoring of Storage and Transportation Temperature Conditions in Red Blood Cell Units: A Cross-Sectional Study," National Center for Biotechnology Information (NCBI), April 2019. Available online. URL: www.ncbi.nlm.nih.gov/pmc/articles/PMC6439098. Accessed July 4, 2023.

"Storing Blood Before Transfusion," National Institute of Health (NIH), April 27, 2015. Available online. URL: https://www.nih.gov/news-events/nih-research-matters/storing-blood-transfusion. Accessed July 4, 2023.

Section 3.5 | **Cord Blood Banking**

Expecting a baby can be a very exciting time for soon-to-be parents. It can also be very confusing, with many decisions to make. One choice prospective parents often face is whether to donate, bank, or discard their baby's cord blood. Did you know that the U.S. Food and Drug Administration (FDA) regulates cord blood? Here is some information for expectant parents about the regulations in place designed to help ensure the safety of cord blood for transplantation.

WHAT IS CORD BLOOD?

Cord blood is the blood contained in the placental blood vessels and umbilical cord, which connects an unborn baby to the mother's womb. Cord blood contains hematopoietic progenitor cells (HPCs). At birth, cord blood can be collected (or "recovered") from the umbilical cord.

WHAT ARE HEMATOPOIETIC PROGENITOR CELLS?

Hematopoietic progenitor cells are blood-forming stem cells. HPCs are found in the bone marrow, peripheral blood, and cord blood. These types of stem cells are routinely used to treat patients with cancers, such as leukemia or lymphoma, and other disorders of the blood and immune systems.

HOW ARE PATIENTS AND DONATED CORD BLOOD UNITS "MATCHED" SO THAT A UNIT OF CORD BLOOD CAN BE USED FOR A PATIENT'S TRANSPLANT?

Human leukocyte antigen (HLA) typing is used to match patients and donors for cord blood transplants. HLAs are proteins found in most cells in the body. A person's immune system uses these proteins as markers to recognize which cells belong in their body and which do not. A close match between the patient's and the donor's HLA markers can reduce the risk that the patient's immune cells will attack the donor's cells or that the donor's immune cells will attack the patient's body after the transplant.

HOW ARE HEMATOPOIETIC PROGENITOR CELLS FROM CORD BLOOD DIFFERENT FROM HEMATOPOIETIC PROGENITOR CELLS FROM OTHER SOURCES?

There is evidence that cord blood HPCs may not require as exact a match as HPCs from the bone marrow or the bloodstream because the antigens in cord blood are less mature. This suggests that transplants involving compatible HPCs from cord blood may be less likely to cause adverse reactions because the donor's cells are less likely to see the patient's cells as foreign bodies and attack them.

WHAT ARE THE OPTIONS FOR CORD BLOOD BANKING?

Cord blood can be donated to a public cord blood bank, where it will be stored for potential future use by anyone who may need it. Alternatively, parents may arrange for the cord blood to be stored in a private cord bank for potential use if it is later needed for treatment of the child from whom it was recovered or for use in first- or second-degree relatives.

You may also wish to consult your health-care provider about the options.

HOW DOES THE FDA REGULATE CORD BLOOD STORED FOR PERSONAL OR FAMILY USE?

Cord blood stored for personal use and for use in first- or second-degree relatives that also meets other criteria in the FDA's regulations does not require approval before use. Private cord banks must still comply with other FDA requirements, including establishment registration and listing, donor screening and testing for infectious diseases (except when used for the original donor), reporting and labeling requirements, and compliance with current good tissue practice regulations.

HOW DOES THE FDA REGULATE CORD BLOOD INTENDED FOR USE IN PATIENTS UNRELATED TO THE DONOR (I.E., CORD BLOOD STORED IN PUBLIC BANKS)?

Cord blood stored for potential future use by a patient unrelated to the donor meets the definition of "drug" under the Food, Drug, and

Cosmetic Act (FDCA) and "biological product" under Section 351 of the Public Health Service Act. Cord blood in this category must meet additional requirements and be licensed under a Biologics License Application (BLA) or subject to an Investigational New Drug (IND) Application before use.

ARE THERE ANY FDA-APPROVED USES FOR CORD BLOOD?

Cord blood can be used in hematopoietic stem cell transplantation procedures in patients with some disorders affecting the hematopoietic (blood-forming) system. For example, cord blood transplants have been used to treat patients with certain blood cancers and some inherited metabolic and immune system disorders.

IF A CORD BLOOD BANK IS REGISTERED WITH THE FDA, DOES THAT MEAN THAT THE CORD BANK IS FDA-APPROVED?

Establishments that perform any of the manufacturing steps for cord blood must register with the FDA and list their products and each of the manufacturing steps they perform. Registration with the FDA does not mean a firm is "endorsed" by the agency; it simply means the firm has notified the FDA that it is performing one or more manufacturing steps.

DOES THE FDA INSPECT FACILITIES THAT STORE CORD BLOOD?

Yes. Registered establishments are subject to FDA inspection to ensure they are complying with the regulations. The inspections of private banks are designed to ensure the prevention of infectious disease transmission.

WHERE CAN YOU GET MORE INFORMATION ABOUT DONATING YOUR BABY'S CORD BLOOD?

To make your baby's cord blood available for use by anyone who needs a cord blood transplant, you may donate it to a public cord blood bank. Information on donating cord blood to a public cord blood bank is also found on the Health Resources and Services Administration (HRSA) website (http://bloodcell.transplant.hrsa.gov/CORD/Options/index.html).

WHERE CAN YOU GET MORE INFORMATION ABOUT BANKING YOUR BABY'S CORD BLOOD?

To make your baby's cord blood available for use by the child from whom it was recovered or for use in first- or second-degree relatives, you may bank it with a private cord blood bank. Information on banking cord blood with a private cord blood bank is also found on the HRSA website (http://bloodcell.transplant.hrsa.gov/CORD/Options/index.html).

For some diseases, such as genetically heritable diseases, in the event that your child would need treatment, it is possible that cord blood would not be recommended for such use.[2]

[2] "Cord Blood Banking—Information for Consumers," U.S. Food and Drug Administration (FDA), March 23, 2018. Available online. URL: www.fda.gov/vaccines-blood-biologics/consumers-biologics/cord-blood-banking-information-consumers. Accessed May 3, 2023.

Chapter 4 | **The Blood Circulatory System**

Chapter Contents

Section 4.1 | Classification and Structure of Blood Vessels

Blood vessels are the channels or conduits through which blood is distributed to body tissues. The vessels make up two closed systems of tubes that begin and end at the heart. One system, the pulmonary vessels, transports blood from the right ventricle to the lungs and back to the left atrium. The other system, the systemic vessels, carries blood from the left ventricle to the tissues in all parts of the body and then returns the blood to the right atrium. Based on their structure and function, blood vessels are classified as either arteries, capillaries, or veins (see Figure 4.1).

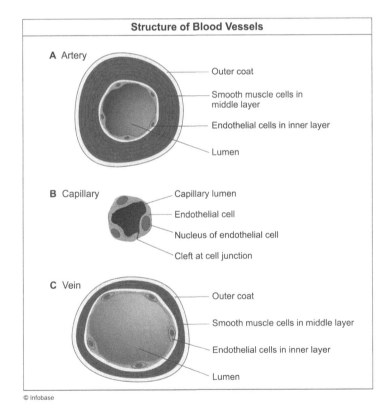

Figure 4.1. Structure of Blood Vessels

Infobase

ARTERIES

Arteries carry blood away from the heart. Pulmonary arteries transport blood that has a low oxygen content from the right ventricle to the lungs. Systemic arteries transport oxygenated blood from the left ventricle to the body tissues. Blood is pumped from the ventricles into large elastic arteries that branch repeatedly into smaller and smaller arteries until the branching results in microscopic arteries called "arterioles." The arterioles play a key role in regulating blood flow into the tissue capillaries. About 10 percent of the total blood volume is in the systemic arterial system at any given time.

The wall of an artery consists of three layers. The innermost layer, the tunica intima (also called the "tunica interna"), is a simple squamous epithelium surrounded by a connective tissue basement membrane with elastic fibers. The middle layer, the tunica media, is primarily smooth muscle and is usually the thickest layer. It not only provides support for the vessel but also changes the vessel diameter to regulate blood flow and blood pressure. The outermost layer, which attaches the vessel to the surrounding tissue, is the tunica externa or tunica adventitia. This layer is connective tissue with varying amounts of elastic and collagenous fibers. The connective tissue in this layer is quite dense where it is adjacent to the tunica media, but it changes to loose connective tissue near the periphery of the vessel.

CAPILLARIES

Capillaries, the smallest and most numerous of the blood vessels, form the connection between the vessels that carry blood away from the heart (arteries) and the vessels that return blood to the heart (veins). The primary function of capillaries is the exchange of materials between the blood and tissue cells.[1]

Roles of Capillaries

In addition to forming the connection between the arteries and veins, capillaries have a vital role in the exchange of gases, nutrients,

[1] Surveillance, Epidemiology, and End Results (SEER) Program, "Classification & Structure of Blood Vessels," National Cancer Institute (NCI), June 30, 2002. Available online. URL: https://training.seer.cancer.gov/anatomy/cardiovascular/blood/classification.html. Accessed May 26, 2023.

and metabolic waste products between the blood and tissue cells. Substances pass through the capillary wall by diffusion, filtration, and osmosis. Oxygen and carbon dioxide move across the capillary wall by diffusion. Fluid movement across a capillary wall is determined by a combination of hydrostatic and osmotic pressure. The net result of the capillary microcirculation created by hydrostatic and osmotic pressure is that substances leave the blood at one end of the capillary and return at the other end (see Figure 4.2).[2]

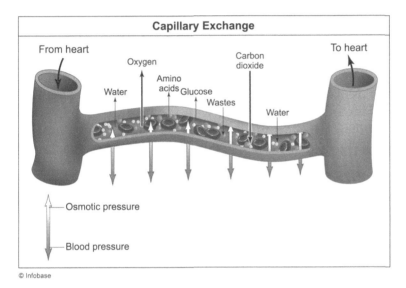

© Infobase

Figure 4.2. Capillary Exchange

Infobase

VEINS

Veins carry blood toward the heart. After blood passes through the capillaries, it enters the smallest veins, called the "venules." From the venules, it flows into progressively larger and larger veins until it reaches the heart. In the pulmonary circuit, the pulmonary veins

[2] Surveillance, Epidemiology, and End Results (SEER) Program, "Physiology of Circulation," National Cancer Institute (NCI), June 30, 2002. Available online. URL: https://training.seer.cancer.gov/anatomy/cardiovascular/blood/physiology.html. Accessed May 30, 2023.

transport blood from the lungs to the left atrium of the heart. This blood has a high oxygen content because it has just been oxygenated in the lungs. Systemic veins transport blood from the body tissue to the right atrium of the heart. This blood has reduced oxygen content because the oxygen has been used for metabolic activities in the tissue cells.

The walls of veins have the same three layers as the arteries. Although all the layers are present, there is less smooth muscle and connective tissue. This makes the walls of veins thinner than those of arteries, which is related to the fact that blood in the veins has less pressure than that in the arteries. Because the walls of the veins are thinner and less rigid than arteries, veins can hold more blood. Almost 70 percent of the total blood volume is in the veins at any given time. Medium and large veins have venous valves, similar to the semilunar valves associated with the heart, that help keep the blood flowing toward the heart. Venous valves are especially important in the arms and legs, where they prevent the backflow of blood in response to the pull of gravity.[3]

Section 4.2 | Circulatory Pathways

The blood vessels of the body are functionally divided into two distinctive circuits: the pulmonary circuit and the systemic circuit (see Figure 4.3). The pump for the pulmonary circuit, which circulates blood through the lungs, is the right ventricle. The left ventricle is the pump for the systemic circuit, which provides the blood supply for the tissue cells of the body.

PULMONARY CIRCUIT

Pulmonary circulation transports oxygen-poor blood from the right ventricle to the lungs, where the blood picks up a new blood supply. Then it returns the oxygen-rich blood to the left atrium.

---

[3] See footnote [1].

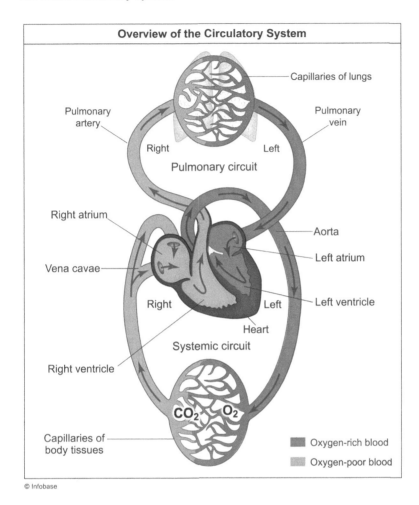

Figure 4.3. Overview of the Circulatory System

Infobase

SYSTEMIC CIRCUIT

Systemic circulation provides the functional blood supply to all body tissues. It carries oxygen and nutrients to the cells and picks up carbon dioxide and waste products. Systemic circulation carries oxygenated blood from the left ventricle, through the arteries, to the capillaries in the tissues of the body. From the tissue capillaries, the deoxygenated blood returns through a system of veins to the right atrium of the heart.

The coronary arteries are the only vessels that branch from the ascending aorta. The brachiocephalic, left common carotid, and left subclavian arteries branch from the aortic arch. The blood supply for the brain is provided by the internal carotid and vertebral arteries. The subclavian arteries provide the blood supply for the upper extremity. The celiac, superior mesenteric, suprarenal, renal, gonadal, and inferior mesenteric arteries branch from the abdominal aorta to supply the abdominal viscera. Lumbar arteries provide blood for the muscles and spinal cord. Branches of the external iliac artery provide the blood supply for the lower extremity. The internal iliac artery supplies the pelvic viscera.

MAJOR SYSTEMIC ARTERIES

All systemic arteries are branches, either directly or indirectly, from the aorta. The aorta ascends from the left ventricle, curves posteriorly and to the left, and then descends through the thorax and abdomen. This geography divides the aorta into three portions: ascending aorta, aortic arch, and descending aorta. The descending aorta is further subdivided into the thoracic aorta and abdominal aorta.

MAJOR SYSTEMIC VEINS

After blood delivers oxygen to the tissues and picks up carbon dioxide, it returns to the heart through a system of veins. The capillaries, where the gaseous exchange occurs, merge into venules, and these converge to form larger and larger veins until the blood reaches either the superior vena cava (SVC) or inferior vena cava (IVC), which drain into the right atrium.

FETAL CIRCULATION

Most circulatory pathways in a fetus are similar to those in an adult, but there are some notable differences because the lungs, gastrointestinal (GI) tract, and kidneys are not functioning before birth. The fetus obtains its oxygen and nutrients from the mother and also depends on maternal circulation to carry away the carbon dioxide and waste products.

The umbilical cord contains two umbilical arteries to carry fetal blood to the placenta and one umbilical vein to carry oxygen- and nutrient-rich blood from the placenta to the fetus. The ductus venosus allows blood to bypass the immature liver in fetal circulation. The foramen ovale and ductus arteriosus are modifications that permit blood to bypass the lungs in fetal circulation.[4]

---

[4] Surveillance, Epidemiology, and End Results (SEER) Program, "Circulatory Pathways," National Cancer Institute (NCI), June 30, 2002. Available online. URL: https://training.seer.cancer.gov/anatomy/cardiovascular/blood/pathways.html. Accessed May 31, 2023.

Chapter 5 | **Maintaining a Healthy Circulatory System**

Every time your heart beats, it pumps blood through vessels, called "arteries," to the rest of your body. Your blood pressure is how hard your blood pushes against the walls of the arteries. If your blood flows at higher than normal pressures, you may have high blood pressure (HBP), also known as "hypertension."

HBP is a major risk factor for heart disease, which is the leading cause of death in the United States. Millions of Americans have HBP, but many people who have it do not know it. That is why it is important to have your blood pressure checked at least once a year.

HBP is a "silent killer."

It does not usually cause symptoms, but it can damage your body over time.

- If your blood pressure stays higher than 130/80 mm Hg for a period of time, it can cause serious health problems such as:
  - heart disease
  - stroke
  - kidney disease
  - dementia
- The only way to know whether you have HBP is to have your blood pressure measured—a process that is simple and painless.

- If you find out you have HBP, a health-care professional can tell you how to prevent serious complications, including disability and premature death.

Some things put us at a greater risk for HBP:
- **Age**. Blood pressure tends to get higher as we get older. But it can affect many of us when we are younger too.
- **Genes**. HBP often runs in families.
- **Sex**. Before the age of 60, more men than women have HBP. After the age of 60, more women than men have it.
- **Race or ethnicity**. While anyone can have HBP, African Americans tend to get it at a younger age. Among Hispanic adults, people of Cuban, Puerto Rican, and Dominican backgrounds are at a higher risk.
- **Lifestyle habits**. Eating too much salt, drinking too much alcohol, being obese, smoking, and not getting enough exercise can raise our blood pressure.

WHAT STEPS CAN YOU TAKE TO LOWER YOUR BLOOD PRESSURE?

- **Set targets**. Work with your doctor to set blood pressure numbers that are healthy for you.
- **Take control**. Make lifestyle changes, such as eating healthy, staying active, and watching your weight. If you smoke, quitting can help prevent heart disease and other complications of HBP.
- **Work together**. Studies show that if you engage in heart-healthy activities with people at home, at work, in your community, or online, you have a better chance of staying motivated.

TAKING THE FIRST STEP TOWARD A HEALTHY BLOOD PRESSURE

Making lifestyle changes now can help keep your blood pressure in a healthy range—whether you have HBP or you are trying to prevent it. You do not have to make big changes all at once. Small steps can get you where you want to go. Here are some ideas to start. If you have elevated blood pressure and your doctor prescribes medications, make sure to take them as directed.[1]

KNOW YOUR NUMBERS
Take steps today to lower your risk for heart disease.

Control Your Cholesterol and Blood Pressure
High cholesterol and HBP can cause heart disease and heart attack. If your cholesterol or blood pressure numbers are high, you can take steps to lower them.

GET YOUR CHOLESTEROL CHECKED
It is important to get your cholesterol checked at least every five years. Some people will need to get it checked more or less often.

GET YOUR BLOOD PRESSURE CHECKED
Starting at the age of 18, get your blood pressure checked regularly. HBP has no symptoms. Get the facts about blood pressure testing.

TALK WITH YOUR DOCTOR
Know Your Family's Health History
Your family history affects your risk for heart disease. Keep track of your family's health and share the information with your doctor or nurse.

Ask Your Doctor about Taking Aspirin Every Day
If you are aged 40–59, taking aspirin every day may lower your risk of heart attack and stroke, but doctors do not recommend it for everyone. Talk with your doctor to find out if taking aspirin is the right choice for you.

---

[1] "Healthy Blood Pressure for Healthy Hearts: Small Steps to Take Control," National Heart, Lung, and Blood Institute (NHLBI), April 16, 2019. Available online. URL: www.nhlbi.nih.gov/sites/default/files/publications/HBP_Infograph_Fact_Sheet_508.pdf. Accessed May 3, 2023.

Talk to Your Doctor about Taking Medicine to Lower Your Risk of Heart Attack and Stroke

Experts recommend that some people aged 40–75 take medicines called "statins" if they are at high risk of heart attack and stroke.

FOOD AND ALCOHOL
Eat Healthy

Eating healthy can help lower your risk of heart disease. A heart-healthy diet includes foods that are low in saturated fat, added sugars, and sodium (salt).

Heart-healthy items include high-fiber foods (whole grains, fruits, and vegetables) and certain fats (such as the fats in olive oil and fish).

Do not forget to make healthy choices when you eat out. For example, ask for a side salad instead of chips or french fries.

Drink Alcohol Only in Moderation

Drinking too much alcohol can increase your risk of heart disease. So, if you choose to drink alcohol, drink only in moderation. That means one drink or less in a day for women and two drinks or less in a day for men.

PHYSICAL ACTIVITY
Get Active

Getting regular physical activity can help prevent heart disease. Adults need at least 150 minutes of moderate-intensity aerobic activity each week. This includes anything that gets your heart beating faster—such as walking, dancing, and biking.

If you are just getting started, take it slow! Try fitting a quick walk into your day. Even five minutes has real health benefits—and you can build up to more activity over time.

Stay at a Healthy Weight

People who are overweight or have obesity are at an increased risk for heart disease, HBP, and type 2 diabetes.

If you are overweight or have obesity, losing 5–10 percent of your body weight can help lower your risk of heart disease. For example, if you weigh 200 pounds, that would mean losing 10–20 pounds.

HEALTHY HABITS
Quit Smoking and Stay Away from Secondhand Smoke

Quitting smoking helps lower your risk of heart disease and heart attack. Call 800-QUIT-NOW (800-784-8669) for free support and to set up your plan for quitting.

Avoiding secondhand smoke is important, too—so keep your home smoke-free. If you have guests who smoke, ask them to smoke outside.

Manage Stress

Managing stress can help prevent serious health problems, such as heart disease, depression, and HBP. Deep breathing and meditation are good ways to relax and manage stress.[2]

---

[2] Office of Disease Prevention and Health Promotion (ODPHP), "Keep Your Heart Healthy," U.S. Department of Health and Human Services (HHS), April 11, 2023. Available online. URL: https://health.gov/myhealthfinder/health-conditions/heart-health/keep-your-heart-healthy#take-action-tab. Accessed May 3, 2023.

Part 2 | Anemia and Related Disorders

Chapter 6 | **Anemia: An Overview**

WHAT IS ANEMIA?

Anemia is a condition that develops when your blood produces a lower-than-normal amount of healthy red blood cells (RBCs). If you have anemia, your body does not get enough oxygen-rich blood. The lack of oxygen can make you feel tired or weak. You may also have shortness of breath, dizziness, headaches, or an irregular heartbeat. According to the Centers for Disease Control and Prevention (CDC), about 3 million people in the United States have anemia.

There are many types of anemia, including the following:
- iron deficiency anemia
- vitamin B_{12} deficiency anemia
- hemolytic anemia

Mild anemia is a common and treatable condition that can develop in anyone. It may come about suddenly or over time and may be caused by your diet, medicines you take, or another medical condition. Anemia can also be chronic, meaning it lasts a long time and may never go away completely. Some types of anemia are inherited. The most common type of anemia is iron deficiency anemia.

WHAT CAUSES ANEMIA?

Some types of anemia are caused by factors you cannot change, such as your family history or your age. Other anemia are caused by factors you can manage, such as eating habits or other health conditions that control how your body makes RBCs.

- **Age**. As you age, your chances of developing anemia increase.
- **Blood loss**. Any condition that causes you to lose a lot of blood increases your risk of anemia. While this can include blood loss during the menstrual cycle, anemia due to bleeding too much from your menstrual cycle is not normal. See your doctor if your periods are heavy. (You need to change your tampon or pad after less than two hours, or you pass clots the size of quarters or larger.) Bleeding can also lead to anemia if you have other risk factors. These include bleeding due to inflammation in the stomach or bowels, bleeding from surgery, bleeding due to a serious injury, or donating blood often.
- **Family history**. If you have a family history of inherited types of anemia, you may have an increased risk.
- **Lifestyle habits**. People who do not get nutrients such as iron, vitamin B_{12}, and folic acid to make healthy RBCs have a higher risk of anemia. Drinking too much alcohol also raises your risk of anemia.
- **Other health conditions**. Chronic (long-term) kidney disease, inflammation from an infection, cancer, or an autoimmune disease can cause your body to make fewer RBCs. Certain medicines or treatments such as chemotherapy for cancer can also raise your risk of anemia.

SYMPTOMS OF ANEMIA

If you have mild anemia, you may not have any symptoms. Symptoms of anemia may develop quickly or slowly, depending on the cause of your anemia. General symptoms that are the same for many types of anemia include the following:

- weakness
- paleness
- tiredness
- chills

- shortness of breath
- headache
- dizziness and fainting
- bleeding
- jaundice, or yellowing of the skin

DIAGNOSIS OF ANEMIA

To diagnose anemia, your doctor may ask you questions about your risk factors and order blood tests or other diagnostic tests. Your doctor may also ask about your medical history, what you eat, and whether other people in your family have been diagnosed with anemia. Your doctor may also do a physical exam to look for symptoms of anemia, such as a pale tongue or brittle nails. If you have anemia, your doctor may ask you to visit a hematologist (a doctor who specializes in blood diseases).

TREATMENT FOR ANEMIA

Treatments for anemia depend on the type you have and how serious it is. For some types of mild-to-moderate anemia, you may need iron supplements, vitamins, or medicines that make your body produce more RBCs. To prevent anemia in the future, your doctor may also suggest healthy eating changes.

CAN YOU PREVENT ANEMIA?

You can take steps to prevent some types of anemia. Your doctor may recommend eating more foods rich in iron or vitamin B_{12}, such as leafy vegetables, meat, milk, and eggs. Your doctor may also talk to you about iron or vitamin B_{12} supplements. If you are a strict vegetarian or vegan, talk to your doctor about how to get all the nutrients you need in your diet.

Anemia that is caused by your genes cannot be prevented. If you plan to have children and have an inherited type of anemia, you can talk to a genetic counselor. A genetic counselor can answer questions about the risk and explain what choices are available.[1]

---

[1] "Anemia," National Heart, Lung, and Blood Institute (NHLBI), March 24, 2022. Available online. URL: www.nhlbi.nih.gov/health/anemia. Accessed May 8, 2023.

Chapter 7 | Anemia due to Inherited Lack of Red Blood Cell Production

Chapter Contents

Section 7.1 | Amegakaryocytic Thrombocytopenia

Amegakaryocytic thrombocytopenia (amega), also sometimes called "congenital amegakaryocytic thrombocytopenia" (CAMT), is a rare, inherited bone marrow failure syndrome (IBMFS) in young children where the bone marrow fails to produce platelets or megakaryocytes. This causes the child's blood not to clot if he or she starts bleeding. Over time, the bone marrow may also cease making red blood cells (RBCs) and neutrophils. Mutation of the amega gene (*MPL*) is the cause of the disease.

About half of the people with IBMFS have characteristic physical findings, including neurologic and cardiac anomalies. Over time, complete failure of the bone marrow to produce other blood products (aplastic anemia) also occurs in nearly half of the children. Males and females are equally affected.[1]

WHAT TYPES OF CANCER ARE INDIVIDUALS WITH AMEGA AT HIGHER RISK OF DEVELOPING?

Individuals with amega are at higher risk of developing leukemia (cancer of the blood and bone marrow).

WHEN CAN AMEGA BE DIAGNOSED?

This can be diagnosed at:
- any time from birth through childhood
- the age younger than one month

HOW IS AMEGA SPECIFICALLY DIAGNOSED?

Amega can be specifically diagnosed by the following:
- clinical findings
- genetic testing

---

[1] "Amegakaryocytic Thrombocytopenia," U.S. Social Security Administration (SSA), August 20, 2020. Available online. URL: https://secure.ssa.gov/poms.nsf/lnx/0423022355. Accessed May 12, 2023.

What Are the Major Findings on Physical Examination?

The major findings of the physical examination are:
- bruises
- bleeding
- tiny spots of bleeding into the skin ("petechiae")

Genetics

Amega is caused by variants in the *MPL* gene and is usually inherited in an autosomal recessive manner. This means that individuals need both copies of the gene variant to have amega.

WHAT IS THE NATURAL PROGRESSION OF BONE MARROW FAILURE IN INDIVIDUALS WITH AMEGA?

Some individuals with amega can live for years without bone marrow failure, while others develop symptoms earlier.

Bone marrow failure means the number of blood cells is too low because the bone marrow has stopped producing enough mature cells.

Individuals typically start with low platelet counts and may progress to low counts in two or more types of blood cells (also known as "aplastic anemia"):
- low RBC count (anemia)
- low platelet count (thrombocytopenia)
- low white blood cell (WBC) count (leukopenia)[2]

Section 7.2 | Diamond-Blackfan Anemia

Diamond-Blackfan anemia is a disorder that primarily affects the bone marrow. People with this condition often also have physical abnormalities affecting various parts of the body.

---

[2] "Other Bone Marrow Failure Syndromes," National Cancer Institute (NCI), July 3, 2019. Available online. URL: https://marrowfailure.cancer.gov/disorders/othersyndromes.html. Accessed May 12, 2023.

The major function of the bone marrow is to produce new blood cells. In Diamond-Blackfan anemia, the bone marrow malfunctions and fails to make enough red blood cells (RBCs), which carry oxygen to the body's tissues. The resulting shortage of RBCs (anemia) usually becomes apparent during the first year of life. Symptoms of anemia include fatigue, weakness, and an abnormally pale appearance (pallor).

SYMPTOMS OF DIAMOND-BLACKFAN ANEMIA

Approximately half of the individuals with Diamond-Blackfan anemia have physical abnormalities. They may have an unusually small head size (microcephaly) and a low frontal hairline, along with distinctive facial features such as wide-set eyes (hypertelorism); droopy eyelids (ptosis); a broad, flat bridge of the nose; small, low-set ears; and a small lower jaw (micrognathia). Affected individuals may also have an opening in the roof of the mouth (cleft palate) with or without a split in the upper lip (cleft lip). They may have a short, webbed neck; shoulder blades that are smaller and higher than usual; and abnormalities of their hands, most commonly malformed or absent thumbs. About one-third of affected individuals have slow growth leading to short stature.

Other features of Diamond-Blackfan anemia may include eye problems such as clouding of the lens of the eyes (cataracts), increased pressure in the eyes (glaucoma), or eyes that do not look in the same direction (strabismus). Affected individuals may also have kidney abnormalities, structural defects of the heart, and, in males, the opening of the urethra on the underside of the penis (hypospadias).

The severity of Diamond-Blackfan anemia may vary, even within the same family. Increasingly, individuals with "nonclassical" Diamond-Blackfan anemia have been identified. This form of the disorder typically has less severe symptoms. For example, some affected individuals have mild anemia beginning later in childhood or in adulthood, while others have some of the physical features but no bone marrow problems.

CAUSES OF DIAMOND-BLACKFAN ANEMIA

Diamond-Blackfan anemia can be caused by mutations in one of many genes, including the *RPL5, RPL11, RPL35A, RPS10, RPS17, RPS19, RPS24,* and *RPS26* genes. These and other genes associated with Diamond-Blackfan anemia provide instructions for making ribosomal proteins, which are components of cellular structures called "ribosomes." Ribosomes process the cell's genetic instructions to create proteins.

Each ribosome is made up of two parts (subunits): the "large" and "small" subunits. The ribosomal proteins produced from the *RPL5, RPL11,* and *RPL35A* genes are among those found in the large subunit. The proteins produced from the *RPS10, RPS17, RPS19, RPS24,* and *RPS26* genes are among those found in the small subunit.

Some ribosomal proteins are involved in the assembly or stability of ribosomes. Others help carry out the ribosome's main function of building new proteins. Studies suggest that some ribosomal proteins may have other functions, such as participating in chemical signaling pathways within the cell, regulating cell division, and controlling the self-destruction of cells (apoptosis).

Approximately 25 percent of individuals with Diamond-Blackfan anemia have mutations in the *RPS19* gene. About 25–35 percent of individuals with this disorder have mutations in the *RPL5, RPL11, RPL35A, RPS10, RPS17, RPS24,* or *RPS26* gene. Mutations in any of these genes are believed to cause problems with ribosome function. Studies indicate that a shortage of functioning ribosomes may increase the self-destruction of blood-forming cells in the bone marrow, resulting in anemia. Abnormal regulation of cell division or inappropriate triggering of apoptosis may contribute to other health problems that affect some people with Diamond-Blackfan anemia. Scientists are working to determine why blood abnormalities and physical problems can vary so much between individuals.

Mutations in many other genes, some of which have not been identified, account for the remaining Diamond-Blackfan anemia cases. While mutations in genes that provide instructions for ribosomal proteins cause most cases of Diamond-Blackfan anemia, gene changes affecting proteins that interact with ribosomal proteins or that play other roles in blood-forming processes have been identified in a few individuals with this disorder.

RISK FACTORS FOR DIAMOND-BLACKFAN ANEMIA

People with Diamond-Blackfan anemia have an increased risk of several serious complications related to their malfunctioning bone marrow. Specifically, they have a higher-than-average chance of developing myelodysplastic syndrome (MDS), which is a disorder in which immature blood cells fail to develop normally. Individuals with Diamond-Blackfan anemia also have an increased risk of developing bone marrow cancer known as "acute myeloid leukemia" (AML), a type of bone cancer called "osteosarcoma," and other cancers.

FREQUENCY OF DIAMOND-BLACKFAN ANEMIA

Diamond-Blackfan anemia affects approximately 5–7 per million newborn babies worldwide.

INHERITANCE OF DIAMOND-BLACKFAN ANEMIA

This condition is inherited in an autosomal dominant pattern, which means one copy of the altered gene in each cell is sufficient to cause the disorder.

In approximately 45 percent of cases, an affected person inherits the mutation from one affected parent. The remaining cases result from new mutations in the gene and occur in people with no history of the disorder in their family.[3]

---

[3] MedlinePlus, "Diamond-Blackfan Anemia," National Institutes of Health (NIH), September 1, 2018. Available online. URL: https://medlineplus.gov/genetics/condition/diamond-blackfan-anemia. Accessed May 12, 2023.

Section 7.3 | **Dyskeratosis Congenita**

Dyskeratosis congenita (DKC) is a disorder that can affect many parts of the body. There are three features that are characteristic of this disorder: fingernails and toenails that grow poorly or are abnormally shaped (nail dystrophy); changes in skin coloring (pigmentation), especially on the neck and chest, in a pattern often described as "lacy"; and white patches inside the mouth (oral leukoplakia).

SIGNS AND SYMPTOMS OF DYSKERATOSIS CONGENITA

People with DKC may also develop pulmonary fibrosis, a condition that causes scar tissue (fibrosis) to build up in the lungs, decreasing the transport of oxygen into the bloodstream. Additional signs and symptoms that occur in some people with DKC include eye abnormalities such as narrow tear ducts that may become blocked, preventing drainage of tears and leading to eyelid irritation; dental problems; hair loss or prematurely gray hair; low bone mineral density (osteoporosis); degeneration (avascular necrosis) of the hip and shoulder joints; or liver disease. Some affected males may have a narrowing (stenosis) of the urethra, which is the tube that carries urine out of the body from the bladder. Urethral stenosis may lead to difficult or painful urination and urinary tract infections (UTIs).

The severity of DKC varies widely among affected individuals. The least severely affected individuals have only a few mild physical features of the disorder and normal bone marrow function. More severely affected individuals have many of the characteristic physical features and experience bone marrow failure, cancer, or pulmonary fibrosis by early adulthood.

While most people with DKC have normal intelligence and development of motor skills, such as standing and walking, developmental delay may occur in some severely affected individuals. In one severe form of the disorder called "Hoyeraal-Hreidarsson syndrome," affected individuals have an unusually small and underdeveloped cerebellum, which is part of the brain that coordinates movement. Another severe variant called "Revesz syndrome" involves abnormalities in the light-sensitive tissue at the back of the eye (retina) in addition to the other symptoms of DKC.

CAUSES OF DYSKERATOSIS CONGENITA

In about half of people with DKC, the disorder is caused by mutations in the *TERT, TERC, DKC1,* or *TINF2* gene. These genes provide instructions for making proteins that help maintain structures known as "telomeres," which are found at the ends of chromosomes. In a small number of individuals with DKC, mutations in other genes involved with telomere maintenance have been identified. Other affected individuals have no mutations in any of the genes currently associated with DKC. In these cases, the cause of the disorder is unknown, but other unidentified genes related to telomere maintenance are likely involved.

Telomeres help protect chromosomes from abnormally sticking together or breaking down (degrading). In most cells, telomeres become progressively shorter as the cell divides. After a certain number of cell divisions, the telomeres become so short that they trigger the cell to stop dividing or self-destruct (undergo apoptosis).

Telomeres are maintained by two important protein complexes called "telomerase" and "shelterin." Telomerase helps maintain normal telomere length by adding small repeated segments of deoxyribonucleic acid (DNA) to the ends of chromosomes each time the cell divides. The main components of telomerase, called "hTR" and "hTERT," are produced from the *TERC* and *TERT* genes, respectively. The hTR component is a ribonucleic acid (RNA) molecule, a chemical cousin of DNA. It provides a template for creating the repeated sequence of DNA that telomerase adds to the ends of chromosomes. The function of the hTERT component is to add the new DNA segment to chromosome ends. The *DKC1* gene provides instructions for making another protein that is important in telomerase function. This protein, called "dyskerin," attaches (binds) to hTR and helps stabilize the telomerase complex.

The shelterin complex helps protect telomeres from the cell's DNA repair process. Without the protection of shelterin, the repair mechanism would sense the chromosome ends as abnormal breaks in the DNA sequence and either attempt to join the ends together or initiate apoptosis. The *TINF2* gene provides instructions for making a protein that is part of the shelterin complex.

TERT, *TERC*, *DKC1*, or *TINF2* gene mutations result in dysfunction of the telomerase or shelterin complexes, leading to impaired maintenance of telomeres and reduced telomere length. Cells that divide rapidly are especially vulnerable to the effects of shortened telomeres. As a result, people with DKC may experience a variety of problems affecting quickly dividing cells in the body, such as cells of the nail beds, hair follicles, skin, lining of the mouth (oral mucosa), and bone marrow.

Breakage and instability of chromosomes resulting from inadequate telomere maintenance may lead to genetic changes that allow cells to divide in an uncontrolled way, resulting in the development of cancer in people with DKC.

RISK FACTORS FOR DYSKERATOSIS CONGENITA

People with DKC have an increased risk of developing several life-threatening conditions. They are especially vulnerable to disorders that impair bone marrow function. These disorders disrupt the ability of the bone marrow to produce new blood cells. Affected individuals may develop aplastic anemia, also known as "bone marrow failure," which occurs when the bone marrow does not produce enough new blood cells. They are also at higher-than-average risk for myelodysplastic syndrome (MDS), a condition in which immature blood cells fail to develop normally; this condition may progress to a form of blood cancer called "leukemia." People with DKC are also at increased risk of developing leukemia, even if they never develop MDS. In addition, they have a higher-than-average risk of developing other cancers, especially cancers of the head, neck, anus, or genitals.

FREQUENCY OF DYSKERATOSIS CONGENITA

The exact prevalence of DKC is unknown. It is estimated to occur in approximately 1 in 1 million people.

INHERITANCE OF DYSKERATOSIS CONGENITA

Dyskeratosis congenita can have different inheritance patterns.

When DKC is caused by *DKC1* gene mutations, it is inherited in an X-linked recessive pattern. The *DKC1* gene is located on the X chromosome, which is one of the two sex chromosomes. In males (who have only one X chromosome), one altered copy of the gene in each cell is sufficient to cause the condition. In females (who have two X chromosomes), a mutation would have to occur in both copies of the gene to cause the disorder. Because it is unlikely that females will have two altered copies of this gene, males are affected by X-linked recessive disorders much more frequently than females. A characteristic of X-linked inheritance is that fathers cannot pass X-linked traits to their sons.

When DKC is caused by mutations in other genes, it can be inherited in an autosomal dominant or autosomal recessive pattern. Autosomal dominant means one copy of the altered gene in each cell is sufficient to cause the disorder. Autosomal recessive means both copies of the gene in each cell have mutations. The parents of an individual with an autosomal recessive condition each carry one copy of the mutated gene, but they typically do not show signs and symptoms of the condition.[4]

Section 7.4 | Fanconi Anemia

Fanconi anemia is a condition that affects many parts of the body. People with this condition may have bone marrow failure, physical abnormalities, organ defects, and an increased risk of certain cancers. Approximately 90 percent of people with Fanconi anemia have impaired bone marrow function that leads to a decrease in the production of all blood cells (aplastic anemia).

SYMPTOMS OF FANCONI ANEMIA

Affected individuals experience extreme tiredness (fatigue) due to low numbers of red blood cells (RBCs; anemia), frequent infections

---

[4] MedlinePlus, "Dyskeratosis Congenita," National Institutes of Health (NIH), March 1, 2014. Available online. URL: https://medlineplus.gov/genetics/condition/dyskeratosis-congenita. Accessed May 12, 2023.

due to low numbers of white blood cells (WBCs; neutropenia), and clotting problems due to low numbers of platelets (thrombocytopenia). People with Fanconi anemia may also develop myelodysplastic syndrome (MDS), a condition in which immature blood cells fail to develop normally.

More than half of people with Fanconi anemia have physical abnormalities. These abnormalities can involve irregular skin coloring such as unusually light-colored skin (hypopigmentation) or café-au-lait spots, which are flat patches on the skin that are darker than the surrounding area. Other possible symptoms of Fanconi anemia include malformed thumbs or forearms and other skeletal problems, including short stature; malformed or absent kidneys and other defects of the urinary tract; gastrointestinal (GI) abnormalities; heart defects; eye abnormalities such as small or abnormally shaped eyes; and malformed ears and hearing loss. People with this condition may have abnormal genitalia or malformations of the reproductive system. As a result, most affected males and about half of the affected females cannot have biological children (infertility). Additional signs and symptoms can include abnormalities of the brain and spinal cord (central nervous system (CNS)), including increased fluid in the center of the brain (hydrocephalus), or an unusually small head size (microcephaly).

CAUSES OF FANCONI ANEMIA

Mutations in at least 15 genes can cause Fanconi anemia. Proteins produced from these genes are involved in a cell process known as the "FA pathway." The FA pathway is turned on (activated) when the process of making new copies of DNA, called "DNA replication," is blocked due to DNA damage. The FA pathway sends certain proteins to the area of damage, which trigger DNA repair, so DNA replication can continue.

The FA pathway is particularly responsive to a certain type of DNA damage known as "interstrand cross-links" (ICLs). ICLs occur when two DNA building blocks (nucleotides) on opposite strands of DNA are abnormally attached or linked together, which stops the process of DNA replication. ICLs can be caused by a buildup of toxic substances produced in the body or by treatment with certain cancer therapy drugs.

Eight proteins associated with Fanconi anemia group together to form a complex known as the "FA core complex." The FA core complex activates two proteins, called "FANCD2" and "FANCI." The activation of these two proteins brings DNA repair proteins to the area of the ICL, so the cross-link can be removed and DNA replication can continue.

Eighty to ninety percent of cases of Fanconi anemia are due to mutations in one of three genes: *FANCA*, *FANCC*, and *FANCG*. These genes provide instructions for producing components of the FA core complex. Mutations in any of the many genes associated with the FA core complex will cause the complex to be nonfunctional and disrupt the entire FA pathway. As a result, DNA damage is not repaired efficiently, and ICLs build up over time. The ICLs stall DNA replication, ultimately resulting in either abnormal cell death due to an inability to make new DNA molecules or uncontrolled cell growth due to a lack of DNA repair processes. Cells that divide quickly, such as bone marrow cells and cells of the developing fetus, are particularly affected. The death of these cells results in a decrease in blood cells and the physical abnormalities characteristic of Fanconi anemia. When the buildup of errors in DNA leads to uncontrolled cell growth, affected individuals can develop acute myeloid leukemia (AML) or other cancers.

RISK FACTORS FOR FANCONI ANEMIA

Individuals with Fanconi anemia have an increased risk of developing a cancer of blood-forming cells in the bone marrow called AML or tumors of the head, neck, skin, GI system, or genital tract. The likelihood of developing one of these cancers in people with Fanconi anemia is between 10 and 30 percent.

FREQUENCY OF FANCONI ANEMIA

Fanconi anemia occurs in 1 in 160,000 individuals worldwide. This condition is more common among people of Ashkenazi Jewish descent, the Roma population of Spain, and Black South Africans.

INHERITANCE OF FANCONI ANEMIA

Fanconi anemia is most often inherited in an autosomal recessive pattern, which means both copies of the gene in each cell have mutations. The parents of an individual with an autosomal recessive condition each carry one copy of the mutated gene, but they typically do not show signs and symptoms of the condition.

Very rarely, this condition is inherited in an X-linked recessive pattern. The gene associated with X-linked recessive Fanconi anemia is located on the X chromosome, which is one of the two sex chromosomes. In males (who have only one X chromosome), one altered copy of the gene in each cell is sufficient to cause the condition. In females (who have two X chromosomes), a mutation would have to occur in both copies of the gene to cause the disorder. Because it is unlikely that females will have two altered copies of this gene, males are affected by X-linked recessive disorders much more frequently than females. A characteristic of X-linked inheritance is that fathers cannot pass X-linked traits to their sons.[5]

Section 7.5 | Shwachman-Diamond Syndrome

Shwachman-Diamond syndrome (SDS) is an inherited condition that affects many parts of the body, particularly the bone marrow, pancreas, and bones.

In SDS, the bone marrow malfunctions and does not make some or all types of white blood cells (WBCs). A shortage of neutrophils, the most common type of WBC, causes a condition called "neutropenia." Most people with SDS have at least occasional episodes of neutropenia, which makes them more vulnerable to infections, often involving the lungs (pneumonia), ears (otitis media (OM)), or skin. Less commonly, bone marrow abnormalities lead to a shortage of red blood cells (RBCs; anemia), which causes fatigue and

---

[5] MedlinePlus, "Fanconi Anemia," National Institutes of Health (NIH), January 1, 2012. Available online. URL: https://medlineplus.gov/genetics/condition/fanconi-anemia/#inheritance. Accessed May 8, 2023.

weakness, or a reduction in the amount of platelets (thrombocytopenia), which can result in easy bruising and abnormal bleeding.

SYMPTOMS OF SHWACHMAN-DIAMOND SYNDROME

Shwachman-Diamond syndrome also affects the pancreas, which is an organ that plays an essential role in digestion. One of this organ's main functions is to produce enzymes that help break down and use nutrients from food. In most infants with SDS, the pancreas does not produce enough of these enzymes. This condition is known as "pancreatic insufficiency." Infants with pancreatic insufficiency have trouble digesting food and absorbing nutrients and vitamins that are needed for growth. As a result, they often have fatty, foul-smelling stools (steatorrhea); are slow to grow and gain weight (failure to thrive); and experience malnutrition. Pancreatic insufficiency often improves with age in people with SDS.

Skeletal abnormalities are another common feature of SDS. Many affected individuals have problems with bone formation and growth, most often affecting the hips and knees. Low bone density is also frequently associated with this condition. Some affected infants are born with a narrow rib cage and short ribs, which can cause life-threatening problems with breathing. The combination of skeletal abnormalities and slow growth results in short stature in most people with this disorder.

CAUSES OF SHWACHMAN-DIAMOND SYNDROME

Mutations in the *SBDS* gene have been identified in about 90 percent of people with the characteristic features of SDS. This gene provides instructions for making a protein that is critical in building ribosomes. Ribosomes are cellular structures that process the cell's genetic instructions to create proteins. *SBDS* gene mutations reduce the amount or impair the function of the SBDS protein. It is unclear how these changes lead to the major signs and symptoms of SDS. Researchers suspect that a shortage of functional SBDS impairs ribosome formation, which may reduce the production of other proteins and alter developmental processes.

Other genes involved in SDS appear to play roles in the assembly or function of ribosomes. Mutations in each of these genes account for a very small percentage of cases of the condition. In some cases, no mutations in any of the genes associated with the condition are found, and the cause of the disorder is unknown.

RISK FACTORS FOR SHWACHMAN-DIAMOND SYNDROME

People with SDS have an increased risk of several serious complications related to their malfunctioning bone marrow. Specifically, they have a higher-than-average chance of developing myelodysplastic syndrome (MDS) and aplastic anemia, which are disorders caused by abnormal blood stem cells, and a cancer of blood-forming tissue known as "acute myeloid leukemia" (AML).

COMPLICATIONS OF SHWACHMAN-DIAMOND SYNDROME

The complications of SDS can affect several other parts of the body, including the liver, heart, endocrine system (which produces hormones), eyes, teeth, and skin. Additionally, studies suggest that SDS may be associated with delayed speech and the delayed development of motor skills such as sitting, standing, and walking.

FREQUENCY OF SHWACHMAN-DIAMOND SYNDROME

Shwachman-Diamond syndrome is a rare condition that is thought to occur in approximately 1 in 80,000 newborns. Because the signs and symptoms are variable and can be mild in some affected individuals, doctors suspect the condition is underdiagnosed.

INHERITANCE OF SHWACHMAN-DIAMOND SYNDROME

Most cases of SDS, including those caused by mutations in the *SBDS* gene, are inherited in an autosomal recessive pattern, which means both copies of the gene in each cell have mutations. Typically, the parents of the affected individual each carry one copy of the mutated gene, but they do not show signs and symptoms of the condition. In some cases, one parent does not carry a copy of the mutated gene. Instead, a new (de novo) mutation occurs in the gene during the formation of reproductive cells (eggs or sperm) in the parent or during early embryonic development.

Rarely, the condition is inherited in an autosomal dominant pattern, which means one copy of the altered gene in each cell is sufficient to cause the disorder. These cases usually result from de novo mutations in the gene and occur in people with no history of the disorder in their family.[6]

[6] MedlinePlus, "Shwachman-Diamond Syndrome," National Institutes of Health (NIH), March 1, 2020. Available online. URL: https://medlineplus.gov/genetics/condition/shwachman-diamond-syndrome. Accessed May 12, 2023.

Chapter 8 | Anemia due to Acquired Lack of Red Blood Cell Production

Chapter Contents

WHAT IS APLASTIC ANEMIA?

Aplastic anemia is a rare but serious blood condition that occurs when your bone marrow cannot make enough new blood cells for your body to work normally. It can develop quickly or slowly, and it can be mild or serious.

WHAT ARE THE SYMPTOMS OF APLASTIC ANEMIA?

Symptoms of aplastic anemia include the following:

- fatigue
- infections that last a long time
- easy bruising or bleeding

WHAT CAUSES APLASTIC ANEMIA?

Aplastic anemia is caused by damage to stem cells inside your bone marrow, which is the sponge-like tissue within your bones. Many diseases and conditions can damage the stem cells in the bone marrow. As a result, the bone marrow makes fewer red blood cells (RBCs), white blood cells (WBCs), and platelets.

The most common cause of bone marrow damage is from your immune system attacking and destroying the stem cells in your bone marrow. This is a type of autoimmune illness, a disease that makes your body attack itself. Other causes of aplastic anemia include some medicines, such as those used in chemotherapy, and exposure to toxins or chemicals in the environment.

You can also inherit the condition in rare cases.

HOW IS APLASTIC ANEMIA DIAGNOSED?

To diagnose aplastic anemia, your doctor will order tests to find out whether you have low numbers of cells in your bone marrow and blood.

HOW IS APLASTIC ANEMIA TREATED?

Treatments for aplastic anemia may include the following:

- blood and bone marrow transplants, which may cure aplastic anemia in some people
- blood transfusions
- medicines to stop your immune system from destroying the stem cells in your bone marrow
- medicines to help your body make new blood cells
- removing or staying away from toxins in your environment

Your doctor will monitor your condition and screen you for blood conditions regularly. If you take medicine that affects your immune system, you will also need to take steps to prevent infection and get annual flu shots.

WHAT HAPPENS IF APLASTIC ANEMIA IS NOT TREATED?

Aplastic anemia can raise your risk of complications such as bleeding, leukemia, or other serious blood conditions. Without treatment, aplastic anemia can lead to serious medical conditions such as an irregular heartbeat and heart failure.

CAN YOU PREVENT APLASTIC ANEMIA?

At this time, there is no way to prevent aplastic anemia.[1]

Section 8.2 | Hemolytic Anemia

WHAT IS HEMOLYTIC ANEMIA?

Hemolytic anemia is a blood condition that occurs when your red blood cells (RBCs) are destroyed faster than they can be replaced. Hemolytic anemia can develop quickly or slowly, and it can be mild or serious.

---

[1] "Aplastic Anemia," National Heart, Lung, and Blood Institute (NHLBI), March 24, 2022. Available online. URL: www.nhlbi.nih.gov/health/anemia/aplastic-anemia. Accessed May 8, 2023.

WHAT ARE THE SYMPTOMS OF HEMOLYTIC ANEMIA?

Symptoms of hemolytic anemia may include tiredness, dizziness, weakness, and a spleen or liver that is larger than normal.

WHAT CAUSES HEMOLYTIC ANEMIA?

Red blood cells develop in the bone marrow, which is the sponge-like tissue inside your bones. Your body normally destroys old or faulty RBCs in the spleen or other parts of your body through a process called "hemolysis." Hemolytic anemia occurs when you have a low number of RBCs due to too much hemolysis in the body.

Certain conditions can cause hemolysis to happen too fast or too often, including the following:

- autoimmune conditions
- bone marrow failure
- complications from blood transfusions
- infections
- inherited blood conditions such as sickle cell disease (SCD) or thalassemia
- some medicines

HOW IS HEMOLYTIC ANEMIA DIAGNOSED?

To diagnose hemolytic anemia, your doctor will do a physical exam and order blood tests. Additional tests may include a urine test, a bone marrow test, or genetic tests.

HOW IS HEMOLYTIC ANEMIA TREATED?

If you have mild hemolytic anemia, you may not have any symptoms or need treatment. For others, hemolytic anemia can often be treated or managed. Treatments may include the following:

- blood transfusions
- medicines
- surgery to remove your spleen
- blood and bone marrow transplants

If your hemolytic anemia is caused by medicines or another health condition, your doctor may change your treatment to manage or stop hemolytic anemia.

WHAT HAPPENS IF HEMOLYTIC ANEMIA IS NOT TREATED?

Serious hemolytic anemia that is not treated or managed can cause irregular heart rhythms, a heart that is larger than normal, and heart failure if the anemia gets severe.[2]

Section 8.3 | Iron Deficiency Anemia

WHAT IS IRON DEFICIENCY ANEMIA?

Iron deficiency anemia is the most common type of anemia, a condition that happens when your body does not make enough healthy red blood cells (RBCs) or the blood cells do not work correctly.

Iron deficiency anemia happens when you do not have enough iron in your body. Your body needs iron to make hemoglobin, the part of the RBC that carries oxygen through your blood to all parts of your body.

WHO GETS IRON DEFICIENCY ANEMIA?

Iron deficiency anemia affects more women than men. The risk of iron deficiency anemia is highest for women during the following stages:

- **Pregnancy**. Iron deficiency anemia affects one in six pregnant women. You need more iron during pregnancy to support your unborn baby's development.
- **Having heavy menstrual periods**. Up to 5 percent of women of childbearing age develop iron deficiency anemia because of heavy bleeding during their periods.

---

[2] "Hemolytic Anemia," National Heart, Lung, and Blood Institute (NHLBI), March 24, 2022. Available online. URL: www.nhlbi.nih.gov/health/anemia/hemolytic-anemia. Accessed May 15, 2023.

Infants, small children, and teens are also at high risk for iron deficiency anemia.

WHAT ARE THE SYMPTOMS OF IRON DEFICIENCY ANEMIA?

Iron deficiency anemia often develops slowly. In the beginning, you may not have any symptoms, or they may be mild. As it gets worse, you may notice one or more of the following symptoms:

- fatigue (very common)
- weakness (very common)
- dizziness
- headaches
- low body temperature
- pale or yellow "sallow" skin
- rapid or irregular heartbeat
- shortness of breath or chest pain, especially with physical activity
- brittle nails
- pica (unusual cravings for ice, very cold drinks, or nonfood items, such as dirt or paper)

If you think you may have iron deficiency anemia, talk to your doctor or nurse.

WHAT CAUSES IRON DEFICIENCY ANEMIA?

Women can have low iron levels for several reasons that include the following:

- **Iron lost through bleeding**. Bleeding can cause you to lose more blood cells and iron than your body can replace. Women may have low iron levels from bleeding caused by:
  - digestive system problems, such as ulcers, colon polyps, or colon cancer
  - regular, long-term use of aspirin and other over-the-counter (OTC) pain relievers
  - donating blood too often or without enough time in between donations for your body to recover

- heavier or longer-than-normal menstrual periods
- uterine fibroids, which are noncancerous growths in the uterus that can cause heavy bleeding
- **Increased need for iron during pregnancy**. During pregnancy, your body needs more iron than normal to support the fetus.
- **Not eating enough food that contains iron**. Your body absorbs the iron in animal-based foods, such as meat, chicken, and fish, two to three times better than the iron in plant-based foods. Vegetarians or vegans, who eat little or no animal-based foods, need to choose other good sources of iron to make sure they get enough. Your body also absorbs iron from plant-based foods better when you eat them with foods that have vitamin C, such as oranges and tomatoes. But most people in the United States get enough iron from food.
- **Problems absorbing iron**. Certain health conditions, such as Crohn's disease or celiac disease, or gastric bypass surgery for weight loss can make it harder for your body to absorb iron from food.

HOW IS IRON DEFICIENCY ANEMIA DIAGNOSED?

Talk to your doctor if you think you might have iron deficiency anemia. Your doctor may do the following:

- Ask you questions about your health history, including how regular or heavy your menstrual periods are. Your doctor may also ask you about any digestive system problems you may have, such as blood in your stool.
- Do a physical exam.
- Talk to you about the foods you eat, the medicines you take, and your family health history.
- Do blood tests. Your doctor will do a complete blood count (CBC). The CBC measures many parts of your blood. If the CBC test shows that you have anemia, your doctor will likely do another blood test to measure the iron levels in your blood and confirm that you have iron deficiency anemia.

If you have iron deficiency anemia, your doctor may want to do other tests to find out what is causing it.

DO YOU NEED TO BE TESTED FOR IRON DEFICIENCY ANEMIA?
Maybe. Talk to your doctor about getting tested as part of your regular health exam if you have heavy menstrual periods or a health problem, such as Crohn's disease or celiac disease.

HOW IS IRON DEFICIENCY ANEMIA TREATED?
Treatment for iron deficiency anemia depends on the cause:
- **Blood loss from a digestive system problem**. If you have an ulcer, your doctor may give you antibiotics or other medicine to treat the ulcer. If your bleeding is caused by a polyp or cancerous tumor, you may need surgery to remove it.
- **Blood loss from heavy menstrual periods**. Your doctor may give you hormonal birth control to help relieve heavy periods. If your heavy bleeding does not get better, your doctor may recommend surgery. Types of surgery to control heavy bleeding include endometrial ablation, which removes or destroys your uterine lining, and a hysterectomy, which removes all or parts of your uterus.
- **Increased need for iron**. If you have problems absorbing iron or have lower iron levels but do not have severe anemia, your doctor may recommend the following:
  - **Iron pills to build up your iron levels as quickly as possible**. Do not take any iron pills without first talking to your doctor or nurse.
  - **Eating more foods that contain iron**. Good sources of iron include meat, fish, eggs, beans, peas, and fortified foods (look for cereals fortified with 100% of the daily value (DV) for iron).
  - **Eating more foods with vitamin C**. Foods rich in vitamin C helps your body absorb iron. Good sources of vitamin C include oranges, broccoli, and tomatoes.

If you have severe bleeding or symptoms of chest pain or shortness of breath, your doctor may recommend iron or RBC transfusions. Transfusions are only for severe iron deficiencies, and they are much less common.

WHAT DO YOU NEED TO KNOW ABOUT IRON PILLS?

Your doctor may recommend iron pills to help build up your iron levels. Do not take these pills without talking to your doctor or nurse first. Taking iron pills can cause side effects, including an upset stomach, constipation, and diarrhea. If taken as a liquid, iron supplements may stain your teeth.

You can reduce side effects from iron pills by taking the following steps:

- Start with half of the recommended dose. Gradually increase to the full dose.
- Take iron in divided doses. For example, if you take two pills daily, take one in the morning with breakfast and the other after dinner.
- Take iron with food (especially something with vitamin C, such as a glass of orange juice, to help your body absorb the iron).
- If one type of iron pill causes side effects, ask your doctor for another type.
- If you take iron as a liquid instead of as a pill, aim it toward the back of your mouth. This will prevent the liquid from staining your teeth. You can also brush your teeth after taking the medicine to help prevent staining.

WHAT CAN HAPPEN IF IRON DEFICIENCY ANEMIA IS NOT TREATED?

If left untreated, iron deficiency anemia can cause serious health problems. Having too little oxygen in the body can damage organs. With anemia, the heart must work harder to make up for the lack of RBCs or hemoglobin. This extra work can harm the heart.

Iron deficiency anemia can also cause problems during pregnancy.

HOW CAN YOU PREVENT IRON DEFICIENCY ANEMIA?

You can help prevent iron deficiency anemia with the following steps:

- **Treat the cause of blood loss.** Talk to your doctor if you have heavy menstrual periods or if you have digestive system problems, such as frequent diarrhea or blood in your stool.
- **Eat foods with iron.** Good sources of iron include lean meat and chicken; dark, leafy vegetables; and beans.
- **Eat and drink foods that help your body absorb iron.** These include orange juice, strawberries, broccoli, or other fruits and vegetables with vitamin C.
- **Make healthy food choices.** Most people who make healthy, balanced food choices get the iron and vitamins their bodies need from the foods they eat.
- **Avoid drinking coffee or tea with meals.** These drinks make it harder for your body to absorb iron.
- **Talk to your doctor if you take calcium pills.** Calcium can make it harder for your body to absorb iron. If you have a hard time getting enough iron, talk to your doctor about the best way to also get enough calcium.

HOW MUCH IRON DO YOU NEED EVERY DAY?

Table 8.1 lists how much iron you need every day. The recommended amounts are listed in milligrams (mg).

Table 8.1. Recommended Amounts of Iron per Day

Age (Years)	Women (mg)	Pregnant Women (mg)	Breastfeeding Women (mg)	Vegetarian Women* (mg)
14–18	15	27	10	27
19–50	18	27	9	32
51 and over	8	NA	NA	14

* Vegetarians need more iron from food than people who eat meat. This is because the body can absorb iron from meat better than from plant-based foods.
Note: NA – Not applicable.
(Source: Adapted from the Institute of Medicine (IOM), Food and Nutrition Board (FNB).)

WHAT FOODS CONTAIN IRON?

Food sources of iron include the following:

- fortified breakfast cereals (18 mg per serving)
- oysters (8 mg per 3-ounce serving)
- canned white beans (8 mg per cup)
- dark chocolate (7 mg per 3-ounce serving)
- beef liver (5 mg per 3-ounce serving)
- spinach (3 mg per ½ cup)
- tofu, firm (3 mg per ½ cup)
- kidney beans (2 mg per ½ cup)
- canned tomatoes (2 mg per ½ cup)
- lean beef (2 mg for a 3-ounce serving)
- baked potato (2 mg for a medium potato)

DO YOU NEED MORE IRON DURING PREGNANCY?

Yes. During pregnancy, your body needs more iron to support your growing baby. In fact, pregnant women need almost twice as much iron as women who are not pregnant. Not getting enough iron during pregnancy raises your risk for premature birth or a low birth weight baby (less than 5½ pounds). Premature birth is the most common cause of infant death. Both premature birth and low birth weight raise your baby's risk for health and developmental problems at birth and during childhood.

If you are pregnant, talk to your doctor about the following steps:

- getting 27 mg of iron every day (Take a prenatal vitamin with iron every day or talk to your doctor about taking an iron supplement (pill).)
- testing for iron deficiency anemia
- testing for iron deficiency anemia four to six weeks after childbirth

DO YOU NEED MORE IRON IF YOU ARE BREASTFEEDING?

No, you do not need more iron during breastfeeding. In fact, you need less iron than before you were pregnant. The amount of iron women need during breastfeeding is 10 mg per day for young mothers aged 14–18 and 9 mg per day for breastfeeding women older than 18.

You need less iron while breastfeeding because you likely will not lose a lot through your menstrual cycle. Many breastfeeding women do not have a period or may have only a light period. Also, if you get enough iron during pregnancy (27 mg a day), your breast milk will supply enough iron for your baby.

DOES MENOPAUSAL HORMONE THERAPY AFFECT HOW MUCH IRON YOU NEED TO TAKE?

It might. If you still get your period and take menopausal hormone therapy (MHT), you may need more iron than women who are postmenopausal and do not take MHT. Talk to your doctor or nurse.

DOES BIRTH CONTROL AFFECT YOUR RISK FOR IRON DEFICIENCY ANEMIA?

It could. Hormonal birth control, such as the pill, the patch, the shot, or the hormonal intrauterine device (IUD), is often used to treat women with heavy menstrual periods. Lighter menstrual periods may reduce your risk for iron deficiency anemia.

Also, the nonhormonal, copper IUD may make your menstrual flow heavier. This raises your risk for iron deficiency anemia.

Talk to your doctor or nurse about your risk for anemia and whether hormonal birth control may help.

YOU ARE A VEGETARIAN. HOW CAN YOU MAKE SURE YOU GET ENOUGH IRON?

You can help make sure you get enough iron by choosing foods that contain iron more often. Vegetarians need more iron from food than people who eat meat. This is because the body can absorb iron from meat better than from plant-based foods.

Vegetarian sources of iron include:
- cereals and bread with added iron
- lentils and beans
- dark chocolate

- dark green leafy vegetables, such as spinach and broccoli
- tofu
- chickpeas
- canned tomatoes

Talk to your doctor or nurse about whether you get enough iron. Most people get enough iron from food.

CAN YOU GET MORE IRON THAN YOUR BODY NEEDS?

Yes, your body can get too much iron. Extra iron can damage the liver, heart, and pancreas. Try to get no more than 45 mg of iron a day unless your doctor prescribes more.

Some people get too much iron because of a condition called "hemochromatosis" that runs in families.

You can also get too much iron from iron pills (if you also get iron from food) or from repeated blood transfusions.[3]

Section 8.4 | Vitamin B$_{12}$ Deficiency Anemia

WHAT IS VITAMIN B$_{12}$ DEFICIENCY ANEMIA?

Vitamin B$_{12}$ deficiency anemia, also known as "cobalamin deficiency," is a condition that develops when your body cannot make enough healthy red blood cells (RBCs) because it does not have enough vitamin B$_{12}$. Your body needs vitamin B$_{12}$ to make healthy RBCs, white blood cells (WBCs), and platelets. Since your body does not produce vitamin B$_{12}$, you have to get it from the foods you eat or from supplements.

You can get vitamin B$_{12}$ deficiency if you cannot absorb vitamin B$_{12}$ due to problems with your gut or if you have pernicious anemia, which makes it difficult to absorb vitamin B$_{12}$ from your intestines.

---

[3] Office on Women's Health (OWH), "Iron Deficiency Anemia," U.S. Department of Health and Human Services (HHS), February 22, 2021. Available online. URL: www.womenshealth.gov/a-z-topics/iron-deficiency-anemia. Accessed May 31, 2023.

Without enough vitamin B_{12}, blood cells do not form properly inside your bone marrow, the sponge-like tissue within your bones. These blood cells die sooner than normal, leading to anemia.

WHAT ARE THE SYMPTOMS OF VITAMIN B_{12} DEFICIENCY ANEMIA?

If you have vitamin B_{12} deficiency anemia, you may have the typical symptoms of anemia at first, such as fatigue, paleness, shortness of breath, headaches, or dizziness. If left untreated, you may start to notice brain and nervous system symptoms. This is because vitamin B_{12} is also needed for your brain and your nerves to work properly.

Your symptoms may include the following:
- tingling feelings or pain
- trouble walking
- uncontrollable muscle movements
- confusion, slower thinking, forgetfulness, and memory loss
- mood or mental changes, such as depression or irritability
- problems with smell or taste
- vision problems
- diarrhea and weight loss
- glossitis, which is a painful, smooth, red tongue

WHAT CAUSES VITAMIN B_{12} DEFICIENCY ANEMIA?

You can develop vitamin B_{12} deficiency anemia if you do not eat enough food with vitamin B_{12}, such as if you follow a strict vegetarian or vegan diet. But this is rare. In the United States, vitamin B_{12} deficiency anemia is most often due to other risk factors.

You can develop vitamin B_{12} deficiency for the following reasons:
- **Lack of the intrinsic factor**. It is a protein made in the stomach, which helps the body absorb vitamin B_{12}. People who have pernicious anemia do not produce the intrinsic factor. Pernicious anemia is more common in people with northern European or African ancestry. You may develop vitamin B_{12} deficiency anemia if your body is not able to absorb enough vitamin B_{12}

from the foods you eat. Older adults are more likely to have digestive problems that make it harder to absorb vitamin B_{12}.

- **Lifestyle habits**. Drinking too much alcohol can make it harder for your body to absorb vitamin B_{12}. For men, this is more than two drinks in a day. For women, it is more than one drink in a day.
- **Medicines**. Taking certain medicines can make it harder for your body to absorb vitamin B_{12} over time. These include some heartburn medicines and metformin to treat diabetes.
- **Medical conditions**. Some medical conditions can raise your risk of vitamin B_{12} deficiency anemia. These include the following:
  - autoimmune diseases, such as celiac disease, type 1 diabetes, and thyroid disease
  - chronic pancreatic disease
  - genetic conditions, such as Imerslünd-Grasbeck syndrome, inherited intrinsic factor deficiency, and inherited transcobalamin deficiency
  - intestinal and digestive conditions, such as ulcerative colitis (UC), Crohn's disease, and *Helicobacter pylori* infection
  - vitiligo
- **Stomach surgery**. Surgery on your stomach or intestines, such as weight loss surgery or gastrectomy, can make it harder for your body to absorb vitamin B_{12}.

HOW MUCH VITAMIN B_{12} DO YOU NEED EACH DAY?

The recommended daily amounts of vitamin B_{12} depend on your age, your sex, and whether you are pregnant or breastfeeding. Your health-care provider can look at your medical history to help determine how much vitamin B_{12} you need each day.

HOW IS VITAMIN B_{12} DEFICIENCY ANEMIA DIAGNOSED?

To screen for vitamin B_{12} deficiency anemia, your health-care provider may order blood tests to see whether you have low hemoglobin or vitamin B_{12} levels. A complete blood count measures hemoglobin. Another blood test measures vitamin B_{12} levels in the blood. You may still have the condition even if your vitamin B_{12} levels are normal.

HOW IS VITAMIN B_{12} DEFICIENCY ANEMIA TREATED?

If your doctor diagnoses you with vitamin B_{12} deficiency anemia, your treatment will depend on the cause and seriousness of your condition. Some people need lifelong treatment.

Different therapies can be used to treat anemia that include the following:

- Vitamin B_{12} medicine can be prescribed by your provider for you to take by mouth or as a nasal spray or a shot. These supplements can help increase the levels of vitamin B_{12} in your body. For serious vitamin B_{12} deficiency anemia, your doctor may recommend vitamin B_{12} shots until your levels are healthy.
- Blood transfusions are recommended to treat serious vitamin B_{12} deficiency anemia in combination with vitamin B_{12} treatment.

Your care provider may also recommend you make some changes to your eating habits to help increase the amount of vitamin B_{12} in your diet.

Some symptoms may take months to improve, depending on how serious they are. Some symptoms related to the brain or the nerves, such as numbness and tingling, may not go away even with treatment.

WHAT HAPPENS IF VITAMIN B_{12} DEFICIENCY ANEMIA IS NOT TREATED?

Vitamin B_{12} deficiency may cause serious complications, such as bleeding, infections, and problems with your brain or nerves that may be permanent. Babies born to mothers who have vitamin B_{12} deficiency may have developmental delays and birth defects of the brain and spinal cord.

HOW DO YOU PREVENT VITAMIN B$_{12}$ DEFICIENCY?

If you are otherwise healthy, maintaining a normal diet enriched in vitamin B$_{12}$ is important.

Foods that are good sources of vitamin B$_{12}$ include the following:

- lean red meat and chicken
- fish, such as catfish and salmon, and seafood, such as clams and oysters
- milk, yogurt, cheese, and fortified vegan milk substitutes
- fortified cereals
- eggs[4]

[4] "Vitamin B$_{12}$ Deficiency Anemia," National Heart, Lung, and Blood Institute (NHLBI), March 24, 2022. Available online. URL: www.nhlbi.nih.gov/health/anemia/vitamin-b12-deficiency-anemia. Accessed May 8, 2023.

Chapter 9 | Inherited Causes of Hemolytic Anemia

Chapter Contents

Section 9.1 | Glucose-6-Phosphate Dehydrogenase Deficiency

Glucose-6-phosphate dehydrogenase deficiency is a genetic disorder that affects red blood cells (RBCs), which carry oxygen from the lungs to tissues throughout the body. In affected individuals, a defect in an enzyme called "glucose-6-phosphate dehydrogenase" causes RBCs to break down prematurely. This destruction of RBCs is called "hemolysis." The most common medical problem associated with glucose-6-phosphate dehydrogenase deficiency is hemolytic anemia, which occurs when RBCs are destroyed faster than the body can replace them.

SYMPTOMS OF GLUCOSE-6-PHOSPHATE DEHYDROGENASE DEFICIENCY

This type of anemia leads to paleness, yellowing of the skin and whites of the eyes (jaundice), dark urine, fatigue, shortness of breath, and a rapid heart rate. In people with glucose-6-phosphate dehydrogenase deficiency, hemolytic anemia is most often triggered by bacterial or viral infections or by certain drugs (such as some antibiotics and medications used to treat malaria). Hemolytic anemia can also occur after eating fava beans or inhaling pollen from fava plants (a reaction called "favism").

Glucose-6-phosphate dehydrogenase deficiency is also a significant cause of mild-to-severe jaundice in newborns. Many people with this disorder, however, never experience any signs or symptoms and are unaware that they have the condition.

CAUSES OF GLUCOSE-6-PHOSPHATE DEHYDROGENASE DEFICIENCY

Glucose-6-phosphate dehydrogenase deficiency results from variants (also called "mutations") in the *G6PD* gene. This gene provides instructions for making an enzyme called "glucose-6-phosphate dehydrogenase." This enzyme is involved in the normal processing of carbohydrates. It also protects RBCs from the effects of potentially harmful molecules called "reactive oxygen species," which are by-products of normal cellular functions. Chemical reactions involving glucose-6-phosphate dehydrogenase produce compounds that prevent reactive oxygen species from building up to toxic levels within RBCs.

If variants in the *G6PD* gene reduce the amount of glucose-6-phosphate dehydrogenase or alter its structure, this enzyme can no longer play its protective role. As a result, reactive oxygen species can accumulate and damage RBCs. Factors such as infections, certain drugs, or ingesting fava beans can increase the levels of reactive oxygen species, causing RBCs to be destroyed faster than the body can replace them. A reduction in the number of RBCs causes the signs and symptoms of hemolytic anemia.

Researchers believe that people who have a *G6PD* variant may be partially protected against malaria, an infectious disease carried by a certain type of mosquito. A reduction in the amount of functional glucose-6-phosphate dehydrogenase appears to make it more difficult for this parasite to invade RBCs. Glucose-6-phosphate dehydrogenase deficiency occurs most frequently in areas of the world where malaria is common.

FREQUENCY OF GLUCOSE-6-PHOSPHATE DEHYDROGENASE DEFICIENCY

An estimated 400 million people worldwide have glucose-6-phosphate dehydrogenase deficiency. This condition occurs most frequently in certain parts of Africa, Asia, the Mediterranean, and the Middle East. It affects about 1 in 10 African American males in the United States.

INHERITANCE OF GLUCOSE-6-PHOSPHATE DEHYDROGENASE DEFICIENCY

Glucose-6-phosphate dehydrogenase deficiency is inherited in an X-linked pattern. A condition is considered X-linked if the altered gene that causes the disorder is located on the X chromosome, one of the two sex chromosomes in each cell. Males have only one X chromosome, and females have two copies of the X chromosome. A characteristic of X-linked inheritance is that fathers cannot pass X-linked traits to their sons.

In females, who have two copies of the X chromosome, one altered copy of the *G6PD* gene in each cell can lead to less severe features of the condition or may cause no signs or symptoms at all. However, many females with one altered copy of this gene have glucose-6-phosphate dehydrogenase deficiency similar to affected males because the X chromosome with the normal copy of the *G6PD* gene is turned off through a process called "X-inactivation." Early in embryonic development in females, one of the two X chromosomes is permanently inactivated in somatic cells (cells other than egg and sperm cells). X-inactivation ensures that females, like males, have only one active copy of the X chromosome in each body cell. Usually, X-inactivation occurs randomly, such that each X chromosome is active in about half of the body cells. Sometimes, X-inactivation is not random, and one X chromosome is active in more than half of cells. When X-inactivation does not occur randomly, it is called "skewed X-inactivation."

Research shows that females with glucose-6-phosphate dehydrogenase deficiency caused by variants in the *G6PD* gene often have skewed X-inactivation, which results in the inactivation of the X chromosome with the normal copy of the *G6PD* gene in most cells of the body. This skewed X-inactivation causes the chromosome with the altered *G6PD* gene to be expressed in more than half of cells. As a result, not enough normal glucose-6-phosphate dehydrogenase enzyme is produced, leading to hemolytic anemia and other signs and symptoms of glucose-6-phosphate dehydrogenase deficiency.[1]

---

[1] MedlinePlus, "Glucose-6-Phosphate Dehydrogenase Deficiency," National Institutes of Health (NIH), April 12, 2023. Available online. URL: https://medlineplus.gov/genetics/condition/glucose-6-phosphate-dehydrogenase-deficiency. Accessed May 11, 2023.

Section 9.2 | **Hereditary Elliptocytosis**

Hereditary elliptocytosis (HE) refers to a group of inherited blood conditions where the red blood cells (RBCs) are abnormally shaped.

WHEN DO SYMPTOMS OF HEREDITARY ELLIPTOCYTOSIS BEGIN?

Symptoms of this disease may start to appear at any time in life.

SYMPTOMS OF HEREDITARY ELLIPTOCYTOSIS

Symptoms vary from very mild to severe and can include fatigue, shortness of breath, gallstones, and yellowing of the skin and eyes (jaundice). Some people with this condition have an enlarged spleen. The following symptoms have been linked to this disease:

- abnormal erythrocyte morphology (any structural abnormality of erythrocytes (RBCs))
- elliptocytosis (the presence of elliptical, cigar-shaped erythrocytes on peripheral blood smear)
- increased red cell osmotic fragility (swelling of the cells that is associated with an accumulation of sodium that exceeds the loss of potassium)
- congenital hemolytic anemia (a form of hemolytic anemia with congenital onset)
- hemolytic anemia (a type of anemia caused by premature destruction of RBCs (hemolysis))
- jaundice (yellow pigmentation of the skin due to bilirubin, which in turn is the result of increased bilirubin concentration in the bloodstream)
- poikilocytosis (the presence of abnormally shaped erythrocytes)
- prolonged neonatal jaundice (Yellowing of skin and other tissues of a newborn infant as a result of increased concentrations of bilirubin in the blood. Neonatal jaundice affects over half of all newborns to some extent in the first week of life. Prolonged neonatal jaundice is said to be present if jaundice persists for

longer than 14 days in term infants and 21 days in preterm infants.)

- reticulocytosis (an elevation in the number of reticulocytes (immature erythrocytes) in the peripheral blood circulation)
- splenomegaly (abnormally increased size of the spleen)
- stomatocytosis (the presence of erythrocytes with a mouth-shaped (stoma) area of central pallor on a peripheral blood smear)
- abdominal pain
- chills
- cholelithiasis (hard, pebble-like deposits that form within the gallbladder)
- frontal bossing (bilateral bulging of the lateral frontal bone prominences with relative sparing of the midline)
- postnatal growth retardation

CAUSES OF HEREDITARY ELLIPTOCYTOSIS

Hereditary elliptocytosis is a genetic disease, which means that it is caused by one or more genes not working correctly. Disease-causing variants, or differences, in the following genes are known to cause this disease: *SPTA1*, *SPTB*, *EPB41*, and *GYPC*.

DIAGNOSIS OF HEREDITARY ELLIPTOCYTOSIS

Diagnosis of this condition is made by looking at the shape of the RBCs under a microscope.

INHERITANCE OF HEREDITARY ELLIPTOCYTOSIS

Hereditary elliptocytosis is caused by a genetic change in the *EPB41*, *SPTA1*, or *SPTB* gene and is inherited in an autosomal dominant pattern. Hereditary pyropoikilocytosis (HPP) is a related condition with more serious symptoms and is inherited in an autosomal recessive pattern. All individuals inherit two copies of most genes. The number of copies of a gene that need to have a disease-causing variant affects the way a disease is inherited. This disease is inherited in the following patterns.

Autosomal Dominant Inheritance

Autosomal means the gene is located on any chromosome except the X or Y chromosome (sex chromosomes). Genes, like chromosomes, usually come in pairs. Dominant means that only one copy of the responsible gene (causal gene) must have a disease-causing change (pathogenic variant) in order for a person to have the disease.

In some cases, a person inherits the pathogenic variant from a parent who has the genetic disease. In other cases, the disease occurs because of a new pathogenic variant (de novo) in the causal gene, and there is no family history of the disease.

Each child of an individual with HE has a 50 percent (one in two) chance of inheriting the variant and the disease.

Typically, children who inherit a dominant variant will have the disease, but they may be more or less severely impacted than their parents.

Sometimes, a person may have a pathogenic variant for HE and show no signs or symptoms of the disease.

Autosomal Recessive Inheritance

Autosomal means the gene is located on any chromosome except the X or Y chromosome (sex chromosomes). Genes, like chromosomes, usually come in pairs. Recessive means that both copies of the responsible gene must have a disease-causing change (pathogenic variant) in order for a person to have the disease.

A person who has HPP receives a gene with a pathogenic variant from each of their parents. Each parent is a carrier that means they have a pathogenic variant in only one copy of the gene. Carriers of HPP usually do not have any symptoms of the disease. When two carriers of HPP have children, there is a 25 percent (one in four) chance of having a child who has the disease.[2]

---

[2] Genetic and Rare Diseases Information Center (GARD), "Hereditary Elliptocytosis," National Center for Advancing Translational Sciences (NCATS), February 2023. Available online. URL: https://rarediseases.info.nih.gov/diseases/6621/hereditary-elliptocytosis. Accessed June 5, 2023.

Section 9.3 | **Hereditary Spherocytosis**

Hereditary spherocytosis (HS) is a condition that affects red blood cells (RBCs). Most newborns with HS have severe anemia although it improves after the first year of life.

SYMPTOMS OF HEREDITARY SPHEROCYTOSIS

People with this condition typically experience a shortage of RBCs (anemia), yellowing of the eyes and skin (jaundice), and an enlarged spleen (splenomegaly). Splenomegaly can occur anytime from early childhood to adulthood. About half of the affected individuals develop hard deposits in the gallbladder called "gallstones," which typically occur from late childhood to mid-adulthood.

There are four forms of HS, which are distinguished by the severity of signs and symptoms. They are known as "the mild form," "the moderate form," "the moderate/severe form," and "the severe form." It is estimated that 20–30 percent of people with HS have the mild form, 60–70 percent have the moderate form, 10 percent have the moderate/severe form, and 3–5 percent have the severe form.

People with the mild form may have very mild anemia or sometimes have no symptoms. People with the moderate form typically have anemia, jaundice, and splenomegaly. Many also develop gallstones. The signs and symptoms of moderate HS usually appear in childhood. Individuals with the moderate/severe form have all the features of the moderate form but also have severe anemia. Those with the severe form have life-threatening anemia that requires frequent blood transfusions to replenish their RBC supply. They also have severe splenomegaly, jaundice, and a high risk of developing gallstones. Some individuals with the severe form have short stature, delayed sexual development, and skeletal abnormalities.

CAUSES OF HEREDITARY SPHEROCYTOSIS

Mutations in at least five genes cause HS. These genes provide instructions for producing proteins that are found on the membranes of RBCs. These proteins transport molecules into and out of cells, attach to other proteins, and maintain cell structure. Some of these proteins allow for cell flexibility; RBCs have to be flexible to travel from the large blood vessels (arteries) to the smaller blood vessels (capillaries). The proteins allow the cell to change shape without breaking when passing through narrow capillaries.

Mutations in RBC membrane proteins result in an overly rigid, misshapen cell. Instead of a flattened disc shape, these cells are spherical. Dysfunctional membrane proteins interfere with the cell's ability to change shape when traveling through the blood vessels. The misshapen RBCs, called "spherocytes," are removed from circulation and taken to the spleen for destruction. Within the spleen, the RBCs break down (undergo hemolysis). The shortage of RBCs in circulation and the abundance of cells in the spleen are responsible for the signs and symptoms of HS.

Mutations in the *ANK1* gene are responsible for approximately half of all cases of HS. The other genes associated with HS each account for a smaller percentage of cases of this condition.

FREQUENCY OF HEREDITARY SPHEROCYTOSIS

Hereditary spherocytosis occurs in 1 in 2,000 individuals of Northern European ancestry. This condition is the most common cause of inherited anemia in that population. The prevalence of HS in people of other ethnic backgrounds is unknown, but it is much less common.

INHERITANCE OF HEREDITARY SPHEROCYTOSIS

In about 75 percent of cases, HS is inherited in an autosomal dominant pattern, which means one copy of the altered gene in each cell is sufficient to cause the disorder. In some cases, an affected person inherits the mutation from one affected parent. Other cases result from new mutations in the gene and occur in people with no history of the disorder in their family.

This condition can also be inherited in an autosomal recessive pattern, which means both copies of the gene in each cell have mutations. The parents of an individual with an autosomal recessive condition each carry one copy of the mutated gene, but they typically do not show signs and symptoms of the condition.[3]

Section 9.4 | Pyruvate Kinase Deficiency

Pyruvate kinase deficiency is an inherited disorder that affects red blood cells (RBCs), which carry oxygen to the body's tissues. People with this disorder have a condition known as "chronic hemolytic anemia," in which RBCs are broken down (undergo hemolysis) prematurely, resulting in a shortage of RBCs (anemia). Specifically, pyruvate kinase deficiency is a common cause of a type of inherited hemolytic anemia called "hereditary nonspherocytic hemolytic anemia." In hereditary nonspherocytic hemolytic anemia, the RBCs do not assume a spherical shape as they do in some other forms of hemolytic anemia.

SYMPTOMS OF PYRUVATE KINASE DEFICIENCY

Chronic hemolytic anemia can lead to unusually pale skin (pallor), yellowing of the eyes and skin (jaundice), extreme tiredness (fatigue), shortness of breath (dyspnea), and a rapid heart rate (tachycardia). An enlarged spleen (splenomegaly), an excess of iron in the blood, and small pebble-like deposits in the gallbladder or bile ducts (gallstones) are also common in this disorder.

In people with pyruvate kinase deficiency, hemolytic anemia and associated complications may range from mild to severe. Some affected individuals have few or no symptoms. Severe cases can be life-threatening in infancy, and such affected individuals may require regular blood transfusions to survive. The symptoms of this disorder may get worse during an infection or pregnancy.

---

[3] MedlinePlus, "Hereditary Spherocytosis," National Institutes of Health (NIH), September 1, 2013. Available online. URL: https://medlineplus.gov/genetics/condition/hereditary-spherocytosis. Accessed May 11, 2023.

CAUSES OF PYRUVATE KINASE DEFICIENCY

Pyruvate kinase deficiency is caused by mutations in the *PKLR* gene. The *PKLR* gene is active in the liver and in RBCs, where it provides instructions for making an enzyme called "pyruvate kinase." The pyruvate kinase enzyme is involved in a critical energy-producing process known as "glycolysis." During glycolysis, the simple sugar glucose is broken down to produce adenosine triphosphate (ATP), the cell's main energy source.

PKLR gene mutations result in reduced pyruvate kinase enzyme function, causing a shortage of ATP in RBCs and increased levels of other molecules produced earlier in the glycolysis process. The abnormal RBCs are gathered up by the spleen and destroyed, causing hemolytic anemia and an enlarged spleen. A shortage of RBCs to carry oxygen throughout the body leads to fatigue, pallor, and shortness of breath. Iron and a molecule called "bilirubin" are released when RBCs are destroyed, resulting in an excess of these substances circulating in the blood. Excess bilirubin in the blood causes jaundice and increases the risk of developing gallstones.

Pyruvate kinase deficiency may also occur as an effect of other blood diseases, such as leukemia. These cases are called "secondary pyruvate kinase deficiency" and are not inherited.

FREQUENCY OF PYRUVATE KINASE DEFICIENCY

Pyruvate kinase deficiency is the most common inherited cause of nonspherocytic hemolytic anemia. More than 500 affected families have been identified, and studies suggest that the disorder may be underdiagnosed because mild cases may not be identified.

Pyruvate kinase deficiency is found in all ethnic groups. Its prevalence has been estimated at 1 in 20,000 people of European descent. It is more common in the Old Order Amish population of Pennsylvania.

INHERITANCE OF PYRUVATE KINASE DEFICIENCY

This condition is inherited in an autosomal recessive pattern, which means both copies of the gene in each cell have mutations. The parents of an individual with an autosomal recessive condition each carry one copy of the mutated gene, but they typically do not show signs and symptoms of the condition.[4]

Section 9.5 | Sickle Cell Disease

WHAT IS SICKLE CELL DISEASE?

Sickle cell disease (SCD) is a group of inherited red blood cell (RBC) disorders that affect hemoglobin, the protein that carries oxygen throughout the body. The condition affects more than 100,000 people in the United States and 20 million people worldwide.

If you have SCD, your RBCs are crescent- or "sickle"-shaped. These cells do not bend or move easily and can block blood flow to the rest of your body.

The blocked blood flow through the body can lead to serious problems, including stroke, eye problems, infections, and episodes of pain called "pain crises." SCD is a lifelong illness.

WHAT IS A "SICKLED CELL"?

Red blood cells with normal hemoglobin are disc-shaped and flexible so that they can move easily through large and small blood vessels to deliver oxygen throughout the body.

Sickled hemoglobin is not like normal hemoglobin. Sickle-shaped RBCs are not flexible and can stick to vessel walls, causing blockages that slow or stop the flow of blood. The abnormal hemoglobin can also cause stiff strands to form within the RBC. These stiff strands can change the shape of the cell, causing the sickled RBC that gives the disease its name. Figure 9.1 shows the difference between a normal RBC and a sickled RBC.

The sickle-shaped cells cannot deliver oxygen to the rest of the body. This can cause attacks of sudden severe pain, called "pain

[4] MedlinePlus, "Pyruvate Kinase Deficiency," National Institutes of Health (NIH), April 1, 2012. Available online. URL: https://medlineplus.gov/genetics/condition/pyruvate-kinase-deficiency. Accessed May 11, 2023.

crises." These pain crises can occur without warning, and a person who has them often needs to go to the hospital for effective treatment.

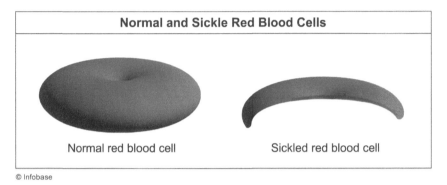

Normal and Sickle Red Blood Cells

Normal red blood cell   Sickled red blood cell

© Infobase

Figure 9.1. Normal and Sickle Red Blood Cells

Infobase

Because sickle cells cannot easily change shape, they also tend to burst apart. Normal RBCs live about 90–120 days, but sickle cells last only 10–20 days. The body is always making new RBCs to replace the old cells. However, in SCD, the body may have trouble keeping up with how fast the cells are being destroyed. Because of this, the number of RBCs is usually lower than in people without SCD. This condition, called "anemia," can cause a person to have less energy.

CAUSES AND RISK FACTORS OF SICKLE CELL DISEASE

Sickle cell disease is inherited, meaning that it runs in families. People who have SCD inherit two faulty hemoglobin genes called "hemoglobin S"—one from each parent.

A person has sickle cell trait when the hemoglobin S gene is inherited from only one parent and a normal hemoglobin gene—hemoglobin A—is inherited from the other. People who have sickle cell trait are generally healthy.

If someone has sickle cell trait, they are a carrier of the hemoglobin S gene. That means they can pass it on when they have a child.

If the child's other parent also has sickle cell trait or another faulty hemoglobin gene, such as beta (β) thalassemia, hemoglobin C, hemoglobin D, or hemoglobin E, that child has a chance of having SCD. That is because the child could inherit a faulty hemoglobin gene from each parent.

Inheritance Pattern for Sickle Cell Disease

Each parent has one normal hemoglobin A gene and one hemoglobin S gene, which means each of their children has:

- a 25 percent, or one in four, chance of inheriting two normal hemoglobin A genes (This child does not have sickle cell trait or disease.)
- a 50 percent, or one in two, chance of inheriting one normal hemoglobin A gene and one hemoglobin S gene (This child has sickle cell trait.)
- a 25 percent, or one in four, chance of inheriting two hemoglobin S genes (This child has SCD.)

It is important to keep in mind that each time this couple has a child, the chances of that child having SCD remain the same. In other words, if the first child has SCD, there is still a 25 percent chance that the second child will also have the disease. Both boys and girls can inherit sickle cell trait, SCD, or normal hemoglobin.

If a person wants to know whether they carry a sickle hemoglobin gene, a doctor can order a blood test to find out.

What Are the Risk Factors?

In the United States, most people who have SCD are of African ancestry or identify themselves as Black:

- About 1 in 13 Black or African American babies is born with sickle cell trait.
- About 1 in every 365 Black or African American babies is born with SCD.

Many people who come from Hispanic, Southern European, Middle Eastern, or Asian Indian backgrounds also have SCD.

About 100,000 people in the United States have SCD.

What Should You Do If You Are at Risk?

People who do not know whether they carry a faulty hemoglobin gene can ask their provider to have their blood tested.

Couples who are planning to have children and know that they are at risk of having a child with SCD may want to meet with a genetic counselor. A genetic counselor can answer questions about the risk and explain the choices that are available.

SYMPTOMS OF SICKLE CELL DISEASE

Sickle cell disease is an inherited disease, which means you are born with it. However, most newborns do not have any problems from the disease until they are about five or six months of age.

The symptoms of SCD can vary from person to person and can change over time. How the disease affects your body over time will determine what kind of symptoms you may have.

Early Symptoms

- a yellowish color of the skin (jaundice) or whites of the eyes (icterus) that occurs when a large number of red cells undergo hemolysis
- extreme tiredness or fussiness from anemia
- painful swelling of the hands and feet, known as "dactylitis"

Know When to Seek Emergency Medical Care

SCD can lead to serious and life-threatening health problems. If you think that you or someone else is having any of the following symptoms or complications, seek medical care or call 911 right away:

- **Symptoms of severe anemia**. These include extreme tiredness (fatigue), shortness of breath, dizziness, or irregular heartbeat. A splenic sequestration crisis or an aplastic crisis can cause severe anemia symptoms. These conditions can be life-threatening.
- **Fever**. All children and adults who have SCD and a fever of more than 101.3 °F, or 38.5 °C, must be seen by

a health-care provider and treated with antibiotics right away. Some people will need to be hospitalized.

- **Symptoms of acute chest syndrome**. These include chest pain, coughing, fever, and shortness of breath. You will need to be admitted to the hospital, where you may receive antibiotics, oxygen therapy, or a blood transfusion.
- **Stroke symptoms**. Warning signs include sudden weakness, numbness on one side of the body, confusion, or trouble speaking, seeing, or walking.
- **Priapism**. If you experience an erection that lasts for four hours or more, go to the hospital to see a hematologist (a doctor who specializes in blood conditions and diseases) and a urologist (a doctor who specializes in treating conditions of the male reproductive and urinary systems).

DIAGNOSIS OF SICKLE CELL DISEASE

If you or your child has symptoms of SCD, your health-care provider may use a number of tests to diagnose the condition.

Blood and Genetic Tests

If you do not know whether you make sickle hemoglobin, you can find out by having your blood tested. You may also have a genetic test performed on your blood. This way, you can learn whether you carry a gene—or have the trait—for sickle hemoglobin that you could pass on to a child.

Genetic testing can help determine which type of SCD you have or can help confirm a diagnosis if results from blood tests are not clear. Genetic testing can also tell whether you have one or two copies of the sickle hemoglobin gene.

Prenatal Screening

Health-care providers can also diagnose SCD before a baby is born. This is done using either a sample of amniotic fluid, the liquid in the sac surrounding a growing embryo, or a sample of tissue taken from the placenta, the organ that attaches the umbilical cord to the womb.

Testing before birth can be done as early as 8–10 weeks into the pregnancy. This testing looks for the sickle hemoglobin gene rather than the abnormal hemoglobin itself. This testing cannot predict the severity of the disease.

Newborn Screening

In newborn screening programs, drops of blood from a heel prick are collected on a special type of paper. The hemoglobin from this blood is then tested in a lab. Newborn screening results are sent to the provider who ordered the test and to your child's health-care provider.

Providers from a special follow-up newborn screening team will contact you directly if your child has SCD. Your child's providers will then retest your child to make sure the diagnosis is correct.

Newborn screening programs also find out whether your baby has the sickle cell trait and is a carrier. If this is the case, counseling will be offered. Remember that when a child has sickle cell trait or SCD, their future siblings or your child's future children may be at risk.

TREATMENT FOR SICKLE CELL DISEASE

A blood and bone marrow transplant is currently the only cure for some patients who have SCD. After early diagnosis, your health-care provider may recommend medicines or transfusions to manage complications, including chronic pain.

Babies who have SCD may see a hematologist, a doctor who specializes in blood diseases such as SCD. For newborns, the first SCD visit should take place before eight weeks of age.

Potential Genetic Therapy Treatments

Genetic therapy involves either restoring a faulty or missing gene or adding a new gene that improves the way the cell works. Researchers take blood or bone marrow from a patient and modify their stem cells in a laboratory using genetic therapies.

Genetic therapies that modify a person's own hematopoietic stem cells may provide a cure for people who have SCD and do not have a well-matched donor. Modified stem cells can be injected into the blood; then the cells travel in the bloodstream to the marrow spaces inside the bones. Once inside the bone marrow, the cells can produce healthy RBCs that do not sickle.[5]

Section 9.6 | **Thalassemia**

WHAT IS THALASSEMIA?

Thalassemia is an inherited blood disorder caused when the body does not make enough of a protein called "hemoglobin," an important part of red blood cells (RBCs). When there is not enough hemoglobin, the body's RBCs do not function properly, and they last shorter periods of time, so there are fewer healthy RBCs traveling in the bloodstream.

RBCs carry oxygen to all the cells of the body. Oxygen is a sort of food that cells use to function. When there are not enough healthy RBCs, there is also not enough oxygen delivered to all the other cells of the body, which may cause a person to feel tired, weak, or short of breath. This is a condition called "anemia." People with thalassemia may have mild or severe anemia. Severe anemia can damage organs and lead to death.

WHAT ARE THE DIFFERENT TYPES OF THALASSEMIA?

When we talk about different "types" of thalassemia, we might be talking about one of two things: the specific part of hemoglobin that is affected (usually either "alpha" or "beta") or the severity of thalassemia, which is noted by words such as trait, carrier, intermedia, or major.

---

[5] "What Is Sickle Cell Disease?" National Heart, Lung, and Blood Institute (NHLBI), July 22, 2022. Available online. URL: www.nhlbi.nih.gov/health/sickle-cell-disease. Accessed June 5, 2023.

Hemoglobin, which carries oxygen to all cells in the body, is made of two different parts, called "alpha" and "beta." When thalassemia is called "alpha" or "beta," this refers to the part of hemoglobin that is not being made. If either the alpha or beta part is not made, there are not enough building blocks to make normal amounts of hemoglobin. Low alpha is called "alpha thalassemia." Low beta is called "beta thalassemia."

When the words "trait," "minor," "intermedia," or "major" are used, these words describe how severe the thalassemia is. A person who has thalassemia trait may not have any symptoms at all or may have only mild anemia, while a person with thalassemia major may have severe symptoms and may need regular blood transfusions.

In the same way that traits for hair color and body structure are passed down from parents to children, thalassemia traits are passed from parents to children. The type of thalassemia that a person has depends on how many and what type of traits for thalassemia a person has inherited, or received, from their parents. For instance, if a person receives a beta thalassemia trait from his or her father and another from his or her mother, he or she will have beta thalassemia major. If a person received an alpha thalassemia trait from his or her mother and the normal alpha parts from his or her father, he or she will have alpha thalassemia trait (also called "alpha thalassemia minor"). Having a thalassemia trait means that you may not have any symptoms, but you may pass that trait on to your children and increase their risk of having thalassemia.

Sometimes, thalassemias have other names, such as Constant Spring, Cooley anemia, or hemoglobin Bart hydrops fetalis. These names are specific to certain thalassemias—for instance, Cooley anemia is the same thing as beta thalassemia major.

HOW DO YOU KNOW IF YOU HAVE THALASSEMIA?

People with moderate and severe forms of thalassemia usually find out about their condition in childhood since they have symptoms of severe anemia early in life. People with less severe forms of thalassemia may only find out because they are having symptoms of anemia or maybe because a doctor finds anemia on a routine blood test or a test done for another reason.

Because thalassemias are inherited, the condition sometimes runs in families. Some people find out about their thalassemia because they have relatives with similar conditions.

People who have family members from certain parts of the world have a higher risk of having thalassemia. Traits for thalassemia are more common in people from Mediterranean countries such as Greece and Turkey and in people from Asia, Africa, and the Middle East. If you have anemia and you also have family members from these areas, your doctor might test your blood further to find out if you have thalassemia.

CAN YOU PREVENT THALASSEMIA?

Because thalassemia is passed from parents to children, it is very hard to prevent. However, if you or your partner knows of family members with thalassemia or if you both have family members from places in the world where thalassemia is common, you can speak to a genetic counselor at www.nsgc.org/page/find-a-genetic-counselor to determine what your risk would be of passing thalassemia to your children.[6]

[6] "What Is Thalassemia?" Centers for Disease Control and Prevention (CDC), April 24, 2023. Available online. URL: www.cdc.gov/ncbddd/thalassemia/facts.html. Accessed May 11, 2023.

Chapter 10 | Acquired Causes of Hemolytic Anemia

Chapter Contents

Section 10.1 | Immune Hemolytic Anemia

Immune hemolytic anemia is a condition in which the body's immune system stops red blood cells (RBCs) from forming or causes them to clump together. Immune complex hemolytic anemia can occur in patients who have chronic lymphocytic leukemia (CLL).[1]

This condition is further classified into autoimmune hemolytic anemia (AIHA), fetal and neonatal alloimmune thrombocytopenia (FNAIT), and drug-induced hemolytic anemia.

AUTOIMMUNE HEMOLYTIC ANEMIA

Autoimmune hemolytic anemia occurs when your immune system makes antibodies that attack your RBCs. This causes a drop in the number of RBCs, leading to hemolytic anemia. Symptoms may include unusual weakness and fatigue with tachycardia and breathing difficulties, jaundice, dark urine, and/or splenomegaly. AIHA can be primary (idiopathic) or result from an underlying disease or medication.

The condition may develop gradually or occur suddenly.

When Do Symptoms of Autoimmune Hemolytic Anemia Begin?

Symptoms of this disease may start to appear at any time in life.

The following symptoms have been linked to this disease:

- abnormal leukocyte morphology (an abnormality of leukocytes)
- autoimmunity (the occurrence of an immune reaction against the organism's own cells or tissues)
- dyspnea (difficult or labored breathing; a subjective feeling only the patient can rate, e.g., on a Borg scale)
- fatigue

---

[1] "Definition of Immune Complex Hemolytic Anemia," National Cancer Institute (NCI), February 3, 2018. Available online. URL: www.cancer.gov/publications/dictionaries/cancer-terms/def/immune-complex-hemolytic-anemia. Accessed June 1, 2023.

- headache
- hemolytic anemia (a type of anemia caused by premature destruction of RBCs (hemolysis))
- muscle weakness
- immunodeficiency
- lymphoma (a cancer originating in lymphocytes and presenting as a solid tumor of lymphoid cells)
- pallor
- abdominal pain
- arrhythmia (Any cardiac rhythm other than the normal sinus rhythm, which may be either of sinus or ectopic origin and either regular or irregular. An arrhythmia may be due to a disturbance in impulse formation or conduction or both.)
- congestive heart failure (The presence of an abnormality of cardiac function that is responsible for the failure of the heart to pump blood at a rate that is commensurate with the needs of the tissues or a state in which abnormally elevated filling pressures are required for the heart to do so. Heart failure is frequently related to a defect in myocardial contraction.)
- splenomegaly (abnormally increased size of the spleen)[2]

FETAL AND NEONATAL ALLOIMMUNE THROMBOCYTOPENIA

Fetal and neonatal alloimmune thrombocytopenia is a blood disorder that affects pregnant women and their babies. FNAIT was first reported in the literature in 1953 and is estimated to occur in as many as 1 in 1,200 live births. FNAIT results in the destruction of platelets in the fetus or infant due to a mismatch between the mother's platelets and those of the baby. Certain molecules (antigens) on the surface of the baby's platelets are recognized as foreign by the mother's immune system. The mother's immune system then creates antibodies that attack and destroy the baby's platelets. Though FNAIT can occur whenever the mother's blood mixes with

---

[2] Genetic and Rare Diseases Information Center (GARD), "Autoimmune Hemolytic Anemia," National Center for Advancing Translational Sciences (NCATS), February 16, 2023. Available online. URL: https://rarediseases.info.nih.gov/diseases/5870/autoimmune-hemolytic-anemia. Accessed June 1, 2023.

that of the baby, it is usually triggered when the mother is exposed to the baby's blood during delivery. Many cases of FNAIT are mild. Signs and symptoms may include a low platelet count (thrombocytopenia) and signs of bleeding into the skin, such as petechiae and purpura. In the most severe cases, FNAIT can cause bleeding episodes that may result in death or long-term disability. Bleeding episodes can occur either during pregnancy or after birth.

When Do Symptoms of Fetal and Neonatal Alloimmune Thrombocytopenia Begin?

Symptoms of this disease may start to appear during pregnancy and as a newborn.

The following symptoms have been linked to this disease:

- **Neonatal alloimmune thrombocytopenia**. Low platelet count associated with maternal platelet-specific alloantibodies.
- **Abnormal bleeding**. An abnormal susceptibility to bleeding, often referred to as a bleeding diathesis. (A bleeding diathesis may be related to vascular, platelet, and coagulation defects.)
- **Cephalohematoma**. Hemorrhage between the skull and periosteum of a newborn resulting from rupture of blood vessels that cross the periosteum.
- **Petechiae**. Pinpoint-sized reddish/purple spots, resembling a rash, that appear just under the skin or a mucous membrane when capillaries have ruptured and some superficial bleeding into the skin has happened. (This term refers to an abnormally increased susceptibility to developing petechiae.)
- **Purpura**. The appearance of red or purple discolorations on the skin that do not blanch on applying pressure. (They are caused by bleeding underneath the skin. This term refers to an abnormally increased susceptibility to developing purpura. Purpura are larger than petechiae.)
- **Spontaneous hematomas**. Spontaneous development of hematomas (hematoma) or bruises without significant trauma.

- **Ecchymosis**. A purpuric lesion that is larger than 1 cm in diameter.
- **Gastrointestinal hemorrhage**. Hemorrhage affecting the gastrointestinal tract.
- **Intracranial hemorrhage**. Hemorrhage occurring within the skull.
- **Melena**. The passage of blackish, tarry feces associated with gastrointestinal hemorrhage. (Melena occurs if the blood remains in the colon long enough for it to be broken down by colonic bacteria. One degradation product, hematin, imbues the stool with a blackish color. Thus, melena generally occurs with bleeding from the upper gastrointestinal tract (e.g., stomach ulcers or duodenal ulcers) since the blood usually remains in the gut for a longer period of time than with lower gastrointestinal bleeding.)
  - **Abnormality of the nervous system**. Including diseases such as Alzheimer disease (AD), neurofibromatosis, Parkinson disease (PD), and other diseases of the nervous system.
  - **Bilateral sensorineural hearing impairment**. A bilateral form of sensorineural hearing impairment.
  - **Blindness**. The condition of having a visual perception below 3/60 and/or a visual field of no greater than 10 degrees in radius around central fixation.
- **Cerebral palsy (CP)**. A group of permanent disorders of the development of movement and posture, causing activity limitation, that are attributed to nonprogressive disturbances that occurred in the developing fetal or infant brain. (The motor disorders of CP are often accompanied by disturbances of sensation, perception, cognition, communication, and behavior; epilepsy; and secondary musculoskeletal problems.)
- **Global developmental delay**. A delay in the achievement of motor or mental milestones in the domains of development of a child, including motor skills, speech and language, cognitive skills, and social and emotional skills. (This term should only be used to describe children younger than five years of age.)

- Subarachnoid hemorrhage. Hemorrhage occurring between the arachnoid mater and the pia mater.[3]

Rhesus Incompatibility in Fetal and Neonatal Alloimmune Thrombocytopenia

When you are pregnant, blood from your baby can cross into your bloodstream, especially during delivery. If you are Rhesus-negative (Rh-negative) and your baby is Rh-positive, your body will react to the baby's blood as a foreign substance. It will create antibodies (proteins) against the baby's blood. These antibodies usually do not cause problems during a first pregnancy.

But Rh incompatibility may cause problems in later pregnancies if the baby is Rh-positive. This is because the antibodies stay in your body once they have formed. The antibodies can cross the placenta and attack the baby's RBCs. The baby could get Rh disease, a serious condition that can cause a serious type of anemia.

Blood tests can tell whether you have Rh factor and whether your body has made antibodies. Injections of a medicine called "Rh immune globulin" can keep your body from making Rh antibodies. It helps prevent the problems of Rh incompatibility. If treatment is needed for the baby, it can include supplements to help the body make RBCs and blood transfusions.[4]

DRUG-INDUCED IMMUNE HEMOLYTIC ANEMIA

Drug-induced immune hemolytic anemia (DIIHA) is a blood disorder caused by medicinal drugs, in which the immune system mistakes the body's RBCs as foreign cells and begins to attack them, resulting in hemolysis.[5] It is normal that the body destroys old RBCs and develops new cells. However, in this case, drugs such as penicillin, quinidine, dapsone, methyldopa, pyridine,

---

[3] Genetic and Rare Diseases Information Center (GARD), "Fetal and Neonatal Alloimmune Thrombocytopenia," National Center for Advancing Translational Sciences (NCATS), February 16, 2023. Available online. URL: https://rarediseases.info.nih.gov/diseases/2295/fetal-and-neonatal-alloimmune-thrombocytopenia. Accessed June 1, 2023.

[4] MedlinePlus, "Rh Incompatibility," National Institutes of Health (NIH), June 19, 2017. Available online. URL: https://medlineplus.gov/rhincompatibility.html. Accessed June 1, 2023.

[5] Todd Gersten, David Zieve, and Brenda Conaway, MedlinePlus, "Drug-Induced Immune Hemolytic Anemia," National Institutes of Health (NIH), January 19, 2021. Available online. URL: medlineplus.gov/ency/article/000578.htm. Accessed July 4, 2023.

levodopa, and levofloxacin cause accelerated destruction of the RBCs.

The onset of DIIHA symptoms is based on whether the RBC destruction occurs during circulation or outside the vascular system, predominantly in the liver and spleen. The most common symptoms are rapid heart rate, dark urine, shortness of breath, pale skin, jaundice, dizziness, fever, confusion, and enlarged liver or spleen.[6]

DIIHA can be diagnosed with blood and urine tests. Certain medicines, such as prednisone, help control mild conditions. Severe symptoms must be treated with blood transfusions. The best treatment for this condition is to stop taking the drug that causes the disorder.[7]

Section 10.2 | Mechanical Hemolytic Anemia

Mechanical hemolytic anemia (MHA) refers to the damage of red blood cells (RBCs) due to repetitive mechanical motions such as marathon running and marching. Although RBCs are flexible, such circumstances cause the cells to shear; this condition is known as "hemoglobinuria."

"March hemoglobinuria" is the term given to the MHA caused by continuous walking or running. The term was coined after the condition was observed in soldiers who marched continuously for long periods.

CAUSES OF MECHANICAL HEMOLYTIC ANEMIA

Apart from the repetitive actions that cause MHA, other factors responsible for this condition are as follows:
- artificial heart valves
- hemodialysis

[6] Amber Yates and Douglas A. Nelson, "Causes and Treatment of Drug-Induced Hemolytic Anemia," Verywell Health, July 7, 2021. Available online. URL: www.verywellhealth.com/drug-induced-hemolytic-anemia-4120830. Accessed July 4, 2023.
[7] See footnote [5].

- preeclampsia
- malignant hypertension
- thrombotic thrombocytopenic purpura (TTP)
- cancer
- chemicals such as arsenic, lead, and snake venom

SYMPTOMS OF MECHANICAL HEMOLYTIC ANEMIA

Symptoms may start mild and gradually get worse or quickly become severe. Some of the symptoms are as follows:

- fatigue
- light-headedness or dizziness
- paleness
- mood swings
- fast heartbeat
- fast breathing or shortness of breath
- jaundice (yellow skin and eyes)
- enlarged spleen
- dark urine
- bleeding from oral, gastrointestinal, or genitourinary tracts

DIAGNOSIS OF MECHANICAL HEMOLYTIC ANEMIA

To diagnose, MHA requires general tests such as a complete blood count (CBC), kidney and liver function, electrolyte levels, reticulocyte count, lactate dehydrogenase levels, and serum haptoglobin levels. In addition, the following tests are performed:

- **Prothrombin time (PT) test**. This test measures the time a blood sample takes to clot.
- **Activated partial thromboplastin time (aPTT) test**. This test also measures the time taken for blood to clot; however, an activator is added, which speeds up the process and narrows the reference range of the results. It is considered more sensitive than a PT test.
- **Fibrinogen test**. This test measures the level of fibrinogen (a blood protein) that is prepared in the liver and helps the blood clot.

TREATMENT FOR MECHANICAL HEMOLYTIC ANEMIA

Mild MHA can be treated with the following:
- iron supplements
- beta-blocker
- erythropoietin
- pentoxifylline

Severe conditions require repeated blood transfusions to replace lost blood or blood components in the body.

References

"Fibrinogen Test," Cleveland Clinic, April 13, 2022. Available online. URL: https://my.clevelandclinic. org/health/diagnostics/22791-fibrinogen-test#:~:text=A%20fibrinogen%20test%20measures%20 your,to%20check%20your%20fibrinogen%20levels. Accessed July 4, 2023.

J. Schiffman Fred and Dalia Samir, "Mechanical Hemolysis," Cancer Therapy Advisor, October 12, 2016. Available online. URL: www.cancertherapyadvisor.com/home/ decision-support-in-medicine/hematology/mechanical-hemolysis-2/. Accessed July 4, 2023.

Muhammad Bader Hammami and Eric B Staros, "Partial Thromboplastin Time, Activated," Medscape, July 2, 2021. Available online. URL: emedicine.medscape.com/ article/2085837-overview#:~:text=Description,in%20 a%20narrower%20reference%20range. Accessed July 4, 2023.

"Types of Hemolytic Anemia," National Heart, Lung, and Blood Institute (NHLBI), April 7, 2011. Available online. URL: www.hoacny.com/patient-resources/blood-disorders/what-hemolytic-anemia/types-hemolytic-anemia. Accessed July 4, 2023.

Wang Jin, et al., "Intractable Mechanical Hemolytic Anemia Complicating Mitral Valve Surgery: A Case Series Study," Biomedcentral.com, March 3, 2020. Available online. URL: bmccardiovascdisord.biomedcentral.com/articles/10.1186/s12872-020-01382-8#Sec2. Accessed July 4, 2023.

Section 10.3 | Paroxysmal Nocturnal Hemoglobinuria

Paroxysmal nocturnal hemoglobinuria (PNH) is an acquired (not inherited) disorder that leads to premature death and impaired production of blood cells. The disorder affects red blood cells (RBCs; erythrocytes), which carry oxygen; white blood cells (WBCs; leukocytes), which protect the body from infections; and platelets (thrombocytes), which are involved in blood clotting. PNH can occur at any age although it is most often diagnosed in young adulthood.

SYMPTOMS OF PAROXYSMAL NOCTURNAL HEMOGLOBINURIA

People with PNH have sudden, recurring episodes of symptoms (paroxysmal symptoms), which may be triggered by stresses on the body, such as infections or physical exertion. During these episodes, RBCs are broken down earlier than they should be (hemolysis). Affected individuals may pass dark-colored urine because of the presence of hemoglobin, the oxygen-carrying protein in the blood. The abnormal presence of hemoglobin in the urine is called "hemoglobinuria." In many, but not all, cases, hemoglobinuria is most noticeable early in the morning, upon passing urine that has accumulated in the bladder during the night (nocturnal).

The premature breakdown of RBCs results in a shortage of these cells in the blood (hemolytic anemia), which can cause signs and symptoms such as fatigue, weakness, abnormally pale skin (pallor), shortness of breath, and an increased heart rate (tachycardia). People with PNH may also be prone to infections because of a shortage of WBCs (leukopenia).

Abnormal platelets associated with PNH can cause problems in the blood clotting process. As a result, people with this disorder may experience abnormal blood clotting (thrombosis), especially in large abdominal veins, or, less often, episodes of severe bleeding (hemorrhage).

CAUSES OF PAROXYSMAL NOCTURNAL HEMOGLOBINURIA

Variants (also known as "mutations") in the *PIGA* gene cause almost all cases of PNH. Variants in the *PIGT* gene cause the rare, inflammatory form of the condition. The proteins produced from both genes are involved in a multistep process that connects particular proteins to the surface of cells. These proteins are attached to the cell by a specialized molecule called "GPI anchor" and are known as "GPI-anchored proteins." The PIG-A protein helps produce the GPI anchor, and the PIG-T protein helps attach the GPI anchor to proteins. Anchored proteins have a variety of roles, including sticking cells to one another, relaying signals into cells, and protecting cells from destruction.

In people with PNH, variants of the *PIGA* gene occur during a person's lifetime and are present only in certain cells. These changes, which are called "somatic variants," are not inherited. In contrast, people with the inflammatory form of the condition inherit one altered copy of the *PIGT* gene. However, for the condition to occur, they need to also acquire a somatic variant that deletes the other copy of the *PIGT* gene and other genes around it.

PNH occurs when a somatic variant of the *PIGA* gene or *PIGT* gene occurs in a blood-forming cell called a "hematopoietic stem cell." Hematopoietic stem cells are found mainly in the bone marrow and give rise to various types of blood cells. These genetic variants severely reduce or eliminate the function of the PIG-A protein or PIG-T protein, respectively, in affected cells. Blood cells that arise from the abnormal stem cells also have the variant and are abnormal. As the abnormal hematopoietic stem cells multiply, more abnormal blood cells are formed alongside normal blood cells produced by normal hematopoietic stem cells.

Cells with no PIG-A protein do not produce the GPI anchor and, therefore, are missing GPI-anchored proteins at the surface. Cells with no PIG-T protein produce the GPI anchor but cannot attach proteins to it. As a result, these cells have the GPI anchor on the surface but no attached proteins. Two important GPI-anchored proteins on RBCs protect them from being broken down by the immune system. Without these proteins, the abnormal RBCs are prematurely destroyed, leading to hemolytic anemia. Studies show that GPI anchors with no attached proteins trigger inflammation in the body, leading to inflammatory features in individuals with PIGT-related PNH. It is unclear how changes in the *PIGA* or *PIGT* gene affect other types of blood cells.

In individuals with either form of PNH, the proportion of abnormal blood cells can vary. It is unclear why the population of cells that grow from the hematopoietic stem cell with a *PIGA* gene variant may be larger than the population of normal cells in some affected individuals and smaller in others. Research suggests that certain abnormal WBCs that are also part of the immune system may mistakenly attack normal blood-forming cells in a malfunction called an "autoimmune process." In addition, abnormal hematopoietic stem cells in people with PNH may be less susceptible than normal cells to a process called "apoptosis," which causes cells to self-destruct when they are damaged or unneeded.

In abnormal blood cells with *PIGT* gene variants, the somatic variant in the *PIGT* gene deletes other nearby genes that control cell growth and development. Researchers suggest that the loss of these genes allows the abnormal cells to grow or survive better than normal cells, increasing the proportion of abnormal blood cells in the body. The proportion of abnormal blood cells affects the severity of the signs and symptoms of PNH, including the risk of hemoglobinuria and thrombosis.

RISK FACTORS FOR PAROXYSMAL NOCTURNAL HEMOGLOBINURIA

Individuals with PNH are at increased risk of developing cancer in blood-forming cells (leukemia). In some cases, people who have or have been treated for another blood disease called "aplastic anemia" may develop PNH. In a small number of affected individuals, the signs and symptoms of PNH disappear on their own.

COMPLICATIONS OF PAROXYSMAL NOCTURNAL HEMOGLOBINURIA

A very rare form of PNH involves abnormal inflammation in addition to the typical features described above. Inflammation is a normal immune system response to injury and foreign invaders (such as bacteria). In people with this rare form of PNH, the immune response is turned on (activated) abnormally and can cause recurrent aseptic meningitis (which is inflammation of the membranes surrounding the brain and spinal cord that is not related to infection); a red, itchy rash (known as "hives" or "urticaria"); joint pain (arthralgia); or inflammatory bowel disease. The inflammatory disorders usually begin earlier than the blood cell problems.

FREQUENCY OF PAROXYSMAL NOCTURNAL HEMOGLOBINURIA

Paroxysmal nocturnal hemoglobinuria is a rare disorder estimated to affect between one and five per million people. The inflammatory form of the disorder is extremely rare and has been identified in a very small number of individuals.

INHERITANCE OF PAROXYSMAL NOCTURNAL HEMOGLOBINURIA

Paroxysmal nocturnal hemoglobinuria is acquired rather than inherited. Most cases result from new variants in the *PIGA* gene and generally occur in people with no previous history of the disorder in their family. This form of the condition is not passed down to the children of affected individuals.

The *PIGA* gene is located on the X chromosome, which is one of the two sex chromosomes. Males have only one X chromosome, and a variant in the only copy of the *PIGA* gene in each cell is sufficient to cause the condition. Females have two X chromosomes. However, early in embryonic development in females, one of the two X chromosomes is permanently inactivated in somatic cells (cells other than egg and sperm cells). This process, called "X-inactivation," ensures that females, like males, have only one active copy of the X chromosome in each body cell. In females, a variant in the active copy of the *PIGA* gene is sufficient to cause the condition.

Acquired Causes of Hemolytic Anemia

The risk of developing PIGT-related PNH follows an autosomal dominant pattern of inheritance, which means one copy of the altered gene in each cell is sufficient to increase a person's chance of developing the condition. Affected individuals inherit one altered copy of the *PIGT* gene from a parent. However, the condition is acquired when a second alteration occurs in the other copy of the *PIGT* gene.[8]

---

[8] MedlinePlus, "Paroxysmal Nocturnal Hemoglobinuria," National Institutes of Health (NIH), February 24, 2022. Available online. URL: https://medlineplus.gov/genetics/condition/paroxysmal-nocturnal-hemoglobinuria. Accessed June 2, 2023.

Chapter 11 | Hemochromatosis: Iron Overload Disorder

Hemochromatosis is a disorder in which extra iron builds up in the body to harmful levels.

Your body needs iron to stay healthy, make red blood cells, build muscle and heart cells, and do the daily tasks that your body and internal organs need to do. However, too much iron is harmful.

The human body typically controls the amount of iron that is absorbed from the diet, increasing the amount when iron is needed and decreasing the amount when iron levels in the body are too high. In hemochromatosis, the body absorbs too much iron from the diet each day.

Without treatment, hemochromatosis can cause iron overload, a buildup of iron that can damage many parts of the body, including the liver, heart, pancreas, endocrine glands, and joints.

ARE THERE DIFFERENT TYPES OF HEMOCHROMATOSIS?

Primary hemochromatosis, also called "hereditary" or "inherited hemochromatosis," is caused by inherited mutations in genes that control how much iron is absorbed from the diet.

Secondary hemochromatosis, also called "secondary iron overload" or "hemosiderosis," is caused by too much iron in the diet or too much iron from blood transfusions, such as transfusions that treat severe anemia.

Neonatal hemochromatosis is a very rare condition caused by injury to the liver of a fetus in the womb. This liver injury causes extra iron to build up in the liver and other organs.

WHAT ARE THE SYMPTOMS OF HEMOCHROMATOSIS?

With the buildup of harmful levels of iron, hemochromatosis can cause symptoms including the following:

- feeling tired or weak
- pain in the joints, particularly in the knees and hands
- loss of interest in sex or erectile dysfunction
- pain in the abdomen over the liver
- darkening of skin color, which may appear gray, metallic, or bronze

With more severe iron overload, people may develop signs and symptoms of complications, such as cirrhosis, diabetes, or heart failure.

Not everyone with hemochromatosis has symptoms, and hemochromatosis may not cause symptoms for many years. Symptoms typically begin after age 40, and on average, women develop symptoms about 10 years later than men.

WHAT CAUSES HEMOCHROMATOSIS?
Primary Hemochromatosis

Mutations in genes that control how the body absorbs iron cause primary hemochromatosis. The most common mutations are in the *HFE* genes and are called "*C282Y*" and "*H63D*."

The important *HFE* mutations are autosomal recessive, meaning that a person must inherit two copies of the *HFE* gene with the mutation to have hemochromatosis. The most common pattern in primary hemochromatosis occurs with two copies of *C282Y*. Two copies of *C282Y* are present in about 85–90 percent of cases of primary hemochromatosis. A less common pattern that leads to milder iron overload is caused by having one copy of *C282Y* and one of *H63D*.

Mutations in other genes that control how the body manages iron levels cause 10–15 percent of cases of primary hemochromatosis.

These rare forms are called "non-HFE hemochromatosis." The most severe forms of non-HFE hemochromatosis are due to mutations in the *HJV* genes or the *HAMP* genes. People with these mutations develop symptoms and complications at a young age and may have cirrhosis and other complications from iron overload in their teenage years.

Secondary Hemochromatosis

Secondary hemochromatosis is caused by excessive iron in the diet or from multiple blood transfusions.

The usual cause of secondary hemochromatosis is blood transfusions given for severe types of anemia, such as sickle cell disease (SCD) or thalassemias. In addition, people with bone marrow failure and severe anemia may require regular blood transfusions given over months or years. Red blood cells (RBCs) are a rich source of iron, and RBCs given by transfusions can lead to a buildup of iron to high levels. The body does not have a good way to get rid of iron.

In the past, iron overload was a common problem in people with kidney failure. However, the use of erythropoietin (EPO) to treat anemia in chronic kidney disease (CKD) in people with kidney failure has lessened the chance of iron overload. EPO helps the body make RBCs, lowering levels of stored iron and reducing the need for blood transfusions.

Iron overload in the liver also occurs in persons with severe liver disease, such as cirrhosis due to alcoholic liver disease or advanced forms of chronic hepatitis B or C. In these situations, the level of iron is high enough to worsen the underlying liver disease.

Iron overload from excess iron in the diet is very rare but can be caused by cooking and brewing alcohol in crude iron pots or skillets. Drinking alcohol in this situation leads to an increase in the absorption of iron and can cause serious iron overload in the liver.

Neonatal Hemochromatosis

Neonatal hemochromatosis is a very rare disease that leads to cirrhosis and liver failure in newborns. In most cases, neonatal hemochromatosis occurs when a pregnant woman's immune system produces antibodies that damage the liver of a fetus, causing iron overload.

A woman who has one child with neonatal hemochromatosis is at risk for having a second or third affected newborn. Doctors can treat women during future pregnancies to help prevent neonatal hemochromatosis.

HOW DO DOCTORS DIAGNOSE HEMOCHROMATOSIS?

Doctors usually diagnose hemochromatosis based on blood test results. Doctors may first suspect hemochromatosis based on a medical and family history, a physical exam, and blood tests.

Medical and Family History

Doctors ask about medical history, including the following:
- symptoms of hemochromatosis, such as feeling tired or weak or pain in the joints
- health problems that may be complications of hemochromatosis, such as diabetes or arthritis

Doctors also ask about any family history of hemochromatosis or health problems such as cirrhosis or diabetes.

Physical Exam

During a physical exam, the doctor will check for signs of hemochromatosis, such as:
- changes in skin color
- enlargement of the liver or spleen
- tenderness in the abdomen over the liver
- tenderness and swelling in the joints

WHAT TESTS DO DOCTORS USE TO DIAGNOSE HEMOCHROMATOSIS?

Blood tests are critical for the diagnosis of hemochromatosis. In some cases, doctors may also order a liver biopsy.

Blood Tests

For a blood test, a health-care professional will take a blood sample from you and send the sample to a lab. Doctors may order blood tests to check:

- levels of iron
- levels of transferrin, the protein that carries iron in the blood
- the ratio of iron to transferrin
- levels of ferritin, the protein that stores iron in the liver

A high ratio of iron to transferrin in the blood may suggest a person has hemochromatosis. A high ferritin level is also typical in people who have hemochromatosis. Doctors may also use blood tests for ferritin levels to see if iron levels are improving with treatment.

Doctors usually order blood tests to check for the gene mutations that cause hemochromatosis. Finding two copies of the *HFE* gene with the C282Y mutation confirms the diagnosis of primary hemochromatosis.

Liver Biopsy

In some cases, doctors will use a liver biopsy to confirm that iron overload is present and that no other liver diseases are present. The liver biopsy also shows whether iron overload has caused scarring or permanent damage to the liver.

During a liver biopsy, a doctor will take small pieces of tissue from the liver. A pathologist will examine the tissue with a microscope. The biopsy can be stained for iron, which will show whether too much iron appears to be present. The biopsy can also be used to measure the actual amount of iron in the liver.

HOW DO DOCTORS TREAT HEMOCHROMATOSIS?

In most cases, doctors treat hemochromatosis with phlebotomy, or drawing about a pint of blood at a time, on a regular schedule. This is the most direct and safe way to lower body stores of iron.

Treatment of hemochromatosis can improve symptoms and prevent complications.

Phlebotomy

Phlebotomy removes extra iron from your blood. Phlebotomy is simple, inexpensive, and safe.

How much blood is drawn and how often depend on your iron levels. Doctors usually start by having a pint of blood drawn once or twice a week for several months. Doctors will order regular blood tests to check iron and ferritin levels.

Phlebotomy is usually done in blood banks, just like routine blood donation. In some cases, blood drawn from people with hemochromatosis may be donated and used in people who need blood transfusions.

After phlebotomy has removed extra iron and blood levels of iron and ferritin return to normal, doctors will reduce phlebotomies to once every one to three months and eventually to two to three times a year. Doctors will continue to order regular blood tests to check iron and ferritin levels.

Other Treatments

People who receive blood transfusions to treat certain types of anemia and develop secondary hemochromatosis cannot have phlebotomy to lower their iron levels. To treat secondary hemochromatosis in these people, doctors prescribe medicines called "chelating agents" that bind to iron and allow it to pass from the body in urine. Chelating agents may be pills taken by mouth or intravenous (IV) medicines, and they do not remove iron as effectively as phlebotomy.

Doctors treat neonatal hemochromatosis in newborns with exchange transfusions—removing blood and replacing it with donor blood—and IV immunoglobulin—a solution of antibodies from healthy people. These treatments do not always work to reverse severe liver damage, and a liver transplant may be needed. Often the newborn's mother or father can serve as a living liver donor. Only a small part of the adult donor liver is needed for transplantation into a newborn.

HOW DO DOCTORS TREAT THE COMPLICATIONS OF HEMOCHROMATOSIS?

Phlebotomy can prevent the complications of hemochromatosis. For people who already have complications, such as cirrhosis, liver failure, or liver cancer, when they are diagnosed with hemochromatosis, phlebotomy may not be able to restore health.

Doctors can treat many complications of cirrhosis with medicines, minor medical procedures, and surgery. People with liver failure or liver cancer usually need a liver transplant to restore health.

CAN YOU PREVENT HEMOCHROMATOSIS?

You cannot prevent inheriting the gene mutations that cause primary hemochromatosis. However, early diagnosis is important since early treatment with phlebotomy can prevent complications of iron overload caused by these gene mutations.

If you have a close relative—a parent, brother or sister, or child—with hemochromatosis, you should be checked for hemochromatosis. Talk with your doctor about testing you and your family members.

Secondary hemochromatosis due to blood transfusion cannot be prevented easily. However, doctors can check iron levels and start treatment with chelating agents early before iron overload causes damage to the liver, joints, and other organs.

If doctors know a pregnant woman is at risk of having an infant with neonatal hemochromatosis due to a family history of the condition, doctors can treat the pregnant woman with IV immunoglobulin to lower the chance that the newborn will have severe iron overload.[1]

---

[1] "Hemochromatosis," National Institute of Diabetes and Digestive and Kidney Diseases (NIDDK), January 2020. Available online. URL: www.niddk.nih.gov/health-information/liver-disease/hemochromatosis/all-content. Accessed May 11, 2023.

Chapter 12 | **Anemia of Inflammation or Chronic Disease**

WHAT IS ANEMIA OF INFLAMMATION?

Anemia of inflammation, also called "anemia of chronic disease" (ACD), is a type of anemia that affects people who have conditions that cause inflammation, such as infections, autoimmune diseases, cancer, and chronic kidney disease (CKD).

In anemia of inflammation, you may have a normal or sometimes increased amount of iron stored in your body tissues, but you have a low level of iron in your blood. Inflammation may prevent your body from using stored iron to make enough healthy red blood cells (RBCs), leading to anemia.

Anemia is a condition in which your blood has fewer RBCs or less hemoglobin than normal.

WHY IS ANEMIA OF INFLAMMATION ALSO CALLED "ANEMIA OF CHRONIC DISEASE?"

Anemia of inflammation is also called "anemia of chronic disease" because this type of anemia commonly occurs in people who have chronic conditions that may be associated with inflammation.

ARE THERE OTHER TYPES OF ANEMIA?

There are many types of anemia. Common types include the following:

- **Iron deficiency anemia**. This is a condition in which the body's stored iron is used up, causing the body to make fewer healthy RBCs. In people with iron deficiency anemia, iron levels are low in both body tissues and the blood. This is the most common type of anemia.
- **Pernicious anemia**. This condition is caused by a lack of vitamin B_{12}.
- **Aplastic anemia**. This is a condition in which the bone marrow does not make enough new RBCs, white blood cells (WBCs), and platelets because the bone marrow's stem cells are damaged.
- **Hemolytic anemia**. This a condition in which RBCs are destroyed earlier than normal.

HOW COMMON IS ANEMIA OF INFLAMMATION?

Anemia of inflammation is the second most common type of anemia after iron deficiency anemia.

WHO IS MORE LIKELY TO HAVE ANEMIA OF INFLAMMATION?

While anemia of inflammation can affect people of any age, older adults are more likely to have this type of anemia because they are more likely to have chronic diseases that cause inflammation. In the United States, about one million people older than the age of 65 have anemia of inflammation.

DOES ANEMIA OF INFLAMMATION LEAD TO OTHER HEALTH PROBLEMS?

Anemia of inflammation is typically mild or moderate, meaning that hemoglobin levels in your blood are lower than normal but not severely low. If your anemia becomes severe, the lack of oxygen in your blood can cause symptoms, such as feeling tired or short of breath. Severe anemia can become life-threatening.

In people who have CKD, severe anemia can increase the chance of developing heart problems.

HOW DO EATING, DIET, AND NUTRITION AFFECT ANEMIA OF INFLAMMATION?

If you have a chronic condition that is causing anemia of inflammation, follow the advice of your doctor or dietitian about healthy eating and nutrition.

WHAT ARE THE SYMPTOMS OF ANEMIA OF INFLAMMATION?

Anemia of inflammation typically develops slowly and may cause few or no symptoms. In fact, you may only experience symptoms of the disease that is causing anemia and not notice additional symptoms.

Symptoms of anemia of inflammation are the same as in any type of anemia and include the following:
- a fast heartbeat
- body aches
- fainting or feeling dizzy or light-headed
- feeling tired or weak
- getting tired easily during or after physical activity
- pale skin
- shortness of breath

WHAT CAUSES ANEMIA OF INFLAMMATION?

Experts think that when you have an infection or disease that causes inflammation, your immune system causes changes in how your body works that may lead to anemia of inflammation.
- Your body may not store and use iron normally.
- Your kidneys may produce less erythropoietin (EPO), a hormone that signals your bone marrow—the spongy tissue inside most of your bones—to make RBCs.
- Your bone marrow may not respond normally to EPO, making fewer RBCs than needed.

- Your RBCs may live for a shorter time than normal, causing them to die faster than they can be replaced.

CHRONIC CONDITIONS THAT CAUSE ANEMIA OF INFLAMMATION

Many different chronic conditions can cause inflammation that leads to anemia, including the following:

- autoimmune diseases, such as rheumatoid arthritis (RA) or lupus
- cancer
- chronic infections, such as human immunodeficiency virus (HIV)/acquired immunodeficiency syndrome (AIDS) and tuberculosis (TB)
- chronic kidney disease (CKD)
- inflammatory bowel diseases (IBDs), such as Crohn's disease or ulcerative colitis (UC)
- other chronic diseases that involve inflammation, such as diabetes and heart failure

In people with certain chronic conditions, anemia may have more than one cause. The following are a few examples:

- Causes of anemia in CKD may include inflammation, low levels of EPO due to kidney damage, or low levels of the nutrients needed to make RBCs. Hemodialysis to treat CKD may also lead to iron deficiency anemia.
- People with IBD may have both iron deficiency anemia due to blood loss and anemia of inflammation.
- In people who have cancer, anemia may be caused by inflammation, blood loss, and cancers that affect or spread to the bone marrow. Cancer treatments, such as chemotherapy and radiation therapy (RT), may also cause or worsen anemia.

OTHER CAUSES OF INFLAMMATION THAT MAY LEAD TO ANEMIA

While anemia of inflammation typically develops slowly, anemia of critical illness is a type of anemia of inflammation that develops quickly in patients who are hospitalized for severe acute infections, trauma, or other conditions that cause inflammation.

In some cases, older adults develop anemia of inflammation that is not related to an underlying infection or chronic disease. Experts think that the aging process may cause inflammation and anemia.

HOW DO HEALTH-CARE PROFESSIONALS DIAGNOSE ANEMIA OF INFLAMMATION?

Health-care professionals use a medical history and blood tests to diagnose anemia of inflammation. If blood test results suggest you have anemia of inflammation, but the cause is unknown, a health-care professional may perform additional tests to look for the cause.

HOW DO HEALTH-CARE PROFESSIONALS TREAT ANEMIA OF INFLAMMATION?

Health-care professionals treat anemia of inflammation by treating the underlying condition and by treating the anemia with medicines and occasionally with blood transfusions.

CAN YOU PREVENT ANEMIA OF INFLAMMATION?

Experts have not yet found a way to prevent anemia of inflammation. For some chronic conditions that cause inflammation, treatments may be available to reduce or prevent the inflammation that can lead to anemia. Talk with your doctor about treatments and follow the treatment plan your doctor recommends.[1]

---

[1] "Anemia of Inflammation or Chronic Disease," National Institute of Diabetes and Digestive and Kidney Diseases (NIDDK), March 2019. Available online. URL: www.niddk.nih.gov/health-information/blood-diseases/anemia-inflammation-chronic-disease. Accessed June 2, 2023.

Chapter 13 | **Managing and Controlling Anemia**

Anemia is a common blood disorder that many people develop at some point in their lives. Many types of anemia are mild and short-term. But the condition can become serious if left untreated for a long time. The good news is that anemia can often be prevented and easily corrected by getting enough iron.

Anemia arises when your body does not have enough healthy red blood cells (RBCs). You may either have too few RBCs, or they may be lacking in an iron-rich protein called "hemoglobin." RBCs are responsible for delivering oxygen throughout your body, and hemoglobin is the protein that carries the oxygen.

When the number of RBCs or your hemoglobin level is too low, your body does not get all of the oxygen it needs, and it can make you feel very tired. You may also have other symptoms such as shortness of breath, dizziness, headaches, pale skin, or cold hands and feet.

The most common type of anemia occurs when your body lacks iron. This condition is called "iron deficiency anemia," and it often arises if you do not have enough iron in your diet. Your body needs iron and other nutrients to make hemoglobin and healthy RBCs. So it is important to get a regular supply of iron as well as vitamin B_{12}, folate, and protein. You can get these nutrients by eating a balanced diet or taking dietary supplements.

Another common cause of iron deficiency anemia is blood loss, which might arise from injury, childbirth, or surgery. Women of childbearing age are at risk for iron deficiency anemia due to blood loss from menstrual periods.

Women also need extra iron during pregnancy. Dr. Harvey Luksenburg, a specialist in blood diseases at the National Institutes of Health (NIH), says that if anemia is not treated during pregnancy, women can give birth to iron-deficient children. This lack of iron can affect a child's growth rate and brain development.

"Women who feel symptoms of sluggishness and fatigue may be iron deficient," Dr. Luksenburg says. "Even if you've lived with it a long time, get it checked. I've seen startling changes when women were put on iron supplements. Some say they've never felt better."

Many people living with anemia may not realize they have it. They might have mild symptoms or none at all. A doctor can determine whether you have anemia by a simple blood test.

Common types of anemia can be prevented and treated by eating iron-rich foods. The best sources are red meat (especially beef and liver), poultry, fish, and shellfish. Other foods high in iron include peas, lentils, beans, tofu, dark green leafy vegetables such as spinach, dried fruits such as prunes and raisins, and iron-fortified cereals and bread.

The NIH researchers are studying how to treat rarer, more severe forms of anemia. Some types can be treated with medicines. Severe cases may require blood transfusions or surgery.

If you do not get enough iron from your food, ask your doctor about taking iron dietary supplements. The body absorbs iron from meat and fish better than that from vegetables. If you are a vegetarian, consult a health-care provider to make sure you are getting enough iron.

Making healthy lifestyle choices, including a nutritious, iron-rich diet, can help prevent common types of anemia, so you can have more energy and feel your best.[1]

---

[1] *NIH News in Health*, "Avoiding Anemia—Boost Your Red Blood Cells," National Institutes of Health (NIH), January 2014. Available online. URL: https://newsinhealth.nih.gov/2014/01/avoiding-anemia. Accessed June 2, 2023.

Part 3 | **Cancer and Other Blood Disorders**

Chapter 14 | Leukemia

Chapter Contents

Section 14.1 | Leukemia: An Overview

WHAT IS LEUKEMIA?

Leukemia is a term for cancers of the blood cells. Leukemia starts in blood-forming tissues such as the bone marrow. Your bone marrow makes the cells that will develop into white blood cells (WBCs), red blood cells (RBCs), and platelets. Each type of cell has a different job:

- WBCs help your body fight infection.
- RBCs deliver oxygen from your lungs to your tissues and organs.
- Platelets help form clots to stop bleeding.

When you have leukemia, your bone marrow makes large numbers of abnormal cells. This problem most often happens with WBCs. These abnormal cells build up in your bone marrow and blood. They crowd out healthy blood cells and make it hard for your cells and blood to do their work.

WHAT ARE THE TYPES OF LEUKEMIA?

There are different types of leukemia. Which type of leukemia you have depends on the type of blood cell that becomes cancer and whether it grows quickly or slowly.

The type of blood cell could be:

- lymphocytes, a type of WBC
- myeloid cells, immature cells that become WBCs, RBCs, or platelets

The different types can grow quickly or slowly:

- Acute leukemia is fast growing. It usually gets worse quickly if it is not treated.
- Chronic leukemia is slow growing. It usually gets worse over a longer period of time.

The main types of leukemia are as follows:

- **Acute lymphocytic leukemia (ALL).** ALL is the most common type of cancer in children but can also affect adults.

- **Acute myeloid leukemia (AML).** AML is more common in older adults but can also affect children.
- **Chronic lymphocytic leukemia (CLL).** CLL is one of the most common types of leukemia in adults, often occurring during or after middle age.
- **Chronic myeloid leukemia (CML).** CML usually occurs in adults during or after middle age.

WHAT CAUSES LEUKEMIA?

Leukemia happens when there are changes in the genetic material (deoxyribonucleic acid (DNA)) in bone marrow cells. The cause of these genetic changes is unknown.

WHO IS AT RISK OF LEUKEMIA?

For the specific types, there are different factors that can raise your risk of getting that type. Overall, your risk of leukemia goes up as you age. It is most common over the age of 60.

WHAT ARE THE SYMPTOMS OF LEUKEMIA?

Some of the symptoms of leukemia may include:
- feeling tired
- fever or night sweats
- easy bruising or bleeding
- weight loss or loss of appetite
- petechiae, which are tiny red dots under the skin (which are caused by bleeding)

Other leukemia symptoms can be different from type to type. Chromic leukemia may not cause symptoms at first.

HOW IS LEUKEMIA DIAGNOSED?

Your health-care provider may use the following ways to diagnose leukemia:
- a physical exam
- a medical history

- blood tests, such as a complete blood count (CBC)
- bone marrow tests (There are two main types: bone marrow aspiration and bone marrow biopsy. Both tests involve removing a sample of bone marrow and bone. The samples are sent to a lab for testing.)
- genetic tests to look for gene and chromosome changes

Once the provider makes a diagnosis, there may be additional tests to see whether the cancer has spread. These include imaging tests and a lumbar puncture, which is a procedure to collect and test cerebrospinal fluid (CSF).

WHAT ARE THE TREATMENTS FOR LEUKEMIA?

The treatments for leukemia depend on which type you have, how severe the leukemia is, your age, your overall health, and other factors. Some possible treatments might include:

- chemotherapy
- radiation therapy
- chemotherapy with stem cell transplant
- targeted therapy, which uses drugs or other substances that attack specific cancer cells with less harm to normal cells[1]

Section 14.2 | Childhood Acute Lymphoblastic Leukemia

WHAT IS CHILDHOOD ACUTE LYMPHOBLASTIC ANEMIA?

Childhood acute lymphoblastic leukemia (also called "acute lymphocytic leukemia" (ALL)) is a cancer of the blood and bone marrow. This type of cancer usually gets worse quickly if it is not treated.

ALL is the most common type of cancer in children.

---

[1] MedlinePlus, "Leukemia," National Institutes of Health (NIH), May 30, 2021. Available online. URL: https://medlineplus.gov/leukemia.html. Accessed May 11, 2023.

LEUKEMIA AND BLOOD STEM CELLS

In a healthy child, the bone marrow makes blood stem cells (immature cells) that become mature blood cells over time. A blood stem cell may become a myeloid stem cell or a lymphoid stem cell.

- A myeloid stem cell becomes one of the three types of mature blood cells:
  - **Red blood cells (RBCs)**. RBCs carry oxygen and other substances to all tissues of the body.
  - **Platelets**. These form blood clots to stop bleeding.
  - **White blood cells (WBCs)**. WBCs fight infection and disease.
- A lymphoid stem cell becomes a lymphoblast cell and then becomes one of the three types of lymphocytes (WBCs):
  - **B lymphocytes**. These WBCs make antibodies to help fight infection.
  - **T lymphocytes**. These WBCs help B lymphocytes make the antibodies that help fight infection.
  - **Natural killer cells**. These WBCs attack cancer cells and viruses.

In a child with ALL, too many stem cells become lymphoblasts, B lymphocytes, or T lymphocytes. The cells do not work as normal lymphocytes and are not able to fight infection very well. These cells are cancer (leukemia) cells. Also, as the number of leukemia cells increases in the blood and bone marrow, there is less room for healthy WBCs, RBCs, and platelets. This may lead to infection, anemia, and easy bleeding.

RISKS OF CHILDHOOD ACUTE LYMPHOBLASTIC LEUKEMIA

Anything that increases your risk of getting a disease is called a "risk factor." Having a risk factor does not mean that you will get cancer; not having risk factors does not mean that you will not get cancer. Talk with your child's doctor if you think your child may be at risk.

Possible risk factors for ALL include the following:
- being exposed to x-rays before birth
- being exposed to radiation

- past treatment with chemotherapy
- having certain genetic conditions, such as:
  - Down syndrome
  - neurofibromatosis type 1 (NF-1)
  - Bloom syndrome (BS)
  - Fanconi anemia
  - ataxia telangiectasia (AT)
  - Li-Fraumeni syndrome (LFS)
  - constitutional mismatch repair deficiency (CMMRD; mutations in certain genes that stop deoxyribonucleic acid (DNA) from repairing itself, which leads to the growth of cancers at an early age)
- having certain changes in chromosomes or genes

SIGNS OF CHILDHOOD ACUTE LYMPHOBLASTIC LEUKEMIA

The following and other signs and symptoms may be caused by childhood ALL or by other conditions. Check with your child's doctor if your child has any of the following symptoms:

- fever
- easy bruising or bleeding
- petechiae (flat, pinpoint, dark-red spots under the skin that are caused by bleeding)
- bone or joint pain
- painless lumps in the neck, underarm, stomach, or groin
- pain or feeling of fullness below the ribs
- weakness, feeling tired, or looking pale
- loss of appetite

DIAGNOSIS OF CHILDHOOD ACUTE LYMPHOBLASTIC LEUKEMIA

The following tests and procedures may be used to diagnose childhood ALL and to find out if leukemia cells have spread to other parts of the body, such as the brain or testicles:

- **Physical exam and history**. This is an exam of the body to check general signs of health, including checking for signs of disease, such as lumps or anything else that seems unusual. A history of the patient's health habits and past illnesses and treatments will also be taken.

- **A complete blood count (CBC) with differential**. This is a procedure in which a sample of blood is drawn and checked for the following:
  - the number of RBCs and platelets
  - the number and type of WBCs
  - the amount of hemoglobin (the protein that carries oxygen) in the RBCs
  - the portion of the sample made up of RBCs
- **Blood chemistry studies**. This is a procedure in which a blood sample is checked to measure the amount of certain substances released into the blood by organs and tissues in the body. An unusual (higher or lower than normal) amount of a substance can be a sign of disease.
- **Bone marrow aspiration and biopsy**. This is the removal of bone marrow and a small piece of bone by inserting a hollow needle into the hip bone or breastbone. A pathologist views the bone marrow and bone under a microscope to look for signs of cancer.

The following tests are done on blood or the bone marrow tissue that is removed:

- **Cytogenetic analysis**. This is a laboratory test in which the cells in a sample of blood or bone marrow are viewed under a microscope to look for certain changes in the chromosomes of lymphocytes. For example, in Philadelphia chromosome–positive ALL, part of one chromosome switches places with part of another chromosome. This is called the "Philadelphia chromosome" (Ph).
- **Immunophenotyping**. This is a laboratory test in which the antigens or markers on the surface of a blood or bone marrow cell are checked to see if they are lymphocytes or myeloid cells. If the cells are malignant lymphocytes (cancer), they are checked to see if they are B lymphocytes or T lymphocytes.

- **Lumbar puncture (LP)**. This is a procedure used to collect a sample of cerebrospinal fluid (CSF) from the spinal column. This is done by placing a needle between two bones in the spine and into the CSF around the spinal cord and removing a sample of the fluid. The sample of CSF is checked under a microscope for signs that leukemia cells have spread to the brain and spinal cord. This procedure is also called an "LP" or "spinal tap." This procedure is done after leukemia is diagnosed to find out if leukemia cells have spread to the brain and spinal cord. Intrathecal chemotherapy is given after the sample of fluid is removed to treat any leukemia cells that may have spread to the brain and spinal cord.
- **Chest x-ray**. This is an x-ray of the organs and bones inside the chest. An x-ray is a type of energy beam that can go through the body and onto film, making a picture of areas inside the body. The chest x-ray is done to see if leukemia cells have formed a mass in the middle of the chest.

FACTORS AFFECTING PROGNOSIS AND TREATMENT OPTIONS

The prognosis (chance of recovery) depends on the following:
- how quickly and how low the leukemia cell count drops after the first month of treatment
- age at the time of diagnosis, sex, race, and ethnic background
- the number of WBCs in the blood at the time of diagnosis
- whether the leukemia cells began from B lymphocytes or T lymphocytes
- whether there are certain changes in the chromosomes or genes of the lymphocytes with cancer
- whether the child has Down syndrome
- whether leukemia cells are found in the CSF
- the child's weight at the time of diagnosis and during treatment

Treatment options depend on the following:
- whether the leukemia cells began from B lymphocytes or T lymphocytes
- whether the child has standard-risk, high-risk, or very high-risk ALL
- the age of the child at the time of diagnosis
- whether there are certain changes in the chromosomes of lymphocytes, such as the Ph
- whether the child was treated with steroids before the start of induction therapy
- how quickly and how low the leukemia cell count drops during treatment

For leukemia that relapses (comes back) after treatment, the prognosis and treatment options depend partly on the following:
- how long it is between the time of diagnosis and when leukemia comes back
- whether leukemia comes back in the bone marrow or in other parts of the body[2]

Section 14.3 | Adult Acute Lymphoblastic Leukemia

WHAT IS ADULT ACUTE LYMPHOBLASTIC LEUKEMIA?

Adult acute lymphoblastic leukemia (also called "acute lymphocytic leukemia" (ALL)) is a cancer of the blood and bone marrow. This type of cancer usually gets worse quickly if it is not treated.

LEUKEMIA AND BLOOD STEM CELLS

Normally, the bone marrow makes blood stem cells (immature cells) that become mature blood cells over time. A blood stem cell may become a myeloid stem cell or a lymphoid stem cell.

---

[2] "Childhood Acute Lymphoblastic Leukemia Treatment (PDQ®)—Patient Version," National Cancer Institute (NCI), September 2, 2022. Available online. URL: www.cancer.gov/types/leukemia/patient/child-all-treatment-pdq. Accessed May 31, 2023.

- A myeloid stem cell becomes one of the three types of mature blood cells:
  - **Red blood cells (RBCs)**. RBCs carry oxygen and other substances to all tissues of the body.
  - **Platelets**. These blood cells form blood clots to stop bleeding.
  - **Granulocytes (white blood cells (WBCs))**. These cells fight infection and disease.
- A lymphoid stem cell becomes a lymphoblast cell and then becomes one of the three types of lymphocytes (WBCs):
  - **B lymphocytes**. These WBCs make antibodies to help fight infection.
  - **T lymphocytes**. These WBCs help B lymphocytes make the antibodies that help fight infection.
  - **Natural killer cells**. These WBCs attack cancer cells and viruses.

In ALL, too many stem cells become lymphoblasts, B lymphocytes, or T lymphocytes. These cells are also called "leukemia cells." These leukemia cells are not able to fight infection very well. Also, as the number of leukemia cells increases in the blood and bone marrow, there is less room for healthy WBCs, RBCs, and platelets. This may cause infection, anemia, and easy bleeding. The cancer can also spread to the central nervous system (brain and spinal cord).

RISKS OF DEVELOPING ACUTE LYMPHOBLASTIC LEUKEMIA

Anything that increases your risk of getting a disease is called a "risk factor." Having a risk factor does not mean that you will get cancer; not having risk factors does not mean that you will not get cancer. Talk with your doctor if you think you may be at risk. Possible risk factors for ALL include the following:

- being male
- being White
- being older than 70 years of age
- having had past treatment with chemotherapy or radiation therapy

- being exposed to high levels of radiation in the environment (such as nuclear radiation)
- having certain genetic disorders, such as Down syndrome

SIGNS AND SYMPTOMS OF ADULT ACUTE LYMPHOBLASTIC LEUKEMIA

The early signs and symptoms of adult ALL may be similar to the flu or other common diseases. Check with your doctor if you have any of the following:

- weakness or feeling tired
- fever or night sweats
- easy bruising or bleeding
- petechiae (flat, pinpoint spots under the skin caused by bleeding)
- shortness of breath
- weight loss or loss of appetite
- pain in the bones or stomach
- pain or feeling of fullness below the ribs
- painless lumps in the neck, underarm, stomach, or groin
- having many infections

The abovementioned and other signs and symptoms may be caused by adult ALL or by other conditions.

DIAGNOSIS OF ADULT ACUTE LYMPHOBLASTIC LEUKEMIA

The following tests and procedures may be used:

- **Physical exam and history**. This is an exam of the body to check general signs of health, including checking for signs of disease, such as infection or anything else that seems unusual. A history of the patient's health habits and past illnesses and treatments will also be taken.
- **A complete blood count (CBC) with differential**. This is a procedure in which a sample of blood is drawn and checked for the following:
  - the number of RBCs and platelets
  - the number and type of WBCs

- the amount of hemoglobin (the protein that carries oxygen) in the RBCs
- the portion of the blood sample made up of RBCs
- **Blood chemistry studies**. This is a procedure in which a blood sample is checked to measure the amount of certain substances released into the blood by organs and tissues in the body. An unusual (higher or lower than normal) amount of a substance can be a sign of disease.
- **Peripheral blood smear**. This is a procedure in which a sample of blood is checked for blast cells, the number and kinds of WBCs, the number of platelets, and changes in the shape of blood cells.
- **Bone marrow aspiration and biopsy**. This is the removal of bone marrow, blood, and a small piece of bone by inserting a hollow needle into the hip bone or breastbone. A pathologist views the bone marrow, blood, and bone under a microscope to look for abnormal cells.

The following tests may be done on the samples of blood or bone marrow tissue that are removed:

- **Cytogenetic analysis**. This is a laboratory test in which the cells in a sample of blood or bone marrow are looked at under a microscope to find out if there are certain changes in the chromosomes of lymphocytes. For example, in Philadelphia chromosome–positive ALL, part of one chromosome switches places with part of another chromosome. This is called the "Philadelphia chromosome" (Ph).
- **Immunophenotyping**. This is a process used to identify cells based on the types of antigens or markers on the surface of the cell. This process is used to diagnose the subtype of ALL by comparing the cancer cells to normal cells of the immune system. For example, a cytochemistry study may test the cells in a sample of tissue using chemicals (dyes) to look for

certain changes in the sample. A chemical may cause a color change in one type of leukemia cell but not in another type of leukemia cell.

FACTORS AFFECTING PROGNOSIS AND TREATMENT OPTIONS

The prognosis (chance of recovery) and treatment options depend on the following:

- the age of the patient
- whether the cancer has spread to the brain or spinal cord
- whether there are certain changes in the genes, including the Ph
- whether the cancer has been treated before or has recurred (come back)[3]

Section 14.4 | Childhood Acute Myeloid Leukemia

WHAT IS CHILDHOOD ACUTE MYELOID LEUKEMIA?

Childhood acute myeloid leukemia (AML) is a cancer of the blood and bone marrow. AML is also called "acute myelogenous leukemia," "acute myeloblastic leukemia," "acute granulocytic leukemia," and "acute nonlymphocytic leukemia." Cancers that are acute usually get worse quickly if they are not treated. Cancers that are chronic usually get worse slowly.

LEUKEMIA AND BLOOD STEM CELLS

Normally, the bone marrow makes blood stem cells (immature cells) that become mature blood cells over time. A blood stem cell may become a myeloid stem cell or a lymphoid stem cell.

---

[3] "Adult Acute Lymphoblastic Leukemia Treatment (PDQ®)—Patient Version," National Cancer Institute (NCI), November 19, 2021. Available online. URL: www.cancer.gov/types/leukemia/patient/adult-all-treatment-pdq#_1. Accessed June 2, 2023.

- A myeloid stem cell becomes one of the three types of mature blood cells:
  - **Red blood cells (RBCs)**. RBCs carry oxygen and other substances to all tissues of the body.
  - **White blood cells (WBCs)**. WBCs fight infection and disease.
  - **Platelets**. These form blood clots to stop bleeding.
- A lymphoid stem cell becomes a white blood cell (WBC).

In AML, the myeloid stem cells usually become a type of immature WBC called "myeloblasts" (or myeloid blasts). The myeloblasts, or leukemia cells, in AML are abnormal and do not become healthy WBCs. The leukemia cells can build up in the blood and bone marrow, so there is less room for healthy WBCs, RBCs, and platelets. When this happens, infection, anemia, or easy bleeding may occur.

The leukemia cells can spread outside the blood to other parts of the body, including the central nervous system (brain and spinal cord), skin, and gums. Sometimes, leukemia cells form a solid tumor called a "granulocytic sarcoma" (GS) or "chloroma."

RISK FACTORS FOR CHILDHOOD ACUTE MYELOID LEUKEMIA

Anything that increases your risk of getting a disease is called a "risk factor." Having a risk factor does not mean that you will get cancer; not having risk factors does not mean that you will not get cancer. Talk with your child's doctor if you think your child may be at risk. The following and other factors may increase the risk of childhood AML, acute promyelocytic leukemia (APL), juvenile myelomonocytic leukemia (JMML), chronic myelogenous leukemia (CML), and myelodysplastic syndrome (MDS):

- having a sister or brother, especially a twin, with leukemia
- being Hispanic
- being exposed to cigarette smoke or alcohol before birth
- having a personal history of aplastic anemia
- having a personal or family history of MDS
- having a family history of AML
- past treatment with chemotherapy or radiation therapy

- being exposed to ionizing radiation or chemicals such as benzene
- having certain syndromes or inherited disorders, such as:
  - Down syndrome
  - aplastic anemia
  - Fanconi anemia
  - neurofibromatosis type 1 (NF-1)
  - Noonan syndrome (NS)
  - Shwachman-Diamond syndrome (SDS)
  - Li-Fraumeni syndrome (LFS)

SIGNS AND SYMPTOMS OF CHILDHOOD ACUTE MYELOID LEUKEMIA

The following and other signs and symptoms may be caused by childhood AML, APL, JMML, CML, MDS, or other conditions. Check with a doctor if your child has any of the following symptoms:

- fever with or without an infection
- night sweats
- shortness of breath
- weakness or feeling tired
- easy bruising or bleeding
- petechiae (flat, pinpoint spots under the skin that is caused by bleeding)
- pain in the bones or joints
- pain or feeling of fullness below the ribs
- painless lumps in the neck, underarm, stomach, groin, or other parts of the body (In childhood AML, these lumps, called "leukemia cutis" (LC), may be blue or purple.)
- painless lumps that are sometimes around the eyes (These lumps, called "chloromas," are sometimes seen in childhood AML and may be blue-green.)
- an eczema-like skin rash

The signs and symptoms of transient abnormal myelopoiesis (TAM) may include the following:

- swelling all over the body
- shortness of breath

- trouble breathing
- weakness or feeling tired
- bleeding a lot, even from a small cut
- petechiae
- pain below the ribs
- skin rash
- jaundice (yellowing of the skin and whites of the eyes)
- headache, trouble seeing, and confusion

Sometimes, TAM does not cause any symptoms at all and is diagnosed after a routine blood test.

DIAGNOSIS OF CHILDHOOD ACUTE MYELOID LEUKEMIA

The following tests and procedures may be used:

- **Physical exam and history**. This is an exam of the body to check general signs of health, including checking for signs of disease, such as lumps or anything else that seems unusual. A history of the patient's health habits and past illnesses and treatments will also be taken.
- **A complete blood count (CBC) with differential**. This is a procedure in which a sample of blood is drawn and checked for the following:
  - the number of RBCs and platelets
  - the number and type of WBCs
  - the amount of hemoglobin (the protein that carries oxygen) in the RBCs
  - the portion of the blood sample made up of RBCs
- **Blood chemistry studies**. This is a procedure in which a blood sample is checked to measure the amount of certain substances released into the blood by organs and tissues in the body. An unusual (higher or lower than normal) amount of a substance can be a sign of disease.
- **Chest x-ray**. This is an x-ray of the organs and bones inside the chest. An x-ray is a type of energy beam that can go through the body and onto film, making a picture of areas inside the body.

- **Biopsy**. This is the removal of cells or tissues so that they can be viewed under a microscope by a pathologist to check for signs of cancer. Biopsies that may be done include the following:
    - **Bone marrow aspiration and biopsy**. This is the removal of bone marrow, blood, and a small piece of bone by inserting a hollow needle into the hip bone or breastbone.
    - **Tumor biopsy**. A biopsy of a chloroma may be done.
    - **Lymph node biopsy**. This is the removal of all or part of a lymph node.
- **Immunophenotyping**. This is a process used to identify cells, based on the types of antigens or markers on the surface of the cell, that may include special staining of the blood and bone marrow cells. This process is used to diagnose the subtype of AML by comparing the cancer cells to normal cells of the immune system.
- **Cytogenetic analysis**. This is a laboratory test in which cells in a sample of blood or bone marrow are viewed under a microscope to look for certain changes in the chromosomes. Changes in the chromosomes include when part of one chromosome is switched with part of another chromosome, part of one chromosome is missing or repeated, or part of one chromosome is turned upside down. The following test is a type of cytogenetic analysis:
    - **Fluorescence in situ hybridization (FISH)**. This is a laboratory technique used to look at genes or chromosomes in cells and tissues. Pieces of deoxyribonucleic acid (DNA) that contain a fluorescent dye are made in the laboratory and added to cells or tissues on a glass slide. When these pieces of DNA bind to specific genes or areas of chromosomes on the slide, they light up when viewed under a microscope with a special light.

- **Molecular testing**. This is a laboratory test to check for certain genes, proteins, or other molecules in a sample of blood or bone marrow. Molecular tests also check for certain changes in a gene or chromosome that may cause or affect the chance of developing AML. A molecular test may be used to help plan treatment, find out how well treatment is working, or make a prognosis.
- **Lumbar puncture (LP)**. This is a procedure used to collect a sample of cerebrospinal fluid (CSF) from the spinal column. This is done by placing a needle between two bones in the spine and into the CSF around the spinal cord and removing a sample of the fluid. The sample of CSF is checked under a microscope for signs that leukemia cells have spread to the brain and spinal cord. This procedure is also called an "LP" or "spinal tap."

FACTORS AFFECTING PROGNOSIS AND TREATMENT OPTIONS OF CHILDHOOD ACUTE MYELOID LEUKEMIA

The prognosis (chance of recovery) and treatment options for childhood AML depend on the following:

- the age of the child when the cancer is diagnosed
- the race or ethnic group of the child
- whether the child is greatly overweight
- the number of WBCs in the blood at diagnosis
- whether AML occurred after previous cancer treatment
- the subtype of AML
- whether there are certain chromosome or gene changes in the leukemia cells
- whether the child has Down syndrome (Most children with AML and Down syndrome can be cured of their leukemia.)
- whether the leukemia is in the central nervous system (brain and spinal cord)
- how quickly leukemia responds to treatment

- whether the AML is newly diagnosed (untreated) or has recurred after treatment
- the length of time since treatment ended for AML that has recurred

The prognosis for childhood APL depends on the following:
- the number of WBCs in the blood at diagnosis
- whether there are certain chromosome or gene changes in the leukemia cells
- whether APL is newly diagnosed or has recurred after treatment

The prognosis and treatment options for JMML depend on the following:
- the age of the child when the cancer is diagnosed
- the type of gene affected and the number of genes that have changed
- how many monocytes (a type of WBC) are in the blood
- how much hemoglobin is in the blood
- whether the JMML is newly diagnosed or has recurred after treatment

The prognosis and treatment options for childhood CML depend on the following:
- how long it has been since the patient was diagnosed
- how many blast cells are in the blood
- whether and how fully the blast cells disappear from the blood and bone marrow after therapy has started
- whether the CML is newly diagnosed or has recurred after treatment

The prognosis and treatment options for MDS depend on the following:
- whether the MDS was caused by the previous cancer treatment
- how low the numbers of RBCs, WBCs, or platelets are
- whether the MDS is newly diagnosed or has recurred after treatment

RECURRING ACUTE MYELOID LEUKEMIA OR MYELODYSPLASTIC SYNDROME

Cancer treatment with certain chemotherapy drugs and/or radiation therapy may cause therapy-related AML (t-AML) or therapy-related MDS (t-MDS). The risk of these therapy-related myeloid diseases depends on the total dose of the chemotherapy drugs used and the radiation dose and treatment field. Some patients also have inherited risk of t-AML and t-MDS. These therapy-related diseases usually occur within seven years after treatment, but they are rare in children.[4]

Section 14.5 | Adult Acute Myeloid Leukemia

WHAT IS ADULT ACUTE MYELOID LEUKEMIA?

Adult acute myeloid leukemia (AML) is a cancer of the blood and bone marrow. This type of cancer usually gets worse quickly if it is not treated. It is the most common type of acute leukemia in adults. AML is also called "acute myelogenous leukemia," "acute myeloblastic leukemia," "acute granulocytic leukemia," and "acute nonlymphocytic leukemia."

LEUKEMIA AND BLOOD STEM CELLS

Normally, the bone marrow makes blood stem cells (immature cells) that become mature blood cells over time. A blood stem cell may become a myeloid stem cell or a lymphoid stem cell.

- A myeloid stem cell becomes one of the three types of mature blood cells:
  - **Red blood cells (RBCs)**. RBCs carry oxygen and other substances to all tissues of the body.

---

[4] "Childhood Acute Myeloid Leukemia/Other Myeloid Malignancies Treatment (PDQ®)—Patient Version," National Cancer Institute (NCI), March 4, 2022. Available online. URL: www.cancer.gov/types/leukemia/patient/child-aml-treatment-pdq. Accessed June 2, 2023.

- **WBCs**. These cells fight infection and disease.
- **Platelets**. These form blood clots to stop bleeding.
- A lymphoid stem cell becomes a white blood cell (WBC).

In AML, the myeloid stem cells usually become a type of immature WBC called "myeloblasts" (or myeloid blasts). The myeloblasts in AML are abnormal and do not become healthy WBCs.
Sometimes, in AML, too many stem cells become abnormal RBCs
or platelets. These abnormal WBCs, RBCs, or platelets are also
called "leukemia cells" or "blasts." Leukemia cells can build up
in the bone marrow and blood, so there is less room for healthy
WBCs, RBCs, and platelets. When this happens, infection, anemia,
or easy bleeding may occur. The leukemia cells can spread outside
the blood to other parts of the body, including the central nervous
system (brain and spinal cord), skin, and gums.

SUBTYPES OF ACUTE MYELOID LEUKEMIA
Most AML subtypes are based on how mature (developed) the
cancer cells are at the time of diagnosis and how different they are
from normal cells.
  Acute promyelocytic leukemia (APL) is a subtype of AML that
occurs when parts of two genes stick together. APL usually occurs
in middle-aged adults. Signs of APL may include both bleeding
and forming blood clots.

RISKS OF ADULT ACUTE MYELOID LEUKEMIA
Anything that increases your risk of getting a disease is called a
"risk factor." Having a risk factor does not mean that you will get
cancer; not having risk factors does not mean that you will not
get cancer. Talk with your doctor if you think you may be at risk.
Possible risk factors for AML include the following:
- being male
- smoking, especially after the age of 60
- having had treatment with chemotherapy or radiation
  therapy in the past
- having had treatment for childhood acute
  lymphoblastic leukemia (ALL) in the past

- being exposed to radiation from an atomic bomb or to the chemical benzene
- having a history of a blood disorder, such as myelodysplastic syndrome

SIGNS AND SYMPTOMS OF ADULT ACUTE MYELOID LEUKEMIA

The early signs and symptoms of adult AML may be similar to those caused by the flu or other common diseases. Check with your doctor if you have any of the following:

- fever
- shortness of breath
- easy bruising or bleeding
- petechiae (flat, pinpoint spots under the skin that are caused by bleeding)
- weakness or feeling tired
- weight loss or loss of appetite

DIAGNOSIS OF ADULT ACUTE MYELOID LEUKEMIA

The following tests and procedures may be used:

- **Physical exam and history**. This is an exam of the body to check general signs of health, including checking for signs of disease, such as lumps or anything else that seems unusual. A history of the patient's health habits and past illnesses and treatments will also be taken.
- **A complete blood count (CBC)**. This is a procedure in which a sample of blood is drawn and checked for the following:
  - the number of RBCs, WBCs, and platelets
  - the amount of hemoglobin (the protein that carries oxygen) in the RBCs
  - the portion of the sample made up of RBCs
- **Peripheral blood smear**. This is a procedure in which a sample of blood is checked for blast cells, the number and kinds of WBCs, the number of platelets, and changes in the shape of blood cells.

- **Bone marrow aspiration and biopsy**. This is the removal of bone marrow, blood, and a small piece of bone by inserting a hollow needle into the hip bone or breastbone. A pathologist views the bone marrow, blood, and bone under a microscope to look for signs of cancer.
- **Cytogenetic analysis**. This is a laboratory test in which the cells in a sample of blood or bone marrow are viewed under a microscope to look for certain changes in the chromosomes. Other tests, such as fluorescence in situ hybridization (FISH), may also be done to look for certain changes in the chromosomes.
- **Immunophenotyping**. This is a process used to identify cells based on the types of antigens or markers on the surface of the cell. This process is used to diagnose the subtype of AML by comparing the cancer cells to normal cells of the immune system. For example, a cytochemistry study may test the cells in a sample of tissue using chemicals (dyes) to look for certain changes in the sample. A chemical may cause a color change in one type of leukemia cell but not in another type of leukemia cell.
- **Reverse transcription-polymerase chain reaction (RT-PCR) test**. A laboratory test in which cells in a sample of tissue are studied using chemicals to look for certain changes in the structure or function of genes. This test is used to diagnose certain types of AML, including APL.

FACTORS AFFECTING PROGNOSIS AND TREATMENT OPTIONS OF ADULT ACUTE MYELOID LEUKEMIA

The prognosis (chance of recovery) and treatment options depend on the following:
- the age of the patient
- the subtype of AML
- whether the patient received chemotherapy in the past to treat a different cancer

- whether there is a history of a blood disorder, such as myelodysplastic syndrome
- whether the cancer has spread to the central nervous system
- whether the cancer has been treated before or recurred (come back)

It is important that acute leukemia be treated right away.[5]

Section 14.6 | Chronic Lymphocytic Leukemia

WHAT IS CHRONIC LYMPHOCYTIC LEUKEMIA?

Chronic lymphocytic leukemia (CLL) is a blood and bone marrow disease that usually gets worse slowly. CLL is one of the most common types of leukemia in adults. It often occurs during or after middle age; it rarely occurs in children.

LEUKEMIA AND BLOOD STEM CELLS

Normally, the body makes blood stem cells (immature cells) that become mature blood cells over time. A blood stem cell may become a myeloid stem cell or a lymphoid stem cell.

- A myeloid stem cell becomes one of the three types of mature blood cells:
  - **Red blood cells (RBCs)**. RBCs carry oxygen and other substances to all tissues of the body.
  - **White blood cells (WBCs)**. WBCs fight infection and disease.
  - **Platelets**. These form blood clots to stop bleeding.

---

[5] "Adult Acute Myeloid Leukemia Treatment (PDQ®)—Patient Version," National Cancer Institute (NCI), August 19, 2022. Available online. URL: www.cancer.gov/types/leukemia/patient/adult-aml-treatment-pdq. Accessed June 2, 2023.

- A lymphoid stem cell becomes a lymphoblast cell and then one of the three types of lymphocytes (WBCs):
  - **B lymphocytes**. These WBCs make antibodies to help fight infection.
  - **T lymphocytes**. These WBCs help B lymphocytes make the antibodies that help fight infection.
  - **Natural killer cells**. These WBCs attack cancer cells and viruses.

In CLL, too many blood stem cells become abnormal lymphocytes and do not become healthy WBCs. The abnormal lymphocytes may also be called "leukemia cells." The lymphocytes are not able to fight infection very well. Also, as the number of lymphocytes increases in the blood and bone marrow, there is less room for healthy WBCs, RBCs, and platelets. This may cause infection, anemia, and easy bleeding.

RISKS OF CHRONIC LYMPHOCYTIC LEUKEMIA

Anything that increases your risk of getting a disease is called a "risk factor." Having a risk factor does not mean that you will get cancer; not having risk factors does not mean that you will not get cancer. Talk with your doctor if you think you may be at risk. Risk factors for CLL include the following:

- being middle-aged or older, male, or White
- a family history of CLL or cancer of the lymph system
- having relatives who are Russian Jews or Eastern European Jews

SIGNS AND SYMPTOMS OF CHRONIC LYMPHOCYTIC LEUKEMIA

Usually, CLL does not cause any signs or symptoms and is found during a routine blood test. Signs and symptoms may be caused by CLL or by other conditions. Check with your doctor if you have any of the following symptoms:

- painless swelling of the lymph nodes in the neck, underarm, stomach, or groin
- feeling very tired
- pain or fullness below the ribs

- fever and infection
- weight loss for no known reason

DIAGNOSIS OF CHRONIC LYMPHOCYTIC LEUKEMIA

The following tests and procedures may be used:

- **Physical exam and history**. This is an exam of the body to check general signs of health, including checking for signs of disease, such as lumps or anything else that seems unusual. A history of the patient's health habits and past illnesses and treatments will also be taken.
- **A complete blood count (CBC) with differential**. This is a procedure in which a sample of blood is drawn and checked for the following:
  - the number of RBCs and platelets
  - the number and type of WBCs
  - the amount of hemoglobin (the protein that carries oxygen) in the RBCs
  - the portion of the blood sample made up of RBCs
- **Immunophenotyping**. This is a laboratory test in which the antigens or markers on the surface of a blood or bone marrow cell are checked to see if they are lymphocytes or myeloid cells. If the cells are malignant lymphocytes (cancer), they are checked to see if they are B lymphocytes or T lymphocytes.
- **Fluorescence in situ hybridization (FISH)**. This is a laboratory technique used to look at genes or chromosomes in cells and tissues. Pieces of deoxyribonucleic acid (DNA) that contain a fluorescent dye are made in the laboratory and added to cells or tissues on a glass slide. When these pieces of DNA bind to specific genes or areas of chromosomes on the slide, they light up when viewed under a microscope with a special light.
- **Flow cytometry**. This is a laboratory test that measures the number of cells in a sample, the percentage of live cells in a sample, and certain characteristics of cells, such as size, shape, and presence of tumor markers

on the cell surface. The cells are stained with a light-sensitive dye, placed in a fluid, and passed in a stream before a laser or other type of light. The measurements are based on how the light-sensitive dye reacts to the light.

- *IgVH* **gene mutation test**. This is a laboratory test done on a bone marrow or blood sample to check for an *IgVH* gene mutation. Patients with an *IgVH* gene mutation have a better prognosis.
- **Bone marrow aspiration and biopsy**. This is the removal of bone marrow, blood, and a small piece of bone by inserting a hollow needle into the hip bone or breastbone. A pathologist views the bone marrow, blood, and bone under a microscope to look for abnormal cells.

FACTORS AFFECTING TREATMENT OPTIONS AND PROGNOSIS OF CHRONIC LYMPHOCYTIC LEUKEMIA

Treatment options depend on the following:

- the stage of the disease
- RBC, WBC, and platelet blood counts
- whether there are signs or symptoms, such as fever, chills, or weight loss
- whether the liver, spleen, or lymph nodes are larger than normal
- the response to initial treatment
- whether CLL has recurred (come back)

The prognosis (chance of recovery) depends on the following:

- whether there is a change in the DNA and the type of change, if there is one
- whether lymphocytes are spread throughout the bone marrow
- the stage of the disease
- whether the CLL gets better with treatment or has recurred

- whether the CLL progresses to lymphoma or prolymphocytic leukemia
- the patient's age and general health[6]

Section 14.7 | Chronic Myelogenous Leukemia

WHAT IS CHRONIC MYELOGENOUS LEUKEMIA?

Chronic myelogenous leukemia (CML; also called "chronic granulocytic leukemia") is a slowly progressing blood and bone marrow disease that usually occurs during or after middle age and rarely occurs in children.

LEUKEMIA AND BLOOD STEM CELLS

Normally, the bone marrow makes blood stem cells (immature cells) that become mature blood cells over time. A blood stem cell may become a myeloid stem cell or a lymphoid stem cell.

- A myeloid stem cell becomes one of the three types of mature blood cells:
  - **Red blood cells (RBCs)**. RBCs carry oxygen and other substances to all tissues of the body.
  - **Platelets**. These blood cells form blood clots to stop bleeding.
  - **Granulocytes (white blood cells (WBCs))**. These cells fight infection and disease.
- A lymphoid stem cell becomes a white blood cell (WBC).

In CML, too many blood stem cells become a type of WBC called "granulocytes." These granulocytes are abnormal and do not become healthy WBCs. They are also called "leukemia cells." The leukemia cells can build up in the blood and bone marrow, so there is less room for healthy WBCs, RBCs, and platelets. When this happens, infection, anemia, or easy bleeding may occur.

---

[6] "Chronic Lymphocytic Leukemia Treatment (PDQ®)—Patient Version," National Cancer Institute (NCI), August 26, 2022. Available online. URL: www.cancer.gov/types/leukemia/patient/cll-treatment-pdq. Accessed June 2, 2023.

CHRONIC MYELOGENOUS LEUKEMIA AND GENE MUTATION

Every cell in the body contains deoxyribonucleic acid (DNA; genetic material) that determines how the cell looks and acts. DNA is contained inside chromosomes. In CML, part of the DNA from one chromosome moves to another chromosome. This change is called the "Philadelphia chromosome" (Ph). It results in the bone marrow making a protein called "tyrosine kinase" that causes too many stem cells to become WBCs (granulocytes or blasts).

The Ph is not passed from the parent to the child.

SIGNS AND SYMPTOMS OF CHRONIC MYELOGENOUS LEUKEMIA

The following and other signs and symptoms may be caused by CML or by other conditions. Check with your doctor if you have any of the following symptoms:

- feeling very tired
- weight loss for no known reason
- night sweats
- fever
- pain or a feeling of fullness below the ribs on the left side

Sometimes, CML does not cause any symptoms at all.

DIAGNOSIS OF CHRONIC MYELOGENOUS LEUKEMIA

The following tests and procedures may be used:

- **Physical exam and history**. This is an exam of the body to check general signs of health, including checking for signs of disease, such as an enlarged spleen. A history of the patient's health habits and past illnesses and treatments will also be taken.
- **A complete blood count (CBC) with differential**. This is a procedure in which a sample of blood is drawn and checked for the following:
  - the number of RBCs and platelets
  - the number and type of WBCs
  - the amount of hemoglobin (the protein that carries oxygen) in the RBCs
  - the portion of the blood sample made up of RBCs

- **Blood chemistry studies.** This is a procedure in which a blood sample is checked to measure the amount of certain substances released into the blood by organs and tissues in the body. An unusual (higher or lower than normal) amount of a substance can be a sign of disease.
- **Bone marrow aspiration and biopsy.** This is the removal of bone marrow, blood, and a small piece of bone by inserting a needle into the hip bone or breastbone. A pathologist views the bone marrow, blood, and bone under a microscope to look for abnormal cells.

One of the following tests may be done on the samples of blood or bone marrow tissue that are removed:

- **Cytogenetic analysis.** This is a test in which cells in a sample of blood or bone marrow are viewed under a microscope to look for certain changes in the chromosomes, such as the Ph.
- **Fluorescence in situ hybridization (FISH).** This is a laboratory technique used to look at genes or chromosomes in cells and tissues. Pieces of DNA that contain a fluorescent dye are made in the laboratory and added to cells or tissues on a glass slide. When these pieces of DNA bind to specific genes or areas of chromosomes on the slide, they light up when viewed under a microscope with a special light.
- **Reverse transcription-polymerase chain reaction (RT-PCR).** This is a laboratory test in which cells in a sample of tissue are studied using chemicals to look for certain changes in the structure or function of genes.

FACTORS AFFECTING PROGNOSIS AND TREATMENT OPTIONS OF CHRONIC MYELOGENOUS LEUKEMIA

The prognosis (chance of recovery) and treatment options depend on the following:

- the patient's age
- the phase of CML

- the amount of blasts in the blood or bone marrow
- the size of the spleen at diagnosis
- the patient's general health[7]

Section 14.8 | Hairy Cell Leukemia

WHAT IS HAIRY CELL LEUKEMIA?

Hairy cell leukemia is a cancer of the blood and bone marrow. This rare type of leukemia gets worse slowly or does not get worse at all. The disease is called "hairy cell leukemia" because the leukemia cells look "hairy" when viewed under a microscope.

LEUKEMIA AND BLOOD STEM CELLS

Normally, the bone marrow makes blood stem cells (immature cells) that become mature blood cells over time. A blood stem cell may become a myeloid stem cell or a lymphoid stem cell.

- A myeloid stem cell becomes one of the three types of mature blood cells:
  - **Red blood cells (RBCs).** RBCs carry oxygen and other substances to all tissues of the body.
  - **White blood cells (WBCs).** WBCs fight infection and disease.
  - **Platelets.** These form blood clots to stop bleeding.
- A lymphoid stem cell becomes a lymphoblast cell and then turns into one of the three types of lymphocytes (WBCs):
  - **B lymphocytes.** These WBCs make antibodies to help fight infection.
  - **T lymphocytes.** These WBCs help B lymphocytes make the antibodies that help fight infection.
  - **Natural killer cells.** These WBCs attack cancer cells and viruses.

[7] "Chronic Myelogenous Leukemia Treatment (PDQ®)—Patient Version," National Cancer Institute (NCI), March 25, 2022. Available online. URL: www.cancer.gov/types/leukemia/patient/cml-treatment-pdq. Accessed June 6, 2023.

In hairy cell leukemia, too many blood stem cells become lymphocytes. These lymphocytes are abnormal and do not become healthy WBCs. They are also called "leukemia cells." The leukemia cells can build up in the blood and bone marrow, so there is less room for healthy WBCs, RBCs, and platelets. This may cause infection, anemia, and easy bleeding. Some of the leukemia cells may collect in the spleen and cause it to swell.

RISKS OF HAIRY CELL LEUKEMIA

Anything that increases your chance of getting a disease is called a "risk factor." Having a risk factor does not mean that you will get cancer; not having risk factors does not mean that you will not get cancer. Talk with your doctor if you think you may be at risk. The cause of hairy cell leukemia is unknown. It occurs more often in older men.

SIGNS AND SYMPTOMS OF HAIRY CELL LEUKEMIA

The following and other signs and symptoms may be caused by hairy cell leukemia or by other conditions. Check with your doctor if you have any of the following symptoms:
- weakness or feeling tired
- fever or frequent infections
- easy bruising or bleeding
- shortness of breath
- weight loss for no known reason
- pain or a feeling of fullness below the ribs
- painless lumps in the neck, underarm, stomach, or groin

DIAGNOSIS OF HAIRY CELL LEUKEMIA

The following tests and procedures may be used:
- **Physical exam and history**. This is an exam of the body to check general signs of health, including checking for signs of disease, such as a swollen spleen, lumps, or anything else that seems unusual. A history of the patient's health habits and past illnesses and treatments will also be taken.

- **A complete blood count (CBC).** This is a procedure in which a sample of blood is drawn and checked for the following:
  - the number of RBCs, WBCs, and platelets
  - the amount of hemoglobin (the protein that carries oxygen) in the RBCs
  - the portion of the sample made up of RBCs
- **Peripheral blood smear.** This is a procedure in which a sample of blood is checked for cells that look "hairy," the number and kinds of WBCs, the number of platelets, and changes in the shape of blood cells.
- **Blood chemistry studies.** This is a procedure in which a blood sample is checked to measure the amount of certain substances released into the blood by organs and tissues in the body. An unusual (higher or lower than normal) amount of a substance can be a sign of disease.
- **Bone marrow aspiration and biopsy.** This is the removal of bone marrow, blood, and a small piece of bone by inserting a hollow needle into the hip bone or breastbone. A pathologist views the bone marrow, blood, and bone under a microscope to look for signs of cancer.
- **Immunophenotyping.** This is a laboratory test in which the antigens or markers on the surface of a blood or bone marrow cell are checked to see what type of cell it is. This test is done to diagnose the specific type of leukemia by comparing the cancer cells to normal cells of the immune system.
- **Flow cytometry.** This is a laboratory test that measures the number of cells in a sample, the percentage of live cells in a sample, and certain characteristics of cells, such as size, shape, and presence of tumor markers on the cell surface. The cells are stained with a light-sensitive dye, placed in a fluid, and passed in a stream before a laser or

other type of light. The measurements are based on how the light-sensitive dye reacts to the light.

- **Cytogenetic analysis**. This is a laboratory test in which cells in a sample of tissue are viewed under a microscope to look for certain changes in the chromosomes.
- **Gene mutation test**. This is a laboratory test done on a bone marrow or blood sample to check for mutations in the *BRAF* gene. A *BRAF* gene mutation is often found in patients with hairy cell leukemia.
- **Computed tomography (CT) scan**. This is a procedure that makes a series of detailed pictures of areas inside the body, taken from different angles. The pictures are made by a computer linked to an x-ray machine. A dye may be injected into a vein or swallowed to help the organs or tissues show up more clearly. This procedure is also called "computerized tomography" or "computerized axial tomography" (CAT). A CT scan of the abdomen may be done to check for swollen lymph nodes or a swollen spleen.

FACTORS AFFECTING TREATMENT OPTIONS AND PROGNOSIS

The treatment options may depend on the following:
- the number of hairy (leukemia) cells and healthy blood cells in the blood and bone marrow
- whether the spleen is swollen
- whether there are signs or symptoms of leukemia, such as infection
- whether the leukemia has recurred (come back) after previous treatment

The prognosis (chance of recovery) depends on the following:
- whether the hairy cell leukemia does not grow or grows so slowly that it does not need treatment
- whether the hairy cell leukemia responds to treatment

Treatment often results in a long-lasting remission (a period during which some or all of the signs and symptoms of the leukemia are gone). If the leukemia returns after it has been in remission, retreatment often causes another remission.[8]

[8] "Hairy Cell Leukemia Treatment (PDQ®)—Patient Version," National Cancer Institute (NCI), April 8, 2022. Available online. URL: www.cancer.gov/types/leukemia/patient/hairy-cell-treatment-pdq. Accessed June 6, 2023.

Chapter 15 | Lymphoma

Chapter Contents

Section 15.1 | Lymphoma: An Overview

WHAT IS LYMPHOMA?

"Lymphoma" is a general term for cancers that start in the lymph system (the tissues and organs that produce, store, and carry white blood cells (WBCs) that fight infections). The two main kinds of lymphoma are as follows:

- **Hodgkin lymphoma (HL).** HL spreads in an orderly manner from one group of lymph nodes to another.
- **Non-Hodgkin lymphoma (NHL).** NHL spreads through the lymphatic system in a nonorderly manner.

HL and NHL can occur in children, teens, and adults.

WHAT CAUSES LYMPHOMA?

Non-Hodgkin lymphoma becomes more common as people get older. Unlike most cancers, rates of HL are highest among teens and young adults (individuals between the ages of 15 and 39) and again among older adults (individuals aged 75 or older). White people are more likely than Black people to develop NHL, and men are more likely than women to develop lymphoma.

Scientists do not fully understand all of the causes of lymphoma, but research has found many links. The following are a few examples:

- Research has shown that people who are infected with human immunodeficiency virus (HIV) are at a much higher risk of developing lymphoma.
- Other viruses, such as the human T-cell lymphotropic virus and Epstein-Barr virus (EBV), have also been linked with certain kinds of lymphoma.
- People exposed to high levels of ionizing radiation have a higher risk of developing NHL.
- Family history has been linked with a higher risk of HL.
- Some studies suggest that specific ingredients in herbicides and pesticides may be linked with lymphoma, but scientists do not know how much is needed to raise the risk of developing lymphoma.

SYMPTOMS OF LYMPHOMA

Symptoms of HL and NHL include swollen lymph nodes, especially in the part of the body where the lymphoma starts to grow. Other symptoms include fever, night sweats, feeling tired, and weight loss.

These symptoms can also come from other conditions. If you have any of them, talk to your doctor.[1]

Section 15.2 | Childhood Hodgkin Lymphoma

Hodgkin lymphoma (HL) most often occurs in adolescents aged 15–19. The treatment for children and adolescents is different from the treatment for adults.

TYPES OF CHILDHOOD HODGKIN LYMPHOMA

- **Classic HL.** This is the most common type of HL. It most often occurs in adolescents. When a sample of lymph node tissue is looked at under a microscope, HL cancer cells, called "Reed-Sternberg cells," may be seen. Classic HL is divided into the following four subtypes based on how the cancer cells look under a microscope:
  - **Nodular-sclerosing HL.** This most often occurs in older children and adolescents. It is common to have a chest mass at diagnosis.
  - **Mixed cellularity HL.** This most often occurs in children younger than 10 years of age. It is linked to a history of Epstein-Barr virus (EBV) infection and often occurs in the lymph nodes of the neck.
  - **Lymphocyte-rich classic HL.** This is rare in children. When a sample of lymph node tissue is looked at under a microscope, there are Reed-Sternberg cells and many normal lymphocytes and other blood cells.

[1] "Lymphoma," Centers for Disease Control and Prevention (CDC), May 29, 2018. Available online. URL: www.cdc.gov/cancer/lymphoma/index.htm. Accessed June 2, 2023.

- **Lymphocyte-depleted HL.** This is rare in children and most often occurs in adults or adults with human immunodeficiency virus (HIV). When a sample of lymph node tissue is looked at under a microscope, there are many large, oddly shaped cancer cells and few normal lymphocytes and other blood cells.
- **Nodular lymphocyte-predominant HL.** This is less common than classic HL. It most often occurs in children younger than 10 years of age. Nodular lymphocyte-predominant HL often occurs as a swollen lymph node in the neck, underarm, or groin. Most individuals do not have any other signs or symptoms of cancer at diagnosis. When a sample of lymph node tissue is looked at under a microscope, the cancer cells are shaped like popcorn.

RISK FACTORS FOR CHILDHOOD HODGKIN LYMPHOMA

Anything that increases your risk of getting a disease is called a "risk factor." Not everyone with one or more of the following risk factors will develop childhood HL, and it will develop in some children who do not have any known risk factors. Talk with your child's doctor if you think your child may be at risk.

Risk factors for childhood HL include the following:
- being infected with the EBV
- being infected with HIV
- having certain diseases of the immune system, such as autoimmune lymphoproliferative syndrome (ALPS)
- having a weakened immune system after an organ transplant or from medicine given after a transplant to stop the organ from being rejected by the body
- having a parent, brother, or sister with a personal history of HL

Being exposed to common infections in early childhood may decrease the risk of HL in children.

SIGNS AND SYMPTOMS OF HODGKIN LYMPHOMA

The signs and symptoms of HL depend on where the cancer forms in the body and the size of the cancer. The following and other signs and symptoms may be caused by childhood HL or by other conditions. Check with your child's doctor if your child has any of the following:

- painless, swollen lymph nodes near the collarbone or in the neck, chest, underarm, or groin
- fever for no known reason
- weight loss for no known reason
- drenching night sweats
- feeling very tired
- anorexia
- itchy skin
- coughing
- trouble breathing, especially when lying down

Fever for no known reason, weight loss for no known reason, and drenching night sweats are called "B symptoms." B symptoms are an important part of staging HL and understanding the patient's chance of recovery.

DIAGNOSIS OF CHILDHOOD HODGKIN LYMPHOMA

Tests and procedures that make pictures of the lymph system and other parts of the body help diagnose childhood HL and show how far the cancer has spread. The process used to find if cancer cells have spread outside the lymph system is called "staging." To plan treatment, it is important to know if cancer has spread to other parts of the body.

These tests and procedures may include the following:

- **Physical exam and health history**. This is an exam of the body to check general signs of health, including checking for signs of disease, such as lumps or anything else that seems unusual. A history of the patient's health habits and past illnesses and treatments will also be taken.

- **Complete blood count (CBC).** This is a procedure in which a sample of blood is drawn and checked for the following:
  - the number of red blood cells (RBCs), white blood cells (WBCs), and platelets
  - the amount of hemoglobin (the protein that carries oxygen) in the RBCs
  - the portion of the blood sample made up of RBCs
- **Blood chemistry studies.** This is a procedure in which a blood sample is checked to measure the amount of certain substances released into the blood, including albumin, by organs and tissues in the body. An unusual (higher or lower than normal) amount of a substance can be a sign of disease.
- **C-reactive protein test.** This is a test in which a blood sample is checked to measure the amount of C-reactive protein in the blood. C-reactive protein is made by the liver and sent to the bloodstream in response to inflammation. A higher-than-normal amount of C-reactive protein in the blood may be a sign of disease.
- **Sedimentation rate.** This is a procedure in which a sample of blood is drawn and checked for the rate at which the RBCs settle to the bottom of the test tube. The sedimentation rate is a measure of how much inflammation is in the body. A higher-than-normal sedimentation rate may be a sign of lymphoma. It is also called "erythrocyte sedimentation rate," "sed rate," or "ESR."
- **Computed tomography (CT) scan.** This is a procedure that makes a series of detailed pictures of areas inside the body, such as the neck, chest, abdomen, or pelvis, taken from different angles. The pictures are made by a computer linked to an x-ray machine. A dye may be injected into a vein or swallowed to help the organs or tissues show up more clearly. This procedure is also called "computerized tomography" or "computerized axial tomography" (CAT).

- **Positron emission tomography (PET) scan**. This procedure is used to find malignant tumor cells in the body. A small amount of radioactive glucose (sugar) is injected into a vein. The PET scanner rotates around the body and makes a picture of where glucose is being used in the body. Malignant tumor cells show up brighter in the picture because they are more active and take up more glucose than normal cells.
- **Magnetic resonance imaging (MRI)**. This test uses a magnet, radio waves, and a computer to make a series of detailed pictures of areas inside the body, such as the lymph nodes. This procedure is also called "nuclear MRI" (NMRI).
- **PET-CT scan or PET-MRI scan**. A procedure that combines the pictures from a PET scan and a CT scan or an MRI. The scans are done at the same time with the same machine. The combined scans give more detailed pictures of areas inside the body than any one scan alone.
- **Chest x-ray**. This is an x-ray of the organs and bones inside the chest. An x-ray is a type of energy beam that can go through the body and onto film, making a picture of areas inside the body.
- **Bone marrow aspiration and biopsy**. This is the removal of bone marrow and a small piece of bone by inserting a hollow needle into the hip bone or breastbone. A pathologist views the bone marrow and bone under a microscope to look for abnormal cells. This procedure is done for patients with advanced disease and/or B symptoms.
- **Lymph node biopsy**. This is the removal of all or part of one or more lymph nodes. The lymph node may be removed during an image-guided CT scan or a thoracoscopy, mediastinoscopy, or laparoscopy. One of the following types of biopsies may be done:
  - **Excisional biopsy**. The removal of an entire lymph node.

- **Incisional biopsy**. The removal of part of a lymph node.
- **Core biopsy**. The removal of tissue from a lymph node using a wide needle.

A pathologist views the lymph node tissue under a microscope to check for cancer cells called "Reed-Sternberg cells." These cells are common in classic HL.

TREATMENT FOR CHILDHOOD HODGKIN LYMPHOMA
The treatment options depend on the following:
- whether there is a low, medium, or high risk the cancer will come back after the treatment
- the child's age
- the risk of long-term side effects

Most children and adolescents with newly diagnosed HL can be cured.[2]

Section 15.3 | Adult Hodgkin Lymphoma

WHAT IS ADULT HODGKIN LYMPHOMA?
Adult Hodgkin lymphoma (HL) is a type of cancer that develops in the lymph system. The lymph system is part of the immune system. It helps protect the body from infection and disease.

RISKS OF ADULT HODGKIN LYMPHOMA
Anything that increases your risk of getting a disease is called a "risk factor." Having a risk factor does not mean that you will get

[2] "Childhood Hodgkin Lymphoma Treatment (PDQ®)–Patient Version," National Cancer Institute (NCI), June 23, 2022. Available online. URL: www.cancer.gov/types/lymphoma/patient/child-hodgkin-treatment-pdq. Accessed May 12, 2023.

cancer; not having risk factors does not mean that you will not get cancer. Talk with your doctor if you think you may be at risk. Risk factors for adult HL include the following:

- **Age**. HL is most common in early adulthood (age 20–39) and in late adulthood (age 65 and older).
- **Being male**. The risk of adult HL is slightly higher in males than that in females.
- **Past Epstein-Barr virus infection**. Having an infection with the Epstein-Barr virus in the teenage years or early childhood increases the risk of HL.
- **A family history of HL**. Having a parent, brother, or sister with HL increases the risk of developing HL.

SIGNS AND SYMPTOMS OF ADULT HODGKIN LYMPHOMA

The following and other signs and symptoms may be caused by adult HL or by other conditions. Check with your doctor if any of the following do not go away:

- painless, swollen lymph nodes in the neck, underarm, or groin
- fever for no known reason
- drenching night sweats
- weight loss for no known reason
- itchy skin
- feeling very tired

DIAGNOSIS OF ADULT HODGKIN LYMPHOMA

The following tests and procedures may be used:

- **Physical exam and history**. This is an exam of the body to check general signs of health, including checking for signs of disease, such as lumps or anything else that seems unusual. A history of the patient's health, including fever, night sweats, weight loss, past illnesses, and treatments, will also be taken.

- **A complete blood count (CBC)**. This is a procedure in which a sample of blood is drawn and checked for the following:
  - the number of red blood cells (RBCs), white blood cells (WBCs), and platelets
  - the amount of hemoglobin (the protein that carries oxygen) in the RBCs
  - the portion of the sample made up of RBCs
- **Blood chemistry studies**. This is a procedure in which a blood sample is checked to measure the amount of certain substances released into the blood by organs and tissues in the body. An unusual (higher or lower than normal) amount of a substance can be a sign of disease.
- **Lactate dehydrogenase (LDH) test**. This is a procedure in which a blood sample is checked to measure the amount of lactic dehydrogenase. An increased amount of LDH in the blood may be a sign of tissue damage, lymphoma, or other diseases.
- **Hepatitis B and hepatitis C test**. This is a procedure in which a sample of blood is checked to measure the amount of hepatitis B virus-specific antigens and/or antibodies and the amounts of hepatitis C virus–specific antibodies. These antigens or antibodies are called "markers." Different markers or combinations of markers are used to determine whether a patient has a hepatitis B or C infection, has had a prior infection or vaccination, or is susceptible to infection.
- **Human immunodeficiency virus (HIV) test**. This is a test to measure the level of HIV antibodies in a sample of blood. Antibodies are made by the body when it is invaded by a foreign substance. A high level of HIV antibodies may mean the body has been infected with HIV.
- **Sedimentation rate**. This is a procedure in which a sample of blood is drawn and checked for the rate at

which the RBCs settle to the bottom of the test tube. The sedimentation rate is a measure of how much inflammation is in the body. A higher-than-normal sedimentation rate may be a sign of lymphoma or another condition. This procedure is also called "erythrocyte sedimentation rate," "sed rate," or "ESR."

- **Computed tomography (CT) scan.** This is a procedure that makes a series of detailed pictures of areas inside the body, such as the neck, chest, abdomen, pelvis, and lymph nodes, taken from different angles. The pictures are made by a computer linked to an x-ray machine. A dye may be injected into a vein or swallowed to help the organs or tissues show up more clearly. This procedure is also called "computerized tomography" or "computerized axial tomography" (CAT).
- **Positron emission tomography–CT (PET-CT) scan.** This is a procedure that combines the pictures from a PET scan and a CT scan. The PET and CT scans are done at the same time on the same machine. The pictures from both scans are combined to make a more detailed picture than either test would make by itself. A PET scan is a procedure to find malignant tumor cells in the body. A small amount of radioactive glucose (sugar) is injected into a vein. The PET scanner rotates around the body and makes a picture of where glucose is being used in the body. Malignant tumor cells show up brighter in the picture because they are more active and take up more glucose than normal cells.
- **Lymph node biopsy.** This is the removal of all or part of a lymph node. A pathologist views the tissue under a microscope to look for cancer cells, especially Reed-Sternberg cells. These cells are common in classic HL.

One of the following types of biopsies may be done:
- **Excisional biopsy.** The removal of an entire lymph node.
- **Incisional biopsy.** The removal of part of a lymph node.
- **Core biopsy.** The removal of tissue from a lymph node using a wide needle.

Other areas of the body, such as the liver, lung, bone, bone marrow, and brain, may also have a sample of tissue removed and checked by a pathologist for signs of cancer.

The following test may be done on the tissue that was removed:

- **Immunophenotyping**. This is a laboratory test used to identify cells based on the types of antigens or markers on the surface of the cell. This test is used to diagnose the specific type of lymphoma by comparing the cancer cells to normal cells of the immune system.

For pregnant women with HL, staging tests that protect the fetus from harmful radiation are used. These include the following:

- **Magnetic resonance imaging (MRI)**. This is a procedure that uses a magnet, radio waves, and a computer to make a series of detailed pictures of areas inside the body. This procedure is also called "nuclear magnetic resonance imaging" (NMRI).
- **Ultrasound exam**. This is a procedure in which high-energy sound waves (ultrasound) are bounced off internal tissues or organs and make echoes. The echoes form a picture of body tissues called a "sonogram."

FACTORS AFFECTING PROGNOSIS AND TREATMENT OPTIONS

The prognosis (chance of recovery) and treatment options depend on the following:

- the patient's signs and symptoms, including whether or not they have B symptoms (fever for no known reason, weight loss for no known reason, or drenching night sweats)
- the stage of the cancer (the size of the cancer tumors and whether the cancer has spread to the abdomen or more than one group of lymph nodes)
- the type of HL
- blood test results
- the patient's age, sex, and general health
- whether the cancer is newly diagnosed, continues to grow during treatment, or has come back after treatment

For HL during pregnancy, treatment options also depend on the following:

- the wishes of the patient
- the age of the fetus

Adult HL can usually be cured if found and treated early.[3]

Section 15.4 | Childhood Non-Hodgkin Lymphoma

WHAT IS CHILDHOOD NON-HODGKIN LYMPHOMA?
Childhood non-Hodgkin lymphoma (NHL) is a type of cancer that forms in the lymph system, which is part of the body's immune system. It helps protect the body from infection and disease.

TYPES OF CHILDHOOD NON-HODGKIN LYMPHOMA
The type of lymphoma is determined by how the cells look under a microscope. The following are the three major types of childhood NHL.

Aggressive Mature B-Cell Non-Hodgkin Lymphoma
Aggressive mature B-cell NHLs include the following:

- **Burkitt and Burkitt-like lymphoma/leukemia.** Burkitt lymphoma and Burkitt leukemia are different forms of the same disease. Burkitt lymphoma/leukemia is an aggressive (fast-growing) disorder of B lymphocytes that is most common in children and young adults. It may form in the abdomen, Waldeyer ring, testicles, bone, bone marrow, skin, or central nervous system (CNS). Burkitt leukemia may start in the lymph nodes as Burkitt lymphoma and then spread to the blood

---

[3] "Adult Hodgkin Lymphoma Treatment (PDQ®)—Patient Version," National Cancer Institute (NCI), December 22, 2022. Available online. URL: www.cancer.gov/types/lymphoma/patient/adult-hodgkin-treatment-pdq. Accessed June 2, 2023.

and bone marrow, or it may start in the blood and bone marrow without forming in the lymph nodes first. Both Burkitt leukemia and Burkitt lymphoma have been linked to infection with the Epstein-Barr virus (EBV) although EBV infection is more likely to occur in patients in Africa than in those in the United States. Burkitt and Burkitt-like lymphoma/leukemia are diagnosed when a sample of tissue is checked and a certain change to the *MYC* gene is found.

- **Diffuse large B-cell lymphoma (DLBCL)**. This is the most common type of NHL. It is a type of B-cell NHL that grows quickly in the lymph nodes. The spleen, liver, bone marrow, and other organs are also often affected. Diffuse large B-cell lymphoma occurs more often in adolescents than in children.
- **Primary mediastinal B-cell lymphoma**. This is a type of lymphoma that develops from B cells in the mediastinum (the area behind the breastbone). It may spread to nearby organs, including the lungs and the sac around the heart. It may also spread to lymph nodes and distant organs, including the kidneys. In children and adolescents, primary mediastinal B-cell lymphoma occurs more often in older adolescents.

Lymphoblastic Lymphoma

Lymphoblastic lymphoma is a type of lymphoma that mainly affects T-cell lymphocytes. It usually forms in the mediastinum. This causes trouble with breathing and/or swallowing, wheezing, or swelling of the head and neck. It may spread to the lymph nodes, bone, bone marrow, skin, CNS, abdominal organs, and other areas. Lymphoblastic lymphoma is very similar to acute lymphoblastic leukemia (ALL).

Anaplastic Large-Cell Lymphoma

Anaplastic large-cell lymphoma is a type of lymphoma that mainly affects T-cell lymphocytes. It usually forms in the lymph nodes, skin, or bone and sometimes forms in the gastrointestinal tract, lungs, tissue that covers the lungs, and muscle. Patients with anaplastic large-cell lymphoma have a receptor, called "CD30," on the surface of their T cells. In many children, anaplastic large-cell lymphoma is marked by changes in the *ALK* gene that makes a protein called "anaplastic lymphoma kinase" (ALK). A pathologist checks for these cells and gene changes to help diagnose anaplastic large-cell lymphoma.

Other Types of Non-Hodgkin Lymphoma

Some types of childhood NHL are less common. These include the following:

- **Pediatric-type follicular lymphoma**. In children, follicular lymphoma occurs mainly in males. It is more likely to be found in one area and does not spread to other places in the body. It usually forms in the tonsils and lymph nodes in the neck, but it may also form in the testicles, kidney, gastrointestinal tract, and salivary gland.
- **Marginal zone lymphoma**. Marginal zone lymphoma is a type of lymphoma that tends to grow and spread slowly and is usually found at an early stage. It may be found in the lymph nodes or in areas outside the lymph nodes. Marginal zone lymphoma found outside the lymph nodes in children is called "mucosa-associated lymphoid tissue (MALT) lymphoma." MALT lymphoma may be linked to *Helicobacter pylori* infection of the gastrointestinal tract and *Chlamydophila psittaci* infection of the conjunctival membrane, which lines the eye.
- **Primary CNS lymphoma**. Primary CNS lymphoma is extremely rare in children.
- **Peripheral T-cell lymphoma**. This is an aggressive (fast-growing) NHL that begins in mature T lymphocytes. The T lymphocytes mature in the thymus gland and travel to other parts of the lymph system, such as the lymph nodes, bone marrow, and spleen.

- **Cutaneous T-cell lymphoma**. This type of lymphoma begins in the skin and can cause the skin to thicken or form a tumor. It is very rare in children, but it is more common in adolescents and young adults. There are different types of cutaneous T-cell lymphoma, such as cutaneous anaplastic large-cell lymphoma, subcutaneous panniculitis-like T-cell lymphoma, gamma-delta T-cell lymphoma, and mycosis fungoides. Mycosis fungoides rarely occurs in children and adolescents.

RISKS OF CHILDHOOD NON-HODGKIN LYMPHOMA

Anything that increases your risk of getting a disease is called a "risk factor." Having a risk factor does not mean that you will get cancer; not having risk factors does not mean that you will not get cancer. Talk with your child's doctor if you think your child may be at risk.

Possible risk factors for childhood NHL include the following:
- being infected with the EBV or human immunodeficiency virus (HIV)
- having a weakened immune system after a transplant or from medicines given after a transplant
- having certain inherited diseases (such as DNA repair defect syndromes, which include ataxia telangiectasia (AT), Nijmegen breakage syndrome, and constitutional mismatch repair deficiency)
- past treatment for cancer

SIGNS OF CHILDHOOD NON-HODGKIN LYMPHOMA

The following signs and other signs may be caused by childhood NHL or by other conditions. Check with a doctor if your child has any of the following:
- trouble breathing
- wheezing
- coughing
- high-pitched breathing sounds

- swelling of the head, neck, upper body, or arms
- trouble swallowing
- painless swelling of the lymph nodes in the neck, underarm, stomach, or groin
- painless lump or swelling in a testicle
- fever for no known reason
- weight loss for no known reason
- night sweats

DIAGNOSIS OF CHILDHOOD NON-HODGKIN LYMPHOMA

The following tests and procedures may be used:

- **Physical exam and history**. This is an exam of the body to check general signs of health, including checking for signs of disease, such as lumps or anything else that seems unusual. A history of the patient's health habits and past illnesses and treatments will also be taken.
- **Blood chemistry studies**. This is a procedure in which a blood sample is checked to measure the amount of certain substances released into the blood by organs and tissues in the body, including electrolytes, lactate dehydrogenase (LDH), uric acid, blood urea nitrogen (BUN), creatinine, and liver function values. An unusual (higher or lower than normal) amount of a substance can be a sign of disease.
- **Liver function tests**. This is a procedure in which a blood sample is checked to measure the amount of certain substances released into the blood by the liver. A higher-than-normal amount of a substance can be a sign of cancer.
- **Computed tomography (CT) scan**. This is a procedure that makes a series of detailed pictures of areas inside the body, taken from different angles. The pictures are made by a computer linked to an x-ray machine. A dye may be injected into a vein or swallowed to help the organs or tissues show up more clearly. This procedure is also called "computerized tomography" or "computerized axial tomography."

- **Positron emission tomography (PET) scan**. This is a procedure to find malignant tumor cells in the body. A small amount of radioactive glucose (sugar) is injected into a vein. The PET scanner rotates around the body and makes a picture of where glucose is being used in the body. Malignant tumor cells show up brighter in the picture because they are more active and take up more glucose than normal cells. Sometimes, a PET scan and a CT scan are done at the same time. If there is any cancer, this increases the chance that it will be found.
- **Magnetic resonance imaging (MRI)**. This is a procedure that uses a magnet, radio waves, and a computer to make a series of detailed pictures of areas inside the body. This procedure is also called "nuclear magnetic resonance imaging" (NMRI).
- **Lumbar puncture (LP)**. This is a procedure used to collect cerebrospinal fluid (CSF) from the spinal column. This is done by placing a needle between two bones in the spine and into the CSF around the spinal cord and removing a sample of the fluid. The sample of CSF is checked under a microscope for signs that the cancer has spread to the brain and spinal cord. This procedure is also called a "spinal tap."
- **Chest x-ray**. This is an x-ray of the organs and bones inside the chest. An x-ray is a type of energy beam that can go through the body and onto film, making a picture of areas inside the body.
- **Ultrasound exam**. This is a procedure in which high-energy sound waves (ultrasound) are bounced off internal tissues or organs and make echoes. The echoes form a picture of body tissues called a "sonogram." The picture can be printed to be looked at later.

Biopsy to Diagnose Childhood Non-Hodgkin Lymphoma

Cells and tissues are removed during a biopsy so that they can be viewed under a microscope by a pathologist to check for signs of cancer. Because treatment depends on the type of NHL, biopsy samples should be checked by a pathologist who has experience in diagnosing childhood NHL.

One of the following types of biopsies may be done:

- **Excisional biopsy**. The removal of an entire lymph node or lump of tissue.
- **Incisional biopsy**. The removal of part of a lump, lymph node, or sample of tissue.
- **Core biopsy**. The removal of tissue or part of a lymph node using a wide needle.
- **Fine-needle aspiration (FNA) biopsy**. The removal of tissue or part of a lymph node using a thin needle.

The procedure used to remove the sample of tissue depends on where the tumor is in the body.

- **Bone marrow aspiration and biopsy**. This is the removal of bone marrow and a small piece of bone by inserting a hollow needle into the hip bone or breastbone.
- **Mediastinoscopy**. This is a surgical procedure to look at the organs, tissues, and lymph nodes between the lungs for abnormal areas. An incision (cut) is made at the top of the breastbone, and a mediastinoscope is inserted into the chest. A mediastinoscope is a thin, tube-like instrument with a light and a lens for viewing. It also has a tool to remove tissue or lymph node samples, which are checked under a microscope for signs of cancer.
- **Anterior mediastinotomy**. This is a surgical procedure to look at the organs and tissues between the lungs and between the breastbone and heart for abnormal areas. An incision is made next to the breastbone, and a mediastinoscope is inserted into the chest. It also has a tool to remove tissue or lymph node samples, which are checked under a microscope for signs of cancer. This is also called the "Chamberlain procedure."
- **Thoracentesis**. This is the removal of fluid from the space between the lining of the chest and the lung

using a needle. A pathologist views the fluid under a microscope to look for cancer cells.

If cancer is found, the following tests may be done to study the cancer cells:

- **Immunohistochemistry**. This is a laboratory test that uses antibodies to check for certain antigens in a sample of tissue. The antibody is usually linked to a radioactive substance or a dye that causes the tissue to light up under a microscope. This type of test may be used to tell the difference between different types of cancer.
- **Flow cytometry**. This is a laboratory test that measures the number of cells in a sample; the percentage of live cells in a sample; and certain characteristics of cells, such as size, shape, and presence of tumor markers on the cell surface. The cells are stained with a light-sensitive dye, placed in a fluid, and passed in a stream before a laser or other type of light. The measurements are based on how the light-sensitive dye reacts to the light.
- **Cytogenetic analysis**. This is a laboratory test in which cells in a sample of tissue are viewed under a microscope to look for certain changes in the chromosomes.
- **Fluorescence in situ hybridization (FISH)**. This is a laboratory test used to look at genes or chromosomes in cells and tissues. Pieces of DNA that contain a fluorescent dye are made in the laboratory and added to cells or tissues on a glass slide. When these pieces of DNA attach to certain genes or areas of chromosomes on the slide, they light up when viewed under a microscope with a special light. This type of test is used to find certain gene changes.
- **Immunophenotyping**. This is a laboratory test used to identify cells based on the types of antigens or markers on the surface of the cell. This test is used to diagnose

specific types of lymphoma by comparing the cancer cells to normal cells of the immune system.

FACTORS AFFECTING PROGNOSIS AND TREATMENT OPTIONS

The prognosis (chance of recovery) and treatment options depend on the following:

- the type of lymphoma
- where the tumor is in the body when the tumor is diagnosed
- the stage of the cancer
- whether there are certain changes in the chromosomes
- the type of initial treatment
- whether the lymphoma responded to the initial treatment
- the patient's age and general health[4]

Section 15.5 | Adult Non-Hodgkin Lymphoma

WHAT IS ADULT NON-HODGKIN LYMPHOMA?

Adult non-Hodgkin lymphoma (NHL) is a type of cancer that forms in the lymph system. The lymph system is part of the immune system. It helps protect the body from infection and disease.

NHL during pregnancy is rare. NHL in pregnant women is the same as the disease in nonpregnant women of childbearing age. However, treatment is different for pregnant women.

RISKS OF ADULT NON-HODGKIN LYMPHOMA

Anything that increases your risk of getting a disease is called a "risk factor." Having a risk factor does not mean that you will get cancer; not having risk factors does not mean that you will not get cancer. Talk with your doctor if you think you may be at risk.

[4] "Childhood Non-Hodgkin Lymphoma Treatment (PDQ®)—Patient Version," National Cancer Institute (NCI), March 3, 2023. Available online. URL: www.cancer.gov/types/lymphoma/patient/child-nhl-treatment-pdq. Accessed June 2, 2023.

The following risk factors and other risk factors may increase the risk of certain types of adult NHL:

- being older, male, or White
- having one of the following medical conditions:
  - an inherited immune disorder (such as hypogammaglobulinemia or Wiskott-Aldrich syndrome)
  - an autoimmune disease (such as rheumatoid arthritis, psoriasis, or Sjögren syndrome)
  - human immunodeficiency virus (HIV)/acquired immunodeficiency syndrome (AIDS)
  - human T-lymphotropic virus type I or Epstein-Barr virus (EBV) infection
  - *Helicobacter pylori* infection
- taking immunosuppressant drugs after an organ transplant

SIGNS AND SYMPTOMS OF ADULT NON-HODGKIN LYMPHOMA

The following signs and symptoms may be caused by adult NHL or by other conditions. Check with your doctor if you have any of the following:

- swelling in the lymph nodes in the neck, underarm, groin, or stomach
- fever for no known reason
- recurring night sweats
- feeling very tired
- weight loss for no known reason
- skin rash or itchy skin
- pain in the chest, abdomen, or bones for no known reason

When fever, night sweats, and weight loss occur together, this group of symptoms is called "B symptoms."

Other signs and symptoms of adult NHL may occur and depend on the following:

- where the cancer forms in the body
- the size of the tumor
- how fast the tumor grows

DIAGNOSIS OF ADULT NON-HODGKIN LYMPHOMA

The following tests and procedures may be used:

- **Physical exam and history**. This is an exam of the body to check general signs of health, including checking for signs of disease, such as lumps or anything else that seems unusual. A history of the patient's health, including fever, night sweats, weight loss, health habits, and past illnesses and treatments, will also be taken.
- **A complete blood count (CBC)**. This is a procedure in which a sample of blood is drawn and checked for the following:
  - the number of red blood cells (RBCs), white blood cells (WBCs), and platelets
  - the amount of hemoglobin (the protein that carries oxygen) in the RBCs
  - the portion of the sample made up of RBCs
- **Blood chemistry studies**. This is a procedure in which a blood sample is checked to measure the amount of certain substances released into the blood by organs and tissues in the body. An unusual (higher or lower than normal) amount of a substance can be a sign of disease.
- **Lactate dehydrogenase (LDH) test**. This is a procedure in which a blood sample is checked to measure the amount of LDH. An increased amount of LDH in the blood may be a sign of tissue damage, lymphoma, or other diseases.
- **Hepatitis B and hepatitis C test**. This is a procedure in which a sample of blood is checked to measure the amount of hepatitis B virus-specific antigens and/or antibodies and the amounts of hepatitis C virus-specific antibodies. These antigens or antibodies are called "markers." Different markers or combinations of markers are used to determine whether a patient has a hepatitis B or C infection, has had a prior infection or vaccination, or is susceptible to infection.

- **Human immunodeficiency test**. This is a test to measure the level of HIV antibodies in a sample of blood. Antibodies are made by the body when it is invaded by a foreign substance. A high level of HIV antibodies may mean that the body has been infected with HIV.
- **Computed tomography (CT) scan**. This is a procedure that makes a series of detailed pictures of areas inside the body, such as the neck, chest, abdomen, pelvis, and lymph nodes, taken from different angles. The pictures are made by a computer linked to an x-ray machine. A dye may be injected into a vein or swallowed to help the organs or tissues show up more clearly. This procedure is also called "computerized tomography" or "computerized axial tomography."
- **Positron emission tomography (PET) scan**. This is a procedure to find malignant tumor cells in the body. A small amount of radioactive glucose (sugar) is injected into a vein. The PET scanner rotates around the body and makes a picture of where glucose is being used in the body. Malignant tumor cells show up brighter in the picture because they are more active and take up more glucose than normal cells.
- **Bone marrow aspiration and biopsy**. This is the removal of bone marrow and a small piece of bone by inserting a needle into the hip bone or breastbone. A pathologist views the bone marrow and bone under a microscope to look for signs of cancer.
- **Lymph node biopsy**. This is the removal of all or part of a lymph node. A pathologist views the tissue under a microscope to check for cancer cells. One of the following types of biopsies may be done:
  - **Excisional biopsy**. The removal of an entire lymph node.
  - **Incisional biopsy**. The removal of part of a lymph node.
  - **Core biopsy**. The removal of part of a lymph node using a wide needle.

If cancer is found, the following tests may be done to study the cancer cells:

- **Immunohistochemistry.** This is a test that uses antibodies to check for certain antigens in a sample of tissue. The antibody is usually linked to a radioactive substance or a dye that causes the tissue to light up under a microscope. This type of test may be used to tell the difference between different types of cancer.
- **Cytogenetic analysis.** This is a laboratory test in which cells in a sample of tissue are viewed under a microscope to look for certain changes in the chromosomes
- **Fluorescence in situ hybridization (FISH).** This is a laboratory test used to look at genes or chromosomes in cells and tissues. Pieces of deoxyribonucleic acid (DNA) that contain a fluorescent dye are made in the laboratory and added to cells or tissues on a glass slide. When these pieces of DNA attach to certain genes or areas of chromosomes on the slide, they light up when viewed under a microscope with a special light. This type of test is used to look for certain genetic markers.
- **Immunophenotyping.** This is a process used to identify cells based on the types of antigens or markers on the surface of the cell. This process is used to diagnose specific types of leukemia and lymphoma by comparing the cancer cells to normal cells of the immune system.

Other tests and procedures may be done depending on the signs and symptoms seen and where the cancer forms in the body.

FACTORS AFFECTING PROGNOSIS AND TREATMENT OPTIONS
The prognosis (chance of recovery) and treatment options depend on the following:
- the stage of the cancer
- the type of NHL
- the amount of LDH in the blood

- whether there are certain changes in the genes
- the patient's age and general health
- whether the lymphoma has just been diagnosed or has recurred (come back)

For NHL during pregnancy, the treatment options also depend on:
- the wishes of the patient
- which trimester of pregnancy the patient is in
- whether the baby can be delivered early

Some types of NHL spread more quickly than others. Most NHLs that occur during pregnancy are aggressive. Delaying treatment of aggressive lymphoma until after the baby is born may lessen the mother's chance of survival. Immediate treatment is often recommended, even during pregnancy.[5]

Section 15.6 | AIDS-Related Lymphoma

WHAT IS AIDS-RELATED LYMPHOMA?

Acquired immunodeficiency syndrome (AIDS) is caused by human immunodeficiency virus (HIV), which attacks and weakens the body's immune system. A weakened immune system is unable to fight infection and disease. People with HIV have an increased risk of infection and lymphoma or other types of cancer. A person with HIV and certain types of infection or cancer, such as lymphoma, is diagnosed as having AIDS. Sometimes, people are diagnosed with AIDS and AIDS-related lymphoma at the same time.

AIDS-related lymphoma is a type of cancer that affects the lymph system. Sometimes, it occurs outside the lymph nodes in the bone marrow, liver, meninges (thin membranes that cover the

[5] "Adult Non-Hodgkin Lymphoma Treatment (PDQ®)—Patient Version," National Cancer Institute (NCI), December 29, 2022. Available online. URL: www.cancer.gov/types/lymphoma/patient/adult-nhl-treatment-pdq. Accessed June 2, 2023.

brain), and gastrointestinal tract. Less often, it may occur in the anus, heart, bile duct, gingiva, and muscles.

TYPES OF AIDS-RELATED LYMPHOMA
Lymphomas are divided into two general types:
- Hodgkin lymphoma (HL)
- non-Hodgkin lymphoma (NHL)

Both NHL and HL may occur in patients with AIDS, but NHL is more common. When a person with AIDS has NHL, it is called "AIDS-related lymphoma." When AIDS-related lymphoma occurs in the central nervous system (CNS), it is called "AIDS-related primary CNS lymphoma."

NHLs are grouped by the way their cells look under a microscope. They may be indolent (slow-growing) or aggressive (fast-growing). AIDS-related lymphomas are aggressive. There are two main types of AIDS-related NHL:
- diffuse large B-cell lymphoma (including B-cell immunoblastic lymphoma)
- Burkitt or Burkitt-like lymphoma

SIGNS OF AIDS-RELATED LYMPHOMA
The following and other signs and symptoms may be caused by AIDS-related lymphoma or by other conditions. Check with your doctor if you have any of the following symptoms:
- weight loss or fever for no known reason
- night sweats
- painless, swollen lymph nodes in the neck, chest, underarm, or groin
- a feeling of fullness below the ribs

DIAGNOSIS OF AIDS-RELATED LYMPHOMA
The following tests and procedures may be used:
- **Physical exam and history**. This is an exam of the body to check general signs of health, including checking for signs of disease, such as lumps or anything

else that seems unusual. A history of the patient's health, including fever, night sweats, weight loss, health habits, and past illnesses and treatments, will also be taken.

- **A complete blood count (CBC).** This is a procedure in which a sample of blood is drawn and checked for the following:
  - the number of red blood cells (RBCs), white blood cells (WBCs), and platelets
  - the amount of hemoglobin (the protein that carries oxygen) in the RBCs
  - the portion of the sample made up of RBCs
- **Blood chemistry studies.** This is a procedure in which a blood sample is checked to measure the amount of certain substances released into the blood by organs and tissues in the body. An unusual (higher or lower than normal) amount of a substance can be a sign of disease.
- **Lactate dehydrogenase (LDH) test.** A procedure in which a blood sample is checked to measure the amount of LDH. An increased amount of LDH in the blood may be a sign of tissue damage, lymphoma, or other diseases.
- **Hepatitis B and hepatitis C test.** This is a procedure in which a sample of blood is checked to measure the amount of hepatitis B virus-specific antigens and/ or antibodies and the amounts of hepatitis C virus– specific antibodies. These antigens or antibodies are called "markers." Different markers or combinations of markers are used to determine whether a patient has a hepatitis B or C infection, has had a prior infection or vaccination, or is susceptible to infection.
- **Human immunodeficiency test.** This is a test to measure the level of HIV antibodies in a sample of blood. Antibodies are made by the body when it is invaded by a foreign substance. A high level of HIV antibodies may mean the body has been infected with HIV.

- **Computed tomography (CT) scan**. This is a procedure that makes a series of detailed pictures of areas inside the body, such as the neck, chest, abdomen, pelvis, and lymph nodes, taken from different angles. The pictures are made by a computer linked to an x-ray machine. A dye may be injected into a vein or swallowed to help the organs or tissues show up more clearly. This procedure is also called "computerized tomography" or "computerized axial tomography" (CAT).
- **Positron emission tomography (PET) scan**. This is a procedure to find malignant tumor cells in the body. A small amount of radioactive glucose (sugar) is injected into a vein. The PET scanner rotates around the body and makes a picture of where glucose is being used in the body. Malignant tumor cells show up brighter in the picture because they are more active and take up more glucose than normal cells.
- **Bone marrow aspiration and biopsy**. This is the removal of bone marrow and a small piece of bone by inserting a hollow needle into the hip bone or breastbone. A pathologist views the bone marrow and bone under a microscope to look for signs of cancer.
- **Lymph node biopsy**. This is the removal of all or part of a lymph node. A pathologist views the tissue under a microscope to look for cancer cells. One of the following types of biopsies may be done:
  - **Excisional biopsy**. The removal of an entire lymph node.
  - **Incisional biopsy**. The removal of part of a lymph node.
  - **Core biopsy**. The removal of tissue from a lymph node using a wide needle.

Other areas of the body, such as the liver, lung, bone, bone marrow, and brain, may also have a sample of tissue removed and checked by a pathologist for signs of cancer.

If cancer is found, the following tests may be done to study the cancer cells:

- **Immunohistochemistry**. This is a test that uses antibodies to check for certain antigens in a sample of tissue. The antibody is usually linked to a radioactive substance or a dye that causes the tissue to light up under a microscope. This type of test may be used to tell the difference between different types of cancer.
- **Cytogenetic analysis**. This is a laboratory test in which cells in a sample of tissue are viewed under a microscope to look for certain changes in the chromosomes.
- **Fluorescence in situ hybridization (FISH)**. This is a laboratory test used to look at genes or chromosomes in cells and tissues. Pieces of deoxyribonucleic acid (DNA) that contain a fluorescent dye are made in the laboratory and added to cells or tissues on a glass slide. When these pieces of DNA attach to certain genes or areas of chromosomes on the slide, they light up when viewed under a microscope with a special light. This type of test is used to look for certain genetic markers.
- **Immunophenotyping**. This is a process used to identify cells based on the types of antigens or markers on the surface of the cell. This process is used to diagnose specific types of leukemia and lymphoma by comparing the cancer cells to normal cells of the immune system.

FACTORS AFFECTING PROGNOSIS AND TREATMENT OPTIONS

The prognosis (chance of recovery) and treatment options depend on the following:

- the stage of the cancer
- the age of the patient
- the number of CD4 lymphocytes (a type of WBC) in the blood
- the number of places in the body lymphoma is found outside the lymph system

- whether the patient has a history of intravenous (IV) drug use
- the patient's ability to carry out regular daily activities[6]

Section 15.7 | Mycosis Fungoides and Sézary Syndrome

WHAT ARE MYCOSIS FUNGOIDES AND SÉZARY SYNDROME?

Normally, the bone marrow makes blood stem cells (immature cells) that become mature blood stem cells over time. A blood stem cell may become a myeloid stem cell or a lymphoid stem cell. A myeloid stem cell becomes a red blood cell (RBC), white blood cell (WBC), or platelet. A lymphoid stem cell becomes a lymphoblast and then one of the three types of lymphocytes (WBCs):

- **B-cell lymphocytes.** These WBCs make antibodies to help fight infection.
- **T-cell lymphocytes.** These WBCs help B lymphocytes make the antibodies that help fight infection.
- **Natural killer cells.** These WBCs attack cancer cells and viruses.

In mycosis fungoides, T-cell lymphocytes become cancerous and affect the skin. When these lymphocytes occur in the blood, they are called "Sézary cells." In Sézary syndrome, cancerous T-cell lymphocytes affect the skin, and a large number of Sézary cells are found in the blood.

SIGNS OF MYCOSIS FUNGOIDES AND SÉZARY SYNDROME

Mycosis fungoides may go through the following phases:

- **Premycotic phase.** A scaly, red rash develops in areas of the body that are not usually exposed to the sun. This rash does not cause symptoms and may last for

[6] "AIDS-Related Lymphoma Treatment (PDQ®)—Patient Version," National Cancer Institute (NCI), October 7, 2022. Available online. URL: www.cancer.gov/types/lymphoma/patient/aids-related-treatment-pdq. Accessed June 2, 2023.

months or years. It is hard to diagnose the rash as mycosis fungoides during this phase.

- **Patch phase**. A thin, reddened, eczema-like rash is developed during this phase.
- **Plaque phase**. Small raised bumps (papules) or hardened lesions on the skin, which may be reddened, are seen in patients with mycosis fungoides.
- **Tumor phase**. Tumors form on the skin. These tumors may develop ulcers, and the skin may get infected.

Check with your doctor if you have any of these signs.

Also, skin all over the body is reddened, itchy, peeling, and painful. There may also be patches, plaques, or tumors on the skin. It is not known if Sézary syndrome is an advanced form of mycosis fungoides or a separate disease.

DIAGNOSIS OF MYCOSIS FUNGOIDES AND SÉZARY SYNDROME

The following tests and procedures may be used:
- **Physical exam and history**. This is an exam of the body to check general signs of health, including checking for signs of disease, such as lumps, the number and type of skin lesions, or anything else that seems unusual. Pictures of the skin and a history of the patient's health habits and past illnesses and treatments will also be taken.
- **A complete blood count (CBC) with differential**. This is a procedure in which a sample of blood is drawn and checked for the following:
  - the number of RBCs and platelets
  - the number and type of WBCs
  - the amount of hemoglobin (the protein that carries oxygen) in the RBCs
  - the portion of the blood sample made up of RBCs
- **Peripheral blood smear**. This is a procedure in which a sample of blood is viewed under a microscope to count different circulating blood cells (RBCs, WBCs, platelets, etc.) and see whether the cells look normal.

- **Skin biopsy**. This is the removal of cells or tissues so that they can be viewed under a microscope to check for signs of cancer. The doctor may remove a growth from the skin, which will be examined by a pathologist. More than one skin biopsy may be needed to diagnose mycosis fungoides.
- **Immunophenotyping**. This is a process used to identify cells based on the types of antigens or markers on the surface of the cell. This process may include special staining of the blood cells. It is used to diagnose specific types of leukemia and lymphoma by comparing the cancer cells to normal cells of the immune system.
- **T-cell receptor (TCR) gene rearrangement test**. This is a laboratory test in which cells in a sample of tissue are checked to see if there is a certain change in the genes. This gene change can lead to too many of one kind of T cells (WBCs that fight infection) to be made.
- **Flow cytometry**. This is a laboratory test that measures the number of cells in a sample of blood, the percentage of live cells in a sample, and certain characteristics of cells, such as size, shape, and the presence of tumor markers on the cell surface. The cells are stained with a light-sensitive dye, placed in a fluid, and passed in a stream before a laser or other type of light. The measurements are based on how the light-sensitive dye reacts to the light.

FACTORS AFFECTING PROGNOSIS AND TREATMENT OPTIONS

The prognosis (chance of recovery) and treatment options depend on the following:

- the stage of the cancer
- the type of lesion (patches, plaques, or tumors)
- the patient's age and gender

Mycosis fungoides and Sézary syndrome are hard to cure. Treatment is usually palliative to relieve symptoms and improve

214

the quality of life. Patients with early-stage disease may live many years.[7]

Section 15.8 | Primary Central Nervous System Lymphoma

WHAT IS PRIMARY CENTRAL NERVOUS SYSTEM LYMPHOMA?

Lymphoma is a disease in which malignant (cancer) cells form in the lymph system. Lymphocytes (carried in the lymph) travel in and out of the central nervous system (CNS). It is thought that some of these lymphocytes become malignant and cause lymphoma to form in the CNS. Primary CNS lymphoma can start in the brain, spinal cord, or meninges (the layers that form the outer covering of the brain). Because the eye is so close to the brain, primary CNS lymphoma can also start in the eye (called "ocular lymphoma").

RISKS OF PRIMARY CENTRAL NERVOUS SYSTEM LYMPHOMA

Anything that increases your chance of getting a disease is called a "risk factor." Having a risk factor does not mean that you will get cancer; not having risk factors does not mean that you will not get cancer. Talk with your doctor if you think you may be at risk.

Primary CNS lymphoma may occur in patients who have acquired immunodeficiency syndrome (AIDS) or other disorders of the immune system or who have had a kidney transplant.

DIAGNOSIS OF PRIMARY CENTRAL NERVOUS SYSTEM LYMPHOMA

The following tests and procedures may be used:
- **Neurological exam**. This includes a series of questions and tests to check the brain, spinal cord, and nerve function. The exam checks a person's mental status, coordination, ability to walk normally, and how well

---

[7] "Mycosis Fungoides (Including Sezary Syndrome) Treatment (PDQ®)—Patient Version," National Cancer Institute (NCI), March 25, 2022. Available online. URL: www.cancer.gov/types/lymphoma/patient/mycosis-fungoides-treatment-pdq#_1. Accessed June 2, 2023.

the muscles, senses, and reflexes work. This may also be called a "neuro exam" or a "neurologic exam."

- **Eye exam with dilated pupil**. This is an exam of the eye in which the pupil is dilated (enlarged) with medicated eye drops to allow the doctor to look through the lens and pupil to the retina. The inside of the eye, including the retina and the optic nerve, is checked. Pictures may be taken over time to keep track of changes in the size of the tumor. There are several types of eye exams that include the following:
  - **Ophthalmoscopy**. This is an exam of the inside of the back of the eye to check the retina and optic nerve using a small magnifying lens and a light.
  - **Slit lamp biomicroscopy**. This is an exam of the inside of the eye to check the retina, optic nerve, and other parts of the eye using a strong beam of light and a microscope.
- **Magnetic resonance imaging (MRI)**. This is a procedure that uses a magnet, radio waves, and a computer to make a series of detailed pictures of areas inside the brain and spinal cord. A substance called "gadolinium" is injected into the patient through a vein. The gadolinium collects around the cancer cells, so they show up brighter in the picture. This procedure is also called "nuclear magnetic resonance imaging" (NMRI).
- **Positron emission tomography (PET) scan**. This is a procedure to find malignant tumor cells in the body. A small amount of radioactive glucose (sugar) is injected into a vein. The PET scanner rotates around the body and makes a picture of where glucose is being used in the body. Malignant tumor cells show up brighter in the picture because they are more active and take up more glucose than normal cells.
- **Lumbar puncture (LP)**. This is a procedure used to collect cerebrospinal fluid (CSF) from the spinal column. This is done by placing a needle between two bones in the spine and into the CSF around the spinal cord and removing a sample of the fluid. The sample of CSF is

checked under a microscope for signs of tumor cells. The sample may also be checked for the amounts of protein and glucose. A higher-than-normal amount of protein or a lower-than-normal amount of glucose may be a sign of a tumor. This procedure is also called a "spinal tap."

- **Stereotactic biopsy**. This is a biopsy procedure that uses a computer and a three-dimensional (3D) scanning device to find a tumor site and guide the removal of tissue so that it can be viewed under a microscope to check for signs of cancer.

The following tests may be done on the samples of tissue that are removed:

- **Flow cytometry**. This is a laboratory test that measures the number of cells in a sample, the percentage of live cells in a sample, and certain characteristics of cells, such as size, shape, and the presence of tumor markers on the cell surface. The cells are stained with a light-sensitive dye, placed in a fluid, and passed in a stream before a laser or other type of light. The measurements are based on how the light-sensitive dye reacts to the light.
- **Immunohistochemistry**. This is a test that uses antibodies to check for certain antigens in a sample of tissue. The antibody is usually linked to a radioactive substance or a dye that causes the tissue to light up under a microscope. This type of test may be used to tell the difference between different types of cancer.
- **Cytogenetic analysis**. This is a laboratory test in which cells in a sample of tissue are viewed under a microscope to look for certain changes in the chromosomes. Other tests, such as fluorescence in situ hybridization (FISH), may also be done to look for certain changes in the chromosomes.
- **A complete blood count (CBC) with differential**. This is a procedure in which a sample of blood is drawn and checked for the following:
  - the number of red blood cells (RBCs) and platelets
  - the number and type of white blood cells (WBCs)

- the amount of hemoglobin (the protein that carries oxygen) in the RBCs
- the portion of the blood sample made up of RBCs
- **Blood chemistry studies**. This is a procedure in which a blood sample is checked to measure the amount of certain substances released into the blood by organs and tissues in the body. An unusual (higher or lower than normal) amount of a substance can be a sign of disease.

FACTORS AFFECTING PROGNOSIS AND TREATMENT OPTIONS

Treatment options depend on the following:
- the stage of the cancer
- where the tumor is in the CNS
- the patient's age and general health
- whether the cancer has just been diagnosed or has recurred (come back)

The prognosis (chance of recovery) depends on the following:
- the patient's age and general health
- the level of certain substances in the blood and CSF
- whether the tumor is in the CNS, eye, or both
- whether the patient has AIDS

Treatment for primary CNS lymphoma works best when the tumor has not spread outside the cerebrum (the largest part of the brain) and the patient is younger than 60 years of age, is able to carry out most daily activities, and does not have AIDS or other diseases that weaken the immune system.[8]

[8] "Primary CNS Lymphoma Treatment (PDQ®)—Patient Version," National Cancer Institute (NCI), May 25, 2023. Available online. URL: www.cancer.gov/types/lymphoma/patient/primary-cns-lymphoma-treatment-pdq. Accessed June 5, 2023.

Section 15.9 | **Waldenström Macroglobulinemia**

WHAT IS WALDENSTRÖM MACROGLOBULINEMIA?

Waldenström macroglobulinemia is a rare blood cell cancer characterized by an excess of abnormal white blood cells (WBCs) in the bone marrow. These abnormal cells have characteristics of both WBCs (lymphocytes) called "B cells" and more mature cells derived from B cells known as "plasma cells." These abnormal cells with both lymphocyte and plasma characteristics are known as "lymphoplasmacytic cells." Due to these cells, Waldenström macroglobulinemia is classified as a lymphoplasmacytic lymphoma. In Waldenström macroglobulinemia, these abnormal cells produce excess amounts of immunoglobulin M (IgM), the largest type of protein known as an "immunoglobulin." The overproduction of this large protein contributes to the condition's name (macroglobulinemia).

CAUSES OF WALDENSTRÖM MACROGLOBULINEMIA

It is not clear what causes Waldenström macroglobulinemia though it is likely to result from a combination of genetic changes. The most common known genetic change associated with this condition is a variant (also called "mutation") in the *MYD88* gene, which is found in more than 90 percent of affected individuals. *CXCR4*, another gene commonly associated with Waldenström macroglobulinemia, is altered in approximately 30 percent of affected individuals (most of whom also have the *MYD88* gene variant).

The proteins produced from the *MYD88* and *CXCR4* genes are both involved in signaling within cells. The MYD88 protein relays signals that help prevent the self-destruction (apoptosis) of cells, thus aiding in cell survival. The CXCR4 protein stimulates signaling pathways inside the cell that help regulate cell growth and division (proliferation) and cell survival. Variants in these genes lead to the production of proteins that are constantly turned on (overactive). Excessive signaling through these overactive proteins allows the survival and proliferation of abnormal cells that should undergo apoptosis, which likely contributes to the accumulation of lymphoplasmacytic cells in Waldenström macroglobulinemia.

Other genetic changes believed to be involved in Waldenström macroglobulinemia have not yet been identified. Studies have found that certain regions of DNA are deleted or added in some people with the condition; however, researchers are unsure which genes in these regions are important for the development of the condition. The variants that cause Waldenström macroglobulinemia are acquired during a person's lifetime and are present only in the abnormal blood cells.

WHO DEVELOPS WALDENSTRÖM MACROGLOBULINEMIA?

Waldenström macroglobulinemia usually begins in a person's 60s and is a slow-growing (indolent) cancer. Some affected individuals have elevated levels of IgM and lymphoplasmacytic cells but no symptoms of the condition; in these cases, the disease is usually found incidentally by a blood test taken for another reason. These individuals are diagnosed with smoldering (or asymptomatic) Waldenström macroglobulinemia. It can be many years before a person with the condition develops noticeable signs and symptoms.

SIGNS AND SYMPTOMS OF WALDENSTRÖM MACROGLOBULINEMIA

The most common signs and symptoms to first appear in people with Waldenström macroglobulinemia are weakness and extreme tiredness (fatigue) caused by a shortage of red blood cells (RBCs; anemia). Affected individuals can also experience general symptoms such as fever, night sweats, and weight loss. Some people with Waldenström macroglobulinemia develop a loss of sensation and weakness in the limbs (peripheral neuropathy). Doctors are unsure why this feature occurs although they speculate that the IgM protein attaches to the protective covering of nerve cells (myelin) and breaks it down. The damaged nerves cannot carry signals normally, leading to neuropathy.

Other features of Waldenström macroglobulinemia are due to the accumulation of lymphoplasmacytic cells in different tissues. For example, accumulation of these cells can lead to an enlarged liver (hepatomegaly), spleen (splenomegaly), or lymph nodes (lymphadenopathy). In the bone marrow, the lymphoplasmacytic cells interfere with normal blood cell development, causing a shortage of healthy blood cells (pancytopenia).

Several other signs and symptoms of Waldenström macroglobulinemia are related to the excess amounts of IgM. Increased IgM can thicken the blood and impair circulation, causing a condition known as "hyperviscosity syndrome." Features related to hyperviscosity syndrome include bleeding in the nose or mouth, blurring or loss of vision, headache, dizziness, and confusion. In some affected individuals, IgM and other immunoglobulins react to cold temperatures to form gel-like clumps that block blood flow in areas exposed to the cold, such as the hands and feet. These clumped proteins are referred to as cryoglobulins, and their clumping causes a condition known as "cryoglobulinemia." Cryoglobulinemia can lead to pain in the hands and feet or episodes of Raynaud phenomenon, in which the fingers and toes turn white or blue in response to cold temperatures. The IgM protein, along with another protein called "amyloid," can build up in organs and interfere with their normal function. This buildup causes a condition called "amyloidosis." Organs that are typically affected by amyloidosis include the heart, kidneys, liver, or spleen. Affected individuals can experience weakness, fatigue, shortness of breath, irregular heartbeat, or joint pain.

FREQUENCY OF WALDENSTRÖM MACROGLOBULINEMIA

Waldenström macroglobulinemia affects an estimated three per million people each year in the United States. Approximately 1,000–1,500 new cases of the condition are diagnosed each year in this country, and White people are more likely to develop Waldenström macroglobulinemia than African Americans. For unknown reasons, the condition occurs twice as often in men than in women.

INHERITANCE OF WALDENSTRÖM MACROGLOBULINEMIA

Waldenström macroglobulinemia is not inherited, and most affected people have no history of the disorder in their family. The condition usually arises from genetic changes in blood cells that are acquired during a person's lifetime (somatic variants), which are not inherited.

Some families seem to have a predisposition to the condition. Approximately 20 percent of people with Waldenström macroglobulinemia have a family member with the condition or another disorder involving abnormal B cells.[9]

---

[9] MedlinePlus, "Waldenström Macroglobulinemia," National Institutes of Health (NIH), April 16, 2019. Available online. URL: https://medlineplus.gov/genetics/condition/waldenstrom-macroglobulinemia. Accessed June 5, 2023.

Chapter 16 | Myeloproliferative Disorders

Chapter Contents

Section 16.1 | Myelodysplastic Syndromes

WHAT ARE MYELODYSPLASTIC SYNDROMES?

Myelodysplastic syndromes (MDSs) are a group of cancers in which immature blood cells in the bone marrow do not mature or become healthy blood cells.

In a healthy person, the bone marrow makes blood stem cells (immature cells) that become mature blood cells over time.

A blood stem cell may become a lymphoid stem cell or a myeloid stem cell.

- A myeloid stem cell becomes one of three types of mature blood cells:
  - **Red blood cells (RBCs)**. RBCs carry oxygen and other substances to all tissues of the body.
  - **Granulocytes (WBCs)**. These cells fight infection and disease.
  - **Platelets**. These blood cells form blood clots to stop bleeding.
- A lymphoid stem cell becomes a white blood cell (WBC).

In a patient with an MDS, the blood stem cells (immature cells) do not become mature RBCs, WBCs, or platelets in the bone marrow. These immature blood cells, called "blasts," do not work the way they should and die either in the bone marrow or soon after they go into the blood. This leaves less room for healthy WBCs, RBCs, and platelets to form in the bone marrow. When there are fewer healthy blood cells, infection, anemia, or easy bleeding may occur.

TYPES OF MYELODYSPLASTIC SYNDROMES

The different types of MDSs are diagnosed based on certain changes in the blood cells and bone marrow:

- **Refractory anemia**. There are too few RBCs in the blood, and the patient has anemia. The number of WBCs and platelets is normal.
- **Refractory anemia with ring sideroblasts**. There are too few RBCs in the blood, and the patient has anemia. The RBCs have too much iron inside the cell. The number of WBCs and platelets is normal.

225

- **Refractory anemia with excess blasts**. There are too few RBCs in the blood, and the patient has anemia. Five to nineteen percent of the cells in the bone marrow are blasts. There may also be changes to the WBCs and platelets. Refractory anemia with excess blasts may progress to acute myeloid leukemia (AML).
- **Refractory cytopenia with multilineage dysplasia**. There are too few of at least two types of blood cells (RBCs, platelets, or WBCs). Less than 5 percent of the cells in the bone marrow are blasts, and less than 1 percent of the cells in the blood are blasts. If RBCs are affected, they may have extra iron. Refractory cytopenia may progress to AML.
- **Refractory cytopenia with unilineage dysplasia**. There are too few of one type of blood cell (RBCs, platelets, or WBCs). There are changes in 10 percent or more of two other types of blood cells. Less than 5 percent of the cells in the bone marrow are blasts, and less than 1 percent of the cells in the blood are blasts.
- **Unclassifiable MDSs**. The numbers of blasts in the bone marrow and blood are normal, and the disease is not one of the other MDS.
- **MDS associated with an isolated del(5q) chromosome abnormality**. There are too few RBCs in the blood, and the patient has anemia. Less than 5 percent of the cells in the bone marrow and blood are blasts. There is a specific change in the chromosome.
- **Chronic myelomonocytic leukemia (CMML)**. CMML is a slowly progressing type of myelodysplastic/ myeloproliferative disease in which too many myelomonocytes (a type of white blood cell) are in the bone marrow, crowding out other normal blood cells, such as other white blood cells, red blood cells, and platelets.

RISKS OF MYELODYSPLASTIC SYNDROMES

Age and past treatment with chemotherapy or radiation therapy affect the risk of an MDS.

Anything that increases a person's chance of getting a disease is called a "risk factor." Not every person with one or more of these risk factors will develop MDSs, and they will develop in people who do not have any known risk factors. Talk with your doctor if you think you may be at risk. Risk factors for MDSs include the following:

- past treatment with chemotherapy or radiation therapy for cancer
- being exposed to certain chemicals, including tobacco smoke, pesticides, fertilizers, and solvents such as benzene
- being exposed to heavy metals, such as mercury or lead

The cause of MDS in most patients is not known.

SIGNS AND SYMPTOMS OF MYELODYSPLASTIC SYNDROMES

Signs and symptoms of an MDS include shortness of breath and feeling tired.

MDSs often do not cause early signs or symptoms. They may be found during a routine blood test. Signs and symptoms may be caused by MDSs or by other conditions. Check with your doctor if you have any of the following symptoms:

- shortness of breath
- weakness or feeling tired
- having skin that is paler than usual
- easy bruising or bleeding
- petechiae (flat, pinpoint spots under the skin caused by bleeding)

DIAGNOSIS OF MYELODYSPLASTIC SYNDROMES

Tests that examine the blood and bone marrow are used to diagnose MDS.

In addition to asking about your personal and family health history and doing a physical exam, your doctor may perform the following tests and procedures:

- **Complete blood count (CBC) with differential**. This is a procedure in which a sample of blood is drawn and checked for the following:
  - the number of RBCs and platelets

- the number and type of WBCs
- the amount of hemoglobin (the protein that carries oxygen) in the RBCs
- the portion of the blood sample made up of RBCs
- **Peripheral blood smear**. This is a procedure in which a sample of blood is checked for changes in the number, type, shape, and size of blood cells and for too much iron in the RBCs.
- **Cytogenetic analysis**. This is a laboratory test in which the chromosomes of cells in a sample of the bone marrow or blood are counted and checked for any changes, such as broken, missing, rearranged, or extra chromosomes. Changes in certain chromosomes may be a sign of cancer. Cytogenetic analysis is used to help diagnose cancer, plan treatment, or find out how well treatment is working.
- **Blood chemistry studies**. This is a procedure in which a blood sample is checked to measure the amount of certain substances, such as vitamin B_{12} and folate, released into the blood by organs and tissues in the body. An unusual (higher or lower than normal) amount of a substance can be a sign of disease.
- **Bone marrow aspiration and biopsy**. This is the removal of the bone marrow, blood, and a small piece of bone by inserting a hollow needle into the hip bone or breastbone. A pathologist views the bone marrow, blood, and bone under a microscope to look for abnormal cells.

The following tests may be done on the sample of tissue that is removed:
- **Immunocytochemistry**. This is a laboratory test that uses antibodies to check for certain antigens (markers) in a sample of a patient's bone marrow. The antibodies are usually linked to an enzyme or a fluorescent dye. After the antibodies bind to the antigen in the sample of the patient's cells, the enzyme or dye is activated, and the antigen can then be seen under a microscope.

This type of test is used to help diagnose cancer and to tell the difference between MDSs, leukemia, and other conditions.

- **Immunophenotyping**. This is a laboratory test that uses antibodies to identify cancer cells based on the types of antigens or markers on the surface of the cells. This test is used to help diagnose specific types of leukemia and other blood disorders.
- **Flow cytometry**. This is a laboratory test that measures the number of cells in a sample, the percentage of live cells in a sample, and certain characteristics of the cells, such as size, shape, and the presence of tumor (or other) markers on the cell surface. The cells from a sample of a patient's blood, bone marrow, or other tissue are stained with a fluorescent dye, placed in a fluid, and then passed one at a time through a beam of light. The test results are based on how the cells that were stained with the fluorescent dye react to the beam of light. This test is used to help diagnose and manage certain types of cancers, such as leukemia and lymphoma.
- **Fluorescence in situ hybridization (FISH)**. This is a laboratory test used to look at and count genes or chromosomes in cells and tissues. Pieces of DNA that contain fluorescent dyes are made in the laboratory and added to a sample of a patient's cells or tissues. When these dyed pieces of DNA attach to certain genes or areas of chromosomes in the sample, they light up when viewed under a fluorescent microscope. The FISH test is used to help diagnose cancer and help plan treatment.

FACTORS AFFECTING PROGNOSIS AND TREATMENT OPTIONS
The prognosis and treatment options depend on the following:
- the number of blast cells in the bone marrow
- whether one or more types of blood cells are affected
- whether the patient has signs or symptoms of anemia, bleeding, or infection
- whether the patient has a low or high risk of leukemia
- certain changes in the chromosomes

- whether the MDS occurred after chemotherapy or radiation therapy for cancer
- the patient's age and general health[1]

Section 16.2 | Myelodysplastic/Myeloproliferative Neoplasms

WHAT ARE MYELODYSPLASTIC/ MYELOPROLIFERATIVE NEOPLASMS?

Myelodysplastic/myeloproliferative neoplasms are a group of diseases in which the bone marrow makes too many white blood cells (WBCs).

Normally, the bone marrow makes blood stem cells (immature cells) that become mature blood cells over time. A blood stem cell may become a myeloid stem cell or a lymphoid stem cell.

- A myeloid stem cell becomes one of three types of mature blood cells:
  - **Red blood cells (RBCs)**. RBCs carry oxygen and other substances to all tissues of the body.
  - **Granulocytes (WBCs)**. These cells fight infection and disease.
  - **Platelets**. These blood cells form blood clots to stop bleeding.
- A lymphoid stem cell becomes a WBC.

Myelodysplastic/myeloproliferative neoplasms have features of both myelodysplastic syndromes and myeloproliferative neoplasms.

In myelodysplastic diseases, the blood stem cells do not mature into healthy RBCs, WBCs, or platelets. The immature blood cells, called "blasts," do not work the way they should and die in the bone marrow or soon after they enter the blood. As a result, there are fewer healthy RBCs, WBCs, and platelets.

---

[1] "Myelodysplastic Syndromes Treatment (PDQ®)—Patient Version," National Cancer Institute (NCI), March 31, 2023. Available online. URL: www.cancer.gov/types/myeloproliferative/patient/myelodysplastic-treatment-pdq. Accessed June 5, 2023.

In myeloproliferative diseases, a greater-than-normal number of blood stem cells become one or more types of blood cells, and the total number of blood cells slowly increases.

TYPES OF MYELODYSPLASTIC/MYELOPROLIFERATIVE NEOPLASMS

The following are the three main types of myelodysplastic/myeloproliferative neoplasms:

- chronic myelomonocytic leukemia (CMML)
- juvenile myelomonocytic leukemia (JMML)
- atypical chronic myelogenous leukemia (CML)

When a myelodysplastic/myeloproliferative neoplasm does not match any of these types, it is called "myelodysplastic/myeloproliferative neoplasm, unclassifiable" (MDS/MPN-UC).

Myelodysplastic/myeloproliferative neoplasms may progress to acute leukemia.

DIAGNOSIS OF MYELODYSPLASTIC/ MYELOPROLIFERATIVE NEOPLASMS

Tests that examine the blood and bone marrow are used to diagnose myelodysplastic/myeloproliferative neoplasms.

The following tests and procedures may be used:

- **Physical exam and health history**. This is an exam of the body to check general signs of health, including checking for signs of disease, such as an enlarged spleen and liver. A history of the patient's health habits and past illnesses and treatments will also be taken.
- **Complete blood count (CBC) with differential**. This is a procedure in which a sample of blood is drawn and checked for the following:
  - the number of RBCs and platelets
  - the number and type of WBCs
  - the amount of hemoglobin (the protein that carries oxygen) in the RBCs
  - the portion of the sample made up of RBCs
- **Peripheral blood smear**. This is a procedure in which a sample of blood is checked for blast cells, the number

and kinds of WBCs, the number of platelets, and changes in the shape of blood cells.

- **Blood chemistry studies**. This is a procedure in which a blood sample is checked to measure the amount of certain substances released into the blood by organs and tissues in the body. An unusual (higher or lower than normal) amount of a substance can be a sign of disease.
- **Bone marrow aspiration and biopsy**. This is the removal of a small piece of bone and bone marrow by inserting a needle into the hip bone or breastbone. A pathologist views both the bone and bone marrow samples under a microscope to look for abnormal cells.

The following tests may be done on the sample of tissue that is removed:

- **Cytogenetic analysis**. This is a laboratory test in which the chromosomes of cells in a sample of the bone marrow or blood are counted and checked for any changes, such as broken, missing, rearranged, or extra chromosomes. Changes in certain chromosomes may be a sign of cancer. Cytogenetic analysis is used to help diagnose cancer, plan treatment, or find out how well treatment is working. The cancer cells in myelodysplastic/myeloproliferative neoplasms do not contain the Philadelphia chromosome that is present in chronic myelogenous leukemia.
- **Immunocytochemistry**. This is a laboratory test that uses antibodies to check for certain antigens (markers) in a sample of a patient's bone marrow. The antibodies are usually linked to an enzyme or a fluorescent dye. After the antibodies bind to the antigen in the sample of the patient's bone marrow, the enzyme or dye is activated, and the antigen can then be seen under a microscope. This type of test is used to help diagnose cancer and to tell the difference between myelodysplastic/myeloproliferative neoplasms, leukemia, and other conditions.

TREATMENT FOR MYELODYSPLASTIC/ MYELOPROLIFERATIVE NEOPLASMS

There are different types of treatment for patients with myelodysplastic/myeloproliferative neoplasms. The following five types of standard treatments are used:

- chemotherapy
- other drug therapy
- stem cell transplant
- supportive care
- targeted therapy

New types of treatment are being tested in clinical trials. Treatment for myelodysplastic/myeloproliferative neoplasms may cause side effects.

Patients may want to think about taking part in a clinical trial. Patients can enter clinical trials before, during, or after starting their cancer treatment. Follow-up tests may be needed.[2]

Section 16.3 | Chronic Myeloproliferative Neoplasms

WHAT ARE CHRONIC MYELOPROLIFERATIVE NEOPLASMS?

Chronic myeloproliferative neoplasms (MPNs) are a group of diseases in which the bone marrow makes too many red blood cells (RBCs), white blood cells (WBCs), or platelets.

Normally, the bone marrow makes blood stem cells (immature cells) that become mature blood cells over time.

A blood stem cell may become a myeloid stem cell or a lymphoid stem cell.

- A myeloid stem cell becomes one of three types of mature blood cells:
  - **RBCs.** These blood cells carry oxygen and other substances to all tissues of the body.

[2] "Myelodysplastic/Myeloproliferative Neoplasms Treatment (PDQ®)—Patient Version," National Cancer Institute (NCI), March 4, 2022. Available online. URL: www.cancer.gov/types/myeloproliferative/patient/mds-mpd-treatment-pdq#_1. Accessed June 5, 2023.

- **Granulocytes (WBCs).** These cells fight infection and disease.
- **Platelets.** These blood cells form blood clots to stop bleeding.
- A lymphoid stem cell becomes a WBC.

In chronic MPNs, too many blood stem cells become one or more types of blood cells. The neoplasms usually get worse slowly as the number of extra blood cells increases.

TYPES OF CHRONIC MYELOPROLIFERATIVE NEOPLASMS

The type of chronic MPN is based on whether too many RBCs, WBCs, or platelets are being made. Sometimes, the body will make too many of more than one type of blood cell, but usually one type of blood cell is affected more than the others. The following are the six types of chronic MPNs:

- chronic myelogenous leukemia
- polycythemia vera
- primary myelofibrosis (also called "chronic idiopathic myelofibrosis")
- essential thrombocythemia
- chronic neutrophilic leukemia
- chronic eosinophilic leukemia

Chronic MPNs sometimes become acute leukemia, in which too many abnormal WBCs are made.

DIAGNOSIS OF CHRONIC MYELOPROLIFERATIVE NEOPLASMS

Tests that examine the blood and bone marrow are used to diagnose chronic MPNs.

The following tests and procedures may be used:

- **Physical exam and health history.** This is an exam of the body to check general signs of health, including checking for signs of disease, such as lumps or anything else that seems unusual. A history of the patient's health habits and past illnesses and treatments will also be taken.

- **Complete blood count (CBC) with differential**. This is a procedure in which a sample of blood is drawn and checked for the following:
  - the number of RBCs and platelets
  - the number and type of WBCs
  - the amount of hemoglobin (the protein that carries oxygen) in the RBCs
  - the portion of the blood sample made up of RBCs
- **Peripheral blood smear**. This is a procedure in which a sample of blood is checked for the following:
  - whether there are RBCs shaped like teardrops
  - the number and kinds of WBCs
  - the number of platelets
  - whether there are blast cells
- **Blood chemistry study**. This is a procedure in which a blood sample is checked to measure the amount of certain substances released into the blood by organs and tissues in the body. An unusual (higher or lower than normal) amount of a substance can be a sign of disease.
- **Bone marrow aspiration and biopsy**. This is the removal of bone marrow, blood, and a small piece of bone by inserting a hollow needle into the hip bone or breastbone. A pathologist views the bone marrow, blood, and bone under a microscope to look for abnormal cells.
- **Cytogenetic analysis**. This is a laboratory test in which the chromosomes of cells in a sample of bone marrow or blood are counted and checked for any changes, such as broken, missing, rearranged, or extra chromosomes. Changes in certain chromosomes may be a sign of cancer. Cytogenetic analysis is used to help diagnose cancer, plan treatment, or find out how well treatment is working.
- **Gene mutation test**. This is a laboratory test done on a bone marrow or blood sample to check for mutations in *JAK2*, *MPL*, or *CALR* genes. A *JAK2* gene mutation

235

is often found in patients with polycythemia vera, essential thrombocythemia, or primary myelofibrosis. *MPL* or *CALR* gene mutations are found in patients with essential thrombocythemia or primary myelofibrosis.[3]

Section 16.4 | Polycythemia Vera

Polycythemia vera is a condition characterized by an increased number of red blood cells (RBCs) in the bloodstream. Affected individuals may also have excess white blood cells (WBCs) and blood clotting cells called "platelets." These extra cells and platelets cause the blood to be thicker than normal. As a result, abnormal blood clots are more likely to form and block the flow of blood through arteries and veins. Polycythemia vera typically develops in adulthood, around the age of 60, although in rare cases, it occurs in children and young adults.

CAUSES OF POLYCYTHEMIA VERA

Mutations in the *JAK2* and *TET2* genes are associated with polycythemia vera. Although it remains unclear exactly what initiates polycythemia vera, researchers believe that it begins when mutations occur in the deoxyribonucleic acid (DNA) of a hematopoietic stem cell. These stem cells are located in the bone marrow and have the potential to develop into RBCs, WBCs, and platelets. *JAK2* gene mutations seem to be particularly important for the development of polycythemia vera, as nearly all affected individuals have a mutation in this gene. The *JAK2* gene provides instructions for making a protein that promotes the growth and division (proliferation) of cells. The JAK2 protein is especially important for controlling the production of blood cells from hematopoietic stem cells.

---

[3] "Chronic Myeloproliferative Neoplasms Treatment (PDQ®)—Patient Version," National Cancer Institute (NCI), January 11, 2023. Available online. URL: www.cancer.gov/types/myeloproliferative/patient/chronic-treatment-pdq#_1. Accessed June 5, 2023.

JAK2 gene mutations result in the production of a JAK2 protein that is constantly turned on (constitutively activated), which increases the production of blood cells and prolongs their survival. With so many extra cells in the bloodstream, abnormal blood clots are more likely to form. Thicker blood also flows more slowly throughout the body, which prevents organs from receiving enough oxygen. Many of the signs and symptoms of polycythemia vera are related to a shortage of oxygen in body tissues.

The function of the *TET2* gene is unknown. Although mutations in the *TET2* gene have been found in approximately 16 percent of people with polycythemia vera, it is unclear what role these mutations play in the development of the condition.

RISK FACTORS OF POLYCYTHEMIA VERA

Individuals with polycythemia vera have an increased risk of deep vein thrombosis (DVT), a type of blood clot that occurs in the deep veins of the arms or legs. If a DVT travels through the bloodstream and lodges in the lungs, it can cause a life-threatening clot known as a "pulmonary embolism" (PE). Affected individuals also have an increased risk of heart attack and stroke caused by blood clots in the heart and brain.

SYMPTOMS OF POLYCYTHEMIA VERA

This condition may not cause any symptoms in its early stages. Some people with polycythemia vera experience headaches, dizziness, ringing in the ears (tinnitus), impaired vision, or itchy skin. Affected individuals frequently have reddened skin because of the extra RBCs. Other complications of polycythemia vera include an enlarged spleen (splenomegaly), stomach ulcers, gout (a form of arthritis caused by a buildup of uric acid in the joints), heart disease, and cancer of blood-forming cells (leukemia).

FREQUENCY OF POLYCYTHEMIA VERA

The prevalence of polycythemia vera varies worldwide. The condition affects an estimated 44–57 per 100,000 individuals in the

United States. For unknown reasons, men develop polycythemia vera more frequently than women.

INHERITANCE OF POLYCYTHEMIA VERA

Most cases of polycythemia vera are not inherited. This condition is associated with genetic changes that are somatic, which means they are acquired during a person's lifetime and are present only in certain cells.

In rare instances, polycythemia vera has been found to run in families. In some of these families, the risk of developing polycythemia vera appears to have an autosomal dominant pattern of inheritance. Autosomal dominant inheritance means that one copy of an altered gene in each cell is sufficient to increase the risk of developing polycythemia vera although the cause of this condition in familial cases is unknown. In these families, people seem to inherit an increased risk of polycythemia vera, not the disease itself.[4]

Section 16.5 | Thrombocythemia and Thrombocytosis

WHAT ARE THROMBOCYTHEMIA AND THROMBOCYTOSIS?

Thrombocythemia and thrombocytosis are conditions that occur when your blood has a higher-than-normal platelet count.

Platelets are tiny blood cells. They are made in your bone marrow along with other kinds of blood cells. When you are injured, platelets stick together to form a plug that seals your wound. This plug is called a "blood clot." Platelets are also called "thrombocytes" because a blood clot is also called a "thrombus." If your platelet count is too high, blood clots can form in your blood vessels. This can block blood flow through your body.

[4] MedlinePlus, "Polycythemia Vera," National Institutes of Health (NIH), July 1, 2013. Available online. URL: https://medlineplus.gov/genetics/condition/polycythemia-vera. Accessed May 12, 2023.

- Thrombocythemia refers to a high platelet count that is not caused by another health condition. This condition is sometimes called "primary" or "essential" thrombocythemia.
- Thrombocytosis refers to a high platelet count caused by another disease or condition. This condition is often called "secondary" or "reactive" thrombocytosis. Thrombocytosis is more common than thrombocythemia.

WHAT CAUSES THROMBOCYTHEMIA?

Thrombocythemia occurs when faulty cells in your bone marrow make too many platelets. Your platelets also do not work properly. The bone marrow is the sponge-like tissue inside the bones. It contains stem cells that develop into platelets and other blood cells. With primary thrombocythemia, a high platelet count may happen alone or with other blood cell disorders. This condition is not common.

Thrombocythemia is most often caused by your genes. Mutations, or changes, in the genes that control how your bone marrow forms platelets may cause thrombocythemia. Examples of such genes include *JAK2*, *CALR*, and *MPL*. Thrombocythemia can be inherited. This means the condition can be passed from parents to children.

Primary thrombocythemia is more common in people aged 50–70, but it can occur at any age. It is more common in women than in men.

WHAT CAUSES THROMBOCYTOSIS?

Thrombocytosis occurs when another disease or condition causes you to have a high platelet count. People who have thrombocytosis have normal platelets and a lower risk of blood clots and bleeding than people who have thrombocythemia. Thrombocytosis is more common than thrombocythemia.

Some conditions that can raise your risk of thrombocytosis are as follows:

- **Anemia**. Iron deficiency anemia and hemolytic anemia can cause thrombocytosis.

- **Cancer**. Many people who have high platelet counts also have cancer—mostly lung, gastrointestinal, breast, or ovarian cancer or lymphoma. Sometimes, a high platelet count is the first sign of cancer.
- **Surgery to remove your spleen**. The spleen is an organ in your upper left abdomen. Normally, your spleen stores platelets. Removing your spleen can raise your platelet count.
- **Inflammation or infections**. Conditions such as connective tissue disorders, inflammatory bowel disease, and tuberculosis (TB) can raise your platelet count.

Your platelet count may be high for only a short time. This can be caused by the following:
- recovery from serious blood loss
- recovery from a very low platelet count caused by drinking too much alcohol and having low levels of vitamin B_{12} or folate
- acute (short-term) infection or inflammation

WHAT HEALTH PROBLEMS CAN THROMBOCYTHEMIA AND THROMBOCYTOSIS CAUSE?

Thrombocythemia and thrombocytosis may cause blood clots, which can block blood flow to your organs. This can lead to the following serious complications:
- venous thromboembolism (VTE)
- stroke and transient ischemic attacks (TIAs)
- reduced blood flow to your heart, which can cause a heart attack
- pregnancy complications

Thrombocytopenia and thrombocytosis can also cause your bone marrow to become scarred or to produce too many blood cells. This may lead to some types of leukemia.

WHAT ARE THE SYMPTOMS OF THROMBOCYTHEMIA AND THROMBOCYTOSIS?

Many people who have thrombocythemia or thrombocytosis do not have symptoms. These conditions might be discovered only after routine blood tests.

The symptoms of a high platelet count are linked to blood clots and bleeding. These symptoms are more common in people who have thrombocythemia.

Blood Clots

In thrombocythemia, blood clots most often develop in the brain, hands, and feet. But the clots can develop anywhere in the body. Blood clots in the brain may cause chronic (long-term) headaches and dizziness. In extreme cases, you may have a TIA or a stroke.

You may have blood clots in the tiny blood vessels of your hands and feet. This can make your hands and feet numb and red. You may have a burning feeling and throbbing pain, mostly in the palms of your hands and the soles of your feet.

Other symptoms of a blood clot are as follows:
- confusion or changes in speech
- migraines
- seizures
- upper body discomfort in one or both of your arms, back, neck, jaw, or abdomen
- shortness of breath and nausea (feeling sick to your stomach)
- weakness
- chest pain
- pregnancy complications

You may also have a spleen that is larger than normal.

You may have a higher chance of a blood clot if you are older, have had blood clots in the past, smoke, or have other health conditions, such as diabetes and high blood pressure (HBP).

241

Bleeding

Bleeding can happen in people who have a very high platelet count. You may have nosebleeds, bruising, bleeding from your mouth or gums, or blood in your stool.

Bleeding occurs when blood clots that develop in thrombocythemia or thrombocytosis use up your body's platelets. This means that not enough platelets are left in your bloodstream to seal off cuts or breaks on the blood vessel walls. Bleeding can also happen if your platelets do not work properly.

Another cause of bleeding in people who have very high platelet counts is a condition called "von Willebrand disease" (VWD). This condition affects how your blood clots.

HOW ARE THROMBOCYTHEMIA AND THROMBOCYTOSIS DIAGNOSED?

To diagnose thrombocythemia or thrombocytosis, your provider will ask about your medical and family history. They will ask about your symptoms and do a physical exam to look for signs of blood clots or bleeding.

Your provider may also order one or more of the following tests:

- **Complete blood count (CBC)**. A CBC measures the levels of red blood cells (RBCs), white blood cells (WBCs), and platelets in your blood.
- **Blood smear**. For this test, some of your blood is put on a slide. A microscope is used to look at your platelets and other blood cells.
- **Bone marrow tests**. These tests check whether your bone marrow is healthy.
- **Genetic testing**. This test checks for mutations, or changes, in genes that control how your body makes platelets.

HOW ARE THROMBOCYTHEMIA AND THROMBOCYTOSIS TREATED?

People who have thrombocythemia with no symptoms often do not need treatment. Other people who have this condition may need medicines or procedures to treat it. Treatment does not cure your condition, but it can help prevent blood clots and serious complications.

Treatment for secondary thrombocytosis depends on its cause. People who have thrombocytosis usually do not need platelet-lowering medicines or procedures. This is because their platelets are usually normal and less likely to cause serious blood clots or bleeding.

Treatment for thrombocythemia may include medicines and procedures.

Medicines to Lower Platelet Counts

You may need one of the following medicines to lower your platelet count:

- **Anagrelide**. This medicine is used to lower platelet counts. It is mostly used when hydroxyurea does not work. Anagrelide also has side effects, such as fluid retention, palpitations, arrhythmias, heart failure, and headaches.
- **Aspirin**. This medicine helps prevent blood clots. It is mostly used in people who have a low risk of blood clots. If you have a high risk of blood clots, you may need to take both aspirin and hydroxyurea.
- **Hydroxyurea**. This platelet-lowering medicine is used to treat cancers and sickle cell disease (SCD), for example.
- **Interferon alfa**. This medicine lowers platelet counts, but it can have serious side effects. Side effects may include a flu-like feeling, decreased appetite, nausea (feeling sick to the stomach), diarrhea, seizures, irritability, and sleepiness.

Procedures

Plateletpheresis is a procedure used to quickly lower your platelet count. This procedure is mostly used for emergencies. For example, if you are having a stroke due to primary thrombocythemia, you may need plateletpheresis.

An intravenous (IV) needle that is connected to a tube is placed in one of your blood vessels to remove blood. The blood goes through a machine that removes platelets from the blood. The remaining blood is then put back into you through an IV line in one of your blood vessels.[5]

[5] "Thrombocythemia and Thrombocytosis," National Heart, Lung, and Blood Institute (NHLBI), March 24, 2022. Available online. URL: www.nhlbi.nih.gov/health/thrombocythemia-thrombocytosis. Accessed May 12, 2023.

Chapter 17 | **Plasma Cell Disorders**

Chapter Contents

WHAT IS AMYLOIDOSIS?

Amyloidosis is a rare disease that occurs when amyloid proteins are deposited in tissues and organs. Amyloid proteins are abnormal proteins the body cannot break down and recycle as it does with normal proteins. When amyloid proteins clump together, they form amyloid deposits. The buildup of these deposits damages organs and tissues.

Amyloidosis can affect different organs and tissues in different people, and it can affect more than one organ at the same time. The symptoms and severity of amyloidosis depend on which organs and tissues are affected. Amyloidosis most frequently affects the kidneys, heart, nervous system, liver, and gastrointestinal tract.

WHAT ARE THE TYPES OF KIDNEY-RELATED AMYLOIDOSIS?

The following four types of amyloidosis most often affect the kidneys:

- **Immunoglobulin light-chain amyloidosis (AL amyloidosis), or primary amyloidosis**. AL amyloidosis affects the kidneys in about two out of three people with this condition.
- **Amyloid A amyloidosis (AA amyloidosis), or secondary amyloidosis**. AA amyloidosis is often associated with certain chronic inflammatory conditions.
- **Leukocyte cell–derived chemotaxin 2 (LECT2) amyloidosis**. LECT2 amyloidosis is a recently discovered form of amyloidosis that most often affects the kidneys and liver.
- **Hereditary amyloidosis**. This amyloidosis can be passed down from a parent to a child through rare gene mutations.

Some people with kidney failure may experience another type of amyloidosis, known as "dialysis-related amyloidosis." This type can affect people receiving dialysis treatment—either hemodialysis or peritoneal dialysis—to treat kidney failure. Dialysis-related amyloidosis causes amyloid proteins to build up in bones, joints, and tendons.

WHAT CAUSES KIDNEY-RELATED AMYLOIDOSIS?

Amyloidosis is caused by an abnormal folding of proteins. These proteins can clump together and form amyloid deposits. The deposits collect in organs and tissues and may lead to organ damage and health problems, including kidney disease. Experts have identified more than 30 different proteins that can form amyloid.

Immunoglobulin Light-Chain Amyloidosis

Plasma cells—a type of blood cell made by stem cells in your bone marrow—can produce abnormal proteins that cannot hold their shape. These abnormal proteins clump together, causing AL amyloidosis.

Amyloid A Amyloidosis

Long-lasting infections or chronic inflammatory conditions, such as rheumatoid arthritis, inflammatory bowel disease, familial Mediterranean fever, and tuberculosis, can trigger a protein to build up and cause AA amyloidosis.

Leukocyte Cell–Derived Chemotaxin 2 Amyloidosis

Researchers do not know exactly what causes the LECT2 protein to form amyloid.

Hereditary Amyloidosis

Genetic mutations passed down in families can cause your body—most often, your liver—to produce amyloid proteins. The amyloid proteins collect in certain parts of your body, such as the kidneys, and cause damage. There are many different types of hereditary amyloidosis, each associated with a different gene mutation and type of protein.

Dialysis-Related Amyloidosis

Dialysis does not remove enough of a protein called "beta-2 micro-globulin" from the blood. Over time, this protein can build up and deposit in bones, joints, and tendons, leading to dialysis-related amyloidosis.

WHO IS MORE LIKELY TO DEVELOP KIDNEY-RELATED AMYLOIDOSIS?

The risk factors for kidney-related amyloidosis depend on the type of amyloidosis.

Immunoglobulin Light-Chain Amyloidosis

AL amyloidosis is most common in people over the age of 65, and the risk of developing AL amyloidosis increases as you get older.

Amyloid A Amyloidosis

AA amyloidosis is most common in people who have experienced a long-lasting infection or chronic inflammatory disorder.

Leukocyte Cell–Derived Chemotaxin 2 Amyloidosis

LECT2 amyloidosis is most common in Hispanic adults, particularly those of Mexican descent.

Hereditary Amyloidosis

Hereditary amyloidosis is more common in people who have a family member with the condition.

Dialysis-Related Amyloidosis

The risk of developing dialysis-related amyloidosis increases the longer you have been on dialysis, the older you are at the start of dialysis treatment, and the more your kidney function has declined.

WHAT ARE THE SYMPTOMS OF KIDNEY-RELATED AMYLOIDOSIS?

When amyloidosis affects your kidneys, the most common symptom is nephrotic syndrome—a group of symptoms that indicate kidney damage. These symptoms include:
- too much protein in your urine
- low levels of protein in your blood
- swelling in parts of your body
- high levels of cholesterol and other fats in your blood

Other signs and symptoms of amyloidosis may include:
- anemia
- fatigue or tiredness
- inflammation in the hands or numbness, tingling, or burning sensation in the hands or feet
- low blood pressure
- shortness of breath
- weight loss

When amyloidosis affects your bones, joints, and tendons—as it does in dialysis-related amyloidosis—symptoms may include:
- bone cysts
- carpal tunnel syndrome (CTS)
- joint pain or stiffness

WHAT ARE THE COMPLICATIONS OF KIDNEY-RELATED AMYLOIDOSIS?

Amyloid that builds up in the kidneys can damage the kidneys and affect the kidneys' ability to filter blood. This damage can cause wastes to build up in your body, which may worsen kidney damage and lead to kidney failure.

HOW DO HEALTH-CARE PROFESSIONALS DIAGNOSE KIDNEY-RELATED AMYLOIDOSIS?

Health-care professionals use your medical and family history, a physical exam, and one or more tests to confirm your diagnosis of amyloidosis, identify the type of amyloidosis, and determine treatment.

What Tests Do Health-Care Professionals Use to Diagnose Kidney-Related Amyloidosis?

Your health-care professional may use one or more of the following tests to diagnose amyloidosis.

LAB TESTS

- **Urinalysis**. This test is used to look for amyloid proteins in the urine and to check for kidney damage.
- **Blood tests**. These tests are used to look for amyloid proteins in the blood and to check how well your kidneys are working.
- **Kidney biopsy**. A kidney biopsy may be performed to look for amyloid deposits in kidney tissue and help identify the type of amyloidosis.

Depending on your symptoms, your health-care professional may suggest other lab tests.

IMAGING TESTS

Health-care professionals may use imaging tests to check for signs of dialysis-related amyloidosis, such as bone cysts, bone lesions, and amyloid deposits in or between bones, joints, tendons, and ligaments.

- **X-rays**. These use a small amount of radiation to create pictures of the inside of your body.
- **Computed tomography (CT) scans.** CT scans use a combination of x-rays and computer technology to create images of the inside of your body.
- **Magnetic resonance imaging (MRI).** MRI uses a magnetic field and radio waves—without radiation—to make pictures of your organs and soft tissues inside your body.
- **Ultrasound.** This uses sound waves to look at structures inside your body.

GENETIC TESTS

Genetic testing can be used to look for specific gene mutations that are known to cause amyloidosis. Your health-care professional may use genetic testing to help identify the type of amyloidosis you have.

251

HOW DO HEALTH-CARE PROFESSIONALS TREAT KIDNEY-RELATED AMYLOIDOSIS?

Treatment for amyloidosis varies depending on the type of amyloidosis you have. Your treatment will focus on slowing the production of amyloid and treating the symptoms of organ damage.

Treatments for amyloidosis can ease your symptoms and improve your quality of life, but there is no cure for the condition.

Immunoglobulin Light-Chain Amyloidosis

Treatment for AL amyloidosis focuses on destroying the abnormal cells responsible for forming amyloid proteins.

- **Chemotherapy treatment**. Your health-care team may prescribe one or more of the following medicines—in some cases, the entire four-drug combination—to help slow or stop the growth of abnormal cells:
    - alkylating agents
    - corticosteroids
    - proteasome inhibitors
    - immunomodulators
- **Autologous stem cell transplant**. An autologous stem cell transplant uses your body's healthy stem cells to replace your damaged stem cells. The healthy stem cells are removed from your blood and stored while you receive chemotherapy treatment to destroy the abnormal stem cells. The healthy stem cells are then put back into your body.

Amyloid A Amyloidosis

Health-care professionals treat AA amyloidosis by treating the underlying chronic inflammatory condition that is causing amyloid buildup in your body.

- **Medicines**. Your health-care professional may prescribe medicines to decrease inflammation, including:
    - biologic agents, such as tumor necrosis factor blockers
    - monoclonal antibodies

- corticosteroids
- nonsteroidal anti-inflammatory drugs (NSAIDs)
- dietary supplements, such as fish oil

Your health-care professional may prescribe antibiotics to help fight infection.

Leukocyte Cell–Derived Chemotaxin 2 Amyloidosis
Researchers have not found a way to treat LECT2 amyloidosis, but your health-care professional may suggest treatments to control your kidney disease and ease symptoms.

Dialysis-Related Amyloidosis
Treatment for dialysis-related amyloidosis focuses on reducing the levels of amyloid in the blood so that less amyloid is deposited in organ tissues.
- **Kidney transplant**. A working transplanted kidney does a better job of preventing amyloid proteins from building up in the blood than dialysis treatment. Some people with kidney failure may be able to have a kidney transplant. However, a kidney transplant is not for everyone.

Hereditary Amyloidosis
Treatment for hereditary amyloidosis focuses on slowing or stopping the production of amyloid. The amyloid protein that causes hereditary amyloidosis is most often produced in the liver. The amyloid is then deposited in other parts of the body, such as the kidneys, heart, and nerves.
- **Liver transplant**. Surgery to remove a diseased liver and replace it with a healthy liver may slow down or stop the progression of amyloidosis. However, a liver transplant is not for everyone. Talk with your health-care professional about whether a liver transplant is right for you.

HOW DO HEALTH-CARE PROFESSIONALS TREAT COMPLICATIONS OF AMYLOIDOSIS?

Your health-care professional may suggest one or more of the following treatments to control your kidney disease and ease your symptoms.

Medicines

Medicines to manage your kidney disease can help you feel better.
- **Angiotensin-converting enzyme (ACE) inhibitors or angiotensin receptor blockers (ARBs)**. ACE and ARBs can lower your blood pressure and slow the progression of kidney disease.
- **Diuretics**. These help the kidneys remove fluid from the blood and reduce swelling in your body.
- **Iron supplements and erythropoiesis-stimulating agents**. These can help your body make more red blood cells and improve anemia.

Kidney Replacement Therapy

When amyloid builds up in the kidneys, the kidneys may become so damaged that they fail. If your kidneys fail, you may consider kidney replacement therapy—hemodialysis, peritoneal dialysis, or a kidney transplant—to help you feel better and live longer.

Surgery

Your health-care professional may suggest surgery to reduce pain and allow your joints to work better. Surgery can also be used to remove tumors or tissue damaged by amyloid deposits.

Supportive Care

Your health-care team may suggest healthy ways to manage stress, such as staying physically active, getting enough sleep, and talking about your feelings with family, friends, or a health-care professional.

CAN YOU PREVENT AMYLOIDOSIS?

Most types of amyloidosis are not preventable, but managing your kidney disease may help you delay or avoid kidney failure.

You may be able to prevent AA amyloidosis if your chronic inflammatory condition is treated early and the inflammation is kept under control. If you have familial Mediterranean fever, your health-care professional may use a medicine called "colchicine" to treat the inflammation and help prevent AA amyloidosis from developing.

HOW DO EATING, DIET, AND NUTRITION AFFECT AMYLOIDOSIS?

Eating, diet, and nutrition have not been shown to play a role in preventing or treating amyloidosis. However, if your kidneys are damaged, you may need to change what you eat to manage your kidney disease. For example, people with kidney disease should limit the amounts of protein, sodium, and phosphorus in their diets. Work with your health-care professional or a registered dietitian to develop a meal plan that includes foods you enjoy eating while maintaining your kidney health.[1]

Section 17.2 | Simple Cryoglobulinemia

Simple cryoglobulinemia occurs when the body makes an abnormal immune system protein called a "cryoglobulin." At temperatures less than 98.6 °F (37 °C; normal body temperature), cryoglobulins become solid or gel-like and can block blood vessels. This causes a variety of health problems.

---

[1] "Amyloidosis & Kidney Disease," National Institute of Diabetes and Digestive and Kidney Diseases (NIDDK), February 2022. Available online. URL: www.niddk.nih.gov/health-information/kidney-disease/amyloidosis. Accessed May 12, 2023.

CAUSES OF SIMPLE CRYOGLOBULINEMIA

The underlying cause is unknown. Simple cryoglobulinemia is typically associated with immune system cancers, such as multiple myeloma or non-Hodgkin lymphoma (NHL).

SYMPTOMS OF SIMPLE CRYOGLOBULINEMIA

Many people with cryoglobulins will not experience any symptoms. The following symptoms have been linked to this disease:

- abnormality of blood and blood-forming tissues (an abnormality of the hematopoietic system)
- purpura (It is the appearance of red or purple discolorations on the skin that do not blanch on applying pressure. They are caused by bleeding underneath the skin. This term refers to an abnormally increased susceptibility to developing purpura. Purpura is larger than petechiae.)
- acral ulceration (a type of digital ulcer that manifests as an open sore on the surface of the skin at the tip of a finger or toe)
- distal peripheral sensory neuropathy
- fatigue (a subjective feeling of tiredness characterized by a lack of energy and motivation)
- localized skin lesion (a lesion of the skin that is located in a specific region rather than being generalized)
- multiple mononeuropathy (a type of peripheral neuropathy that happens when there is damage to two or more different nerve areas characterized by peripheral neuropathy of both the motor and sensory nerves of at least two different nerve trunks, in which different nerves are affected either simultaneously or sequentially)
- peripheral neuropathy (It is a term for any disorder of the peripheral nervous system. The main clinical features used to classify peripheral neuropathy are distribution, type (mainly demyelinating versus mainly axonal), duration, and course.)

- Raynaud phenomenon (It is a condition that causes the blood vessels in the extremities to narrow, restricting blood flow. The episodes or "attacks" usually affect the fingers and toes.)
- sensorimotor neuropathy (a rare, genetic, demyelinating hereditary motor and sensory neuropathy disorder characterized by slowly progressive, mild-to-moderate, distal muscle weakness and atrophy of the upper and lower limbs and variable distal sensory impairment associated with variable hyperextensible skin and age-related macular degeneration)
- abnormality of the kidney
- arthralgia (joint pain)
- arthritis (inflammation of a joint)
- B-cell lymphoma (a type of lymphoma that originates in B-cells)
- hypertension
- membranoproliferative glomerulonephritis (It is a type of glomerulonephritis characterized by diffuse mesangial cell proliferation and the thickening of capillary walls due to subendothelial extension of the mesangium. The term membranoproliferative glomerulonephritis is often employed to denote a general pattern of glomerular injury seen in a variety of disease processes that share a common pathogenetic mechanism, rather than to describe a single disease entity.)
- mesangial hypercellularity (increased numbers of mesangial cells per glomerulus, defined as more than three nuclei fully surrounded by the matrix in one or more mesangial areas, not including perihilar region, on a standard 3-micron-thick tissue section, best evaluated on periodic acid–Schiff (PAS) stain)
- multiple myeloma (a malignant plasma cell tumor growing within the soft tissue or within the skeleton)
- paresthesia (abnormal sensations such as tingling, pricking, or numbness of the skin with no apparent physical cause)

- renal insufficiency (a reduction in the level of performance of the kidneys in areas of function comprising the concentration of urine, removal of wastes, the maintenance of electrolyte balance, homeostasis of blood pressure, and calcium metabolism)
- spontaneous pain sensation (a kind of neuropathic pain that occurs without an identifiable trigger)
- vascular skin abnormality
- vasculitis (inflammation of blood vessels)
- weight loss
- abdominal pain (an unpleasant sensation characterized by physical discomfort (such as pricking, throbbing, or aching) and perceived to originate in the abdomen)
- abnormal heart morphology (any structural anomaly of the heart)
- abnormal lung morphology (any structural anomaly of the lung)
- abnormality of the gastrointestinal tract (an abnormality of the gastrointestinal tract)
- chronic lymphatic leukemia (A chronic lymphocytic/lymphatic/lymphoblastic leukemia (CLL) is a neoplastic disease characterized by proliferation and accumulation (blood, marrow, and lymphoid organs) of morphologically mature but immunologically dysfunctional lymphocytes. A CLL is always a B-cell lymphocytic leukemia, as there are no reports of cases of T-cell lymphocytic leukemias.)
- complement deficiency (an immunodeficiency defined by the absent or suboptimal functioning of one of the complement system proteins)
- congestive heart failure (The presence of an abnormality of cardiac function is responsible for the failure of the heart to pump blood at a rate that is commensurate with the needs of the tissues or a state in which abnormally elevated filling pressures are required for the heart to do so. Heart failure

is frequently related to a defect in myocardial contraction.)

- cranial nerve paralysis
- functional motor deficit
- gastrointestinal hemorrhage (hemorrhage affecting the gastrointestinal tract)
- headache (cephalgia, or pain sensed in various parts of the head, not confined to the area of distribution of any nerve)
- morphological central nervous system abnormality
- myocardial infarction (necrosis of the myocardium caused by an obstruction of the blood supply to the heart and often associated with chest pain, shortness of breath, palpitations, and anxiety, as well as characteristic electrocardiogram (ECG or EKG) findings and elevation of serum markers, including creatine kinase–myocardial band fraction and troponin)
- nephritis (the presence of inflammation affecting the kidney)
- nephrotic syndrome (It is a collection of findings resulting from glomerular dysfunction with an increase in glomerular capillary wall permeability associated with pronounced proteinuria. Nephrotic syndrome refers to the constellation of clinical findings that result from severe renal loss of protein, with proteinuria and hypoalbuminemia, edema, and hyperlipidemia.)
- pericarditis (inflammation of the sac-like covering around the heart (pericardium))
- progressive neurologic deterioration
- rheumatoid factor positive (the presence in the serum of an autoantibody directed against the fragment crystallizable (Fc) portion of immunoglobulin G (IgG))
- seizure
- stroke (sudden impairment of blood flow to a part of the brain due to occlusion or rupture of an artery to the brain)
- viral hepatitis (inflammation of the liver due to infection with a virus)

DIAGNOSIS OF SIMPLE CRYOGLOBULINEMIA

It is diagnosed based on the results of a clinical exam and the presence of cryoglobulins in the blood.[2]

Section 17.3 | Gamma-Heavy-Chain Disease

Gamma-heavy-chain disease (GHCD) affects the growth of cells in the immune system. GHCD is one of three different types of heavy-chain disease. People with this disease make an abnormal form of the gamma heavy chain, a protein used to make antibodies. This abnormal protein is overproduced by the body and can lead to abnormal cell growth.

WHAT CAUSES GAMMA-HEAVY-CHAIN DISEASE?

The cause of GHCD is unknown, but about one-third of people with this condition have an autoimmune disease.

WHO IS AT RISK OF GAMMA-HEAVY-CHAIN DISEASE?

Gamma-heavy-chain disease mainly affects older adults with symptoms that may include swollen lymph nodes, an enlarged liver and spleen, and anemia.

SYMPTOMS OF GAMMA-HEAVY-CHAIN DISEASE

Some people with GHCD have no symptoms, while others have many symptoms and can develop an aggressive form of lymphoma. The following symptoms have been linked to this disease:
- abnormal lymphocyte morphology
- abnormality of bone marrow cell morphology (an anomaly of the form or number of cells in the bone marrow)

---

[2] Genetic and Rare Diseases Information Center (GARD), "Simple Cryoglobulinemia," National Center for Advancing Translational Sciences (NCATS), February 2023. Available online. URL: https://rarediseases.info.nih.gov/diseases/6217/cryoglobulinemia. Accessed June 6, 2023.

- fatigue
- anemia
- hepatomegaly (abnormally increased size of the liver)
- lymphadenopathy (enlargement (swelling) of a lymph node)
- neoplasm of the tongue (a tumor (abnormal growth of tissue) of the tongue)
- skin rash
- splenomegaly (abnormally increased size of the spleen)
- abnormal palate morphology (any abnormality of the palate, i.e., of the roof of the mouth)
- autoimmune hemolytic anemia (an autoimmune form of hemolytic anemia)
- autoimmune thrombocytopenia (the presence of thrombocytopenia, in combination with the detection of antiplatelet antibodies)
- autoimmunity (the occurrence of an immune reaction against the organism's own cells or tissues)
- dysphagia (difficulty in swallowing)
- osteolysis (the destruction of bone through bone resorption with removal or loss of calcium)
- peripheral neuropathy (It is a term for any disorder of the peripheral nervous system. The main clinical features used to classify peripheral neuropathy are distribution, type (mainly demyelinating versus mainly axonal), duration, and course.)
- recurrent respiratory infections (an increased susceptibility to respiratory infections as manifested by a history of recurrent respiratory infections)
- rheumatoid arthritis (RA; inflammatory changes in the synovial membranes and articular structures with widespread fibrinoid degeneration of the collagen fibers in mesenchymal tissues, as well as atrophy and rarefaction of bony structures)

WHEN DO SYMPTOMS OF GAMMA-HEAVY-CHAIN DISEASE BEGIN?
Symptoms of this disease may start to appear in adulthood.

DIAGNOSIS OF GAMMA-HEAVY-CHAIN DISEASE

Diagnosis is based on finding high levels of the gamma heavy chain in the blood, urine, and bone marrow.[3]

Section 17.4 | Plasma Cell Neoplasms

WHAT ARE PLASMA CELLS?

Plasma cells develop from B lymphocytes (B cells), a type of white blood cell (WBC) that is made in the bone marrow. Normally, when bacteria or viruses enter the body, some of the B cells will change into plasma cells. The plasma cells make antibodies to fight bacteria and viruses in order to stop infection and disease.

WHAT ARE PLASMA CELL NEOPLASMS?

Plasma cell neoplasms are diseases in which abnormal plasma cells or myeloma cells form tumors in the bones or soft tissues of the body. The plasma cells also make an antibody protein, called "M protein," that is not needed by the body and does not help fight infection. These antibody proteins build up in the bone marrow and can cause the blood to thicken or can damage the kidneys.

TYPES OF PLASMA CELL NEOPLASMS
Monoclonal Gammopathy of Undetermined Significance

In this type of plasma cell neoplasm, less than 10 percent of the bone marrow is made up of abnormal plasma cells, and there is no cancer. The abnormal plasma cells make M protein, which is sometimes found during a routine blood or urine test. In most

---

[3] Genetic and Rare Diseases Information Center (GARD), "Gamma Heavy Chain Disease," National Center for Advancing Translational Sciences (NCATS), February 2023. Available online. URL: https://rarediseases.info.nih.gov/diseases/10346/gamma-heavy-chain-disease. Accessed June 6, 2023.

patients, the amount of M protein stays the same, and there are no signs, symptoms, or health problems.

In some patients, monoclonal gammopathy of undetermined significance (MGUS) may later become a more serious condition, such as amyloidosis, or cause problems with the kidneys, heart, or nerves. MGUS can also become cancer, such as multiple myeloma, lymphoplasmacytic lymphoma, or chronic lymphocytic leukemia.

Plasmacytoma

In this type of plasma cell neoplasm, the abnormal plasma cells (myeloma cells) are in one place and form one tumor called a "plasmacytoma." Sometimes, plasmacytoma can be cured. The following are the two types of plasmacytoma:

- **Isolated plasmacytoma of the bone**. In this plasmacytoma, one plasma cell tumor is found in the bone, less than 10 percent of the bone marrow is made up of plasma cells, and there are no other signs of cancer. Plasmacytoma of the bone often becomes multiple myeloma.
- **Extramedullary plasmacytoma**. In this plasmacytoma, one plasma cell tumor is found in soft tissue, but not in the bone or the bone marrow. Extramedullary plasmacytomas commonly form in tissues of the throat, tonsil, and paranasal sinuses.

Signs and symptoms depend on where the tumor is.
- In bone, the plasmacytoma may cause pain or broken bones.
- In soft tissue, the tumor may press on nearby areas and cause pain or other problems. For example, a plasmacytoma in the throat can make it hard to swallow.

Multiple Myeloma

In multiple myeloma, abnormal plasma cells (myeloma cells) build up in the bone marrow and form tumors in many bones of the body. These tumors may keep the bone marrow from making enough healthy blood cells. Normally, the bone marrow makes stem cells (immature cells) that become three types of mature blood cells:

- **Red blood cells (RBCs)**. RBCs carry oxygen and other substances to all tissues of the body.
- **WBCs**. These blood cells fight infection and disease.
- **Platelets**. These form blood clots to stop bleeding.

As the number of myeloma cells increases, fewer RBCs, WBCs, and platelets are made. The myeloma cells also damage and weaken the bone.

Sometimes, multiple myeloma does not cause any signs or symptoms. This is called "smoldering multiple myeloma" (SMM). It may be found when a blood or urine test is done for another condition. Signs and symptoms may be caused by multiple myeloma or other conditions. Check with your doctor if you have any of the following:

- bone pain, especially in the back or ribs
- bones that break easily
- fever for no known reason or frequent infections
- easy bruising or bleeding
- trouble breathing
- weakness of the arms or legs
- feeling very tired

A tumor can damage the bone and cause hypercalcemia (too much calcium in the blood). This can affect many organs in the body, including the kidneys, nerves, heart, muscles, and digestive tract, and cause serious health problems.

Hypercalcemia may cause the following signs and symptoms:

- loss of appetite
- nausea or vomiting
- feeling thirsty
- frequent urination
- constipation
- feeling very tired
- muscle weakness
- restlessness
- confusion or trouble thinking

MULTIPLE MYELOMA AND AMYLOIDOSIS

In rare cases, multiple myeloma can cause peripheral nerves (nerves that are not in the brain or spinal cord) and organs to fail. This may be caused by a condition called "amyloidosis." Antibody proteins build up and stick together in peripheral nerves and organs, such as the kidneys and heart. This can cause the nerves and organs to become stiff and unable to work the way they should.

Amyloidosis may cause the following signs and symptoms:
- feeling very tired
- purple spots on the skin
- enlarged tongue
- diarrhea
- swelling caused by fluid in your body's tissues
- tingling or numbness in your legs and feet

RISKS OF PLASMA CELL NEOPLASMS

Anything that increases your risk of getting a disease is called a "risk factor." Having a risk factor does not mean that you will get cancer; not having risk factors does not mean that you will not get cancer. Talk with your doctor if you think you may be at risk.

Plasma cell neoplasms are most common in people who are middle-aged or older. For multiple myeloma and plasmacytoma, other risk factors include the following:
- being Black
- being male
- having a personal history of MGUS or plasmacytoma
- being exposed to radiation or certain chemicals

DIAGNOSIS OF MULTIPLE MYELOMA AND OTHER PLASMA CELL NEOPLASMS

The following tests and procedures may be used:
- **Physical exam and history**. This is an exam of the body to check general signs of health, including checking for signs of disease, such as lumps or anything else that seems unusual. A history of the patient's health habits and past illnesses and treatments will also be taken.

- **Blood and urine immunoglobulin studies**. This is a procedure in which a blood or urine sample is checked to measure the amount of certain antibodies (immunoglobulins). For multiple myeloma, beta-2-microglobulin, M protein, free light-chains, and other proteins made by the myeloma cells are measured. A higher-than-normal amount of these substances can be a sign of disease.
- **Bone marrow aspiration and biopsy**. This is the removal of bone marrow, blood, and a small piece of bone by inserting a hollow needle into the hip bone or breastbone. A pathologist views the bone marrow, blood, and bone under a microscope to look for abnormal cells.

The following test may be done on the sample of tissue removed during the bone marrow aspiration and biopsy:
- **Cytogenetic analysis**. This is a test in which cells in a sample of bone marrow are viewed under a microscope to look for certain changes in the chromosomes. Other tests, such as fluorescence in situ hybridization (FISH) and flow cytometry, may also be done to look for certain changes in the chromosomes.
- **Skeletal bone survey**. In a skeletal bone survey, x-rays of all the bones in the body are taken. The x-rays are used to find areas where the bone is damaged. An x-ray is a type of energy beam that can go through the body and onto film, making a picture of areas inside the body.
- **Complete blood count (CBC) with differential**. This is a procedure in which a sample of blood is drawn and checked for the following:
  - the number of RBCs and platelets
  - the number and type of WBCs
  - the amount of hemoglobin (the protein that carries oxygen) in the RBCs
  - the portion of the blood sample made up of RBCs

- **Blood chemistry studies**. This is a procedure in which a blood sample is checked to measure the amount of certain substances, such as calcium or albumin, released into the blood by organs and tissues in the body. An unusual (higher or lower than normal) amount of a substance can be a sign of disease.
- **Twenty-four-hour urine test**. This is a test in which urine is collected for 24 hours to measure the amounts of certain substances. An unusual (higher or lower than normal) amount of a substance can be a sign of disease in the organ or tissue that makes it. A higher-than-normal amount of protein may be a sign of multiple myeloma.
- **Magnetic resonance imaging (MRI)**. This is a procedure that uses a magnet, radio waves, and a computer to make a series of detailed pictures of areas inside the body. This procedure is also called "nuclear magnetic resonance imaging" (NMRI). An MRI of the spine and pelvis may be used to find areas where the bone is damaged.
- **Positron emission tomography (PET) scan**. This is a procedure to find malignant tumor cells in the body. A small amount of radioactive glucose (sugar) is injected into a vein. The PET scanner rotates around the body and makes a picture of where glucose is being used in the body. Malignant tumor cells show up brighter in the picture because they are more active and take up more glucose than normal cells.
- **Computed tomography (CT) scan**. This is a procedure that makes a series of detailed pictures of areas inside the body, such as the spine, taken from different angles. The pictures are made by a computer linked to an x-ray machine. A dye may be injected into a vein or swallowed to help the organs or tissues show up more clearly. This procedure is also called "computerized tomography" or "computerized axial tomography."

- **PET-CT scan**. This is a procedure that combines the pictures from a PET scan and a CT scan. The PET and CT scans are done at the same time with the same machine. The combined scans give more detailed pictures of areas inside the body, such as the spine, than either scan gives by itself.

FACTORS AFFECTING TREATMENT OPTIONS AND PROGNOSIS

Treatment options depend on the following:
- the type of plasma cell neoplasm
- the age and general health of the patient
- whether there are signs, symptoms, or health problems, such as kidney failure or infection, related to the disease
- whether the cancer responds to initial treatment or recurs

The prognosis (chance of recovery) depends on the following:
- the type of plasma cell neoplasm
- the stage of the disease
- whether a certain immunoglobulin (antibody) is present
- whether there are certain genetic changes
- whether the kidney is damaged
- whether the cancer responds to initial treatment or recurs (comes back)[4]

[4] "Plasma Cell Neoplasms (Including Multiple Myeloma) Treatment (PDQ®)—Patient Version," National Cancer Institute (NCI), May 12, 2023. Available online. URL: www.cancer.gov/types/myeloma/patient/myeloma-treatment-pdq#_1. Accessed June 6, 2023.

Chapter 18 | **White Blood Cell Disorders**

Chapter Contents

Section 18.1 | Hypereosinophilic Syndrome

WHAT IS HYPEREOSINOPHILIC SYNDROME?

Hypereosinophilic syndrome (HES) refers to a rare group of conditions that are associated with persistent eosinophilia with evidence of organ involvement. Although any organ system can be involved in HES, the heart, central nervous system, skin, and respiratory tract are the most commonly affected. The condition was originally thought to be idiopathic, or of unknown cause. However, recent advances in diagnostic testing have allowed a cause to be identified in approximately a quarter of cases. Management varies based on the severity of the condition and whether or not an underlying cause has been identified but generally includes imatinib or corticosteroids as an initial treatment.

CAUSES OF HYPEREOSINOPHILIC SYNDROME

When the term "hypereosinophilic syndrome" was originally coined in 1975, the condition was thought to be idiopathic, or of an unknown cause. At present, in approximately 75 percent of cases, the underlying cause still remains unknown. However, recent advances in diagnostic techniques have led researchers to believe that some people affected by HES may have eosinophilia due to a variety of causes, including the following:

- **Myeloproliferative HES**. Myeloproliferative neoplasms (MPNs) or other disorders that affect the bone marrow (myeloproliferative disorders).
- **Lymphocytic HES**. Increased production of interleukin-5 (a protein produced by certain types of white blood cells (WBCs)).
- **Familial HES**. A change (mutation) in an unknown gene passed down through a family.

SYMPTOMS OF HYPEREOSINOPHILIC SYNDROME

The signs and symptoms of HES can vary significantly depending on which parts of the body are affected (see Table 18.1).

Table 18.1. Symptoms of Hypereosinophilic Syndrome in Different Parts of the Body

Affected Body System	Symptoms
Skin	• rashes • itching • edema
Lung	• asthma • cough • difficulty breathing • recurrent upper respiratory infections • pleural effusion
Gastrointestinal system	• abdominal pain • vomiting • diarrhea
Musculoskeletal system	• arthritis • muscle inflammation • muscle aches • joint pain
Nervous system	• vertigo • paresthesia • speech impairment • visual disturbances
Heart	• congestive heart failure • cardiomyopathy • pericardial effusion • myocarditis
Blood	• deep venous thrombosis (DVT) • anemia

Affected people can also experience a variety of nonspecific symptoms, such as fever, weight loss, night sweats, and fatigue.

INHERITANCE OF HYPEREOSINOPHILIC SYNDROME

Although most cases of HES are not inherited, some cases do appear to be passed down through a family. In these families, the exact underlying genetic cause is unknown, but the genetic mutation is thought to be inherited in an autosomal dominant manner.

In autosomal dominant conditions, an affected person only needs a mutation in one copy of the responsible gene in each cell. In some cases, an affected person inherits the mutation from an affected parent. Other cases may result from new (de novo) mutations in the gene. These cases occur in people with no history of the disorder in their family. A person with an autosomal dominant condition has a 50 percent chance with each pregnancy of passing along the altered gene to his or her child.[1]

Section 18.2 | Langerhans Cell Histiocytosis

WHAT IS LANGERHANS CELL HISTIOCYTOSIS?
Langerhans cell histiocytosis (LCH) is a disorder in which excess immune system cells called "Langerhans cells" build up in the body. Langerhans cells, which help regulate the immune system, are normally found throughout the body, especially in the skin, lymph nodes, spleen, lungs, liver, and bone marrow. In LCH, excess immature Langerhans cells usually form tumors called "granulomas." Many researchers now consider LCH to be a form of cancer, but this classification remains controversial.

In approximately 80 percent of affected individuals, one or more granulomas develop in the bones, causing pain and swelling. The granulomas, which usually occur in the skull or the long bones of the arms or legs, may cause the bone to fracture.

CAUSES OF LANGERHANS CELL HISTIOCYTOSIS
Somatic mutations in the *BRAF* gene have been identified in the Langerhans cells of about half of individuals with LCH. Somatic gene mutations are acquired during a person's lifetime and are present only in certain cells. These changes are not inherited.

---

[1] Genetic and Rare Diseases Information Center (GARD), "Hypereosinophilic Syndrome," National Center for Advancing Translational Sciences (NCATS), February 2023. Available online. URL: https://rarediseases.info.nih.gov/diseases/2804/hypereosinophilic-syndrome. Accessed June 6, 2023.

The *BRAF* gene provides instructions for making a protein that is normally switched on and off in response to signals that control cell growth and development. Somatic mutations cause the BRAF protein in affected cells to be continuously active and to transmit messages to the nucleus even in the absence of these chemical signals. The overactive protein may contribute to the development of LCH by allowing the Langerhans cells to grow and divide uncontrollably.

Changes in other genes have also been identified in the Langerhans cells of some individuals with LCH. Some researchers believe that additional factors, such as viral infections and environmental toxins, may also influence the development of this complex disorder.

SIGNS AND SYMPTOMS OF LANGERHANS CELL HISTIOCYTOSIS

Granulomas also frequently occur in the skin, appearing as blisters, reddish bumps, or rashes, which can be mild to severe. The pituitary gland may also be affected; this gland is located at the base of the brain and produces hormones that control many important body functions. Without hormone supplementation, affected individuals may experience delayed or absent puberty or an inability to have children (infertility). In addition, pituitary gland damage may result in the production of excessive amounts of urine (diabetes insipidus) and dysfunction of another gland called the "thyroid." Thyroid dysfunction can affect the rate of chemical reactions in the body (metabolism), body temperature, skin and hair texture, and behavior.

In 15–20 percent of cases, LCH affects the lungs, liver, or blood-forming (hematopoietic) system; damage to these organs and tissues may be life-threatening. Lung involvement, which appears as swelling of the small airways (bronchioles) and blood vessels of the lungs, results in stiffening of the lung tissue, breathing problems, and increased risk of infection. Hematopoietic involvement, which occurs when the Langerhans cells crowd out blood-forming cells in the bone marrow, leads to a general reduction in the number of blood cells (pancytopenia). Pancytopenia results in fatigue due to low numbers of red blood cells (RBCs; anemia), frequent infections due to low numbers of white blood cells (WBCs; neutropenia), and clotting problems due to low numbers of platelets (thrombocytopenia).

Other signs and symptoms that may occur in LCH, depending on which organs and tissues have Langerhans cell deposits, include swollen lymph nodes, abdominal pain, yellowing of the skin and whites of the eyes (jaundice), delayed puberty, protruding eyes, dizziness, irritability, and seizures. About 1 in 50 affected individuals experiences deterioration of neurological function (neurodegeneration).

COMPLICATIONS OF LANGERHANS CELL HISTIOCYTOSIS

The severity of LCH and its signs and symptoms vary widely among affected individuals. Certain presentations or forms of the disorder were formerly considered to be separate diseases. Older names that were sometimes used for forms of LCH include eosinophilic granuloma, Hand-Schüller-Christian disease (HSCD), and Letterer-Siwe disease (LESD).

In many people with LCH, the disorder eventually goes away with appropriate treatment. It may even disappear on its own, especially if the disease occurs only in the skin. However, some complications of the condition, such as diabetes insipidus or other effects of tissue and organ damage, may be permanent.

DIAGNOSIS OF LANGERHANS CELL HISTIOCYTOSIS

Langerhans cell histiocytosis is often diagnosed in childhood, usually between the ages of two and three, but can appear at any age. Most individuals with adult-onset LCH are current or past smokers; in about two-thirds of adult-onset cases, the disorder affects only the lungs.

FREQUENCY OF LANGERHANS CELL HISTIOCYTOSIS

Langerhans cell histiocytosis is a rare disorder. Its prevalence is estimated at 1–2 in 100,000 people.

INHERITANCE OF LANGERHANS CELL HISTIOCYTOSIS

Langerhans cell histiocytosis is usually not inherited and typically occurs in people with no history of the disorder in their family.

A few families with multiple cases of LCH have been identified, but the inheritance pattern is unknown.[2]

Section 18.3 | Lymphocytopenia

Lymphopenia (also called "lymphocytopenia") is a disorder in which your blood does not have enough white blood cells (WBCs) called "lymphocytes." Lymphocytes play a protective role in your immune system.

The following are the three types of lymphocytes. All lymphocytes help protect you from infection, but they have different functions.

- **B lymphocytes**. These lymphocytes are made in the bone marrow. These cells make antibodies to help you get better when you are sick (humoral immunity). They may also protect you from future illness.
- **T lymphocytes**. These cells develop in the thymus gland, an organ in the chest that is part of the lymphatic system. T cells can kill virus-infected cells or cancer cells and signal other cells to help destroy viruses (cellular immunity). T cells also help B cells form antibodies.
- **Natural killer cells**. These cells develop in the bone marrow, thymus, and liver; these are immune cells that contain enzymes to kill cancer cells or cells infected with a virus.

Infections can be life-threatening when people have no T or B cells, as in severe combined immunodeficiency (SCID). In adults,

[2] MedlinePlus, "Langerhans Cell Histiocytosis," National Institutes of Health (NIH), October 1, 2017. Available online. URL: https://medlineplus.gov/genetics/condition/langerhans-cell-histiocytosis. Accessed May 12, 2023.

about 20–40 percent of the WBCs in the body are lymphocytes. These cells help protect your body from infection. If you have low numbers of lymphocytes (lymphopenia), you are at a higher risk of infection.

CAUSES OF LYMPHOPENIA
Sometimes, the cause of lymphopenia is not known.

RISK FACTORS FOR LYMPHOPENIA
The main risk factor for lymphopenia worldwide is poor nutrition. Your risk of lymphopenia is higher if you have one of the diseases, conditions, or factors that can cause a low lymphocyte count. These conditions can be acquired or inherited.

Inherited Conditions That Can Lead to Lymphopenia
- ataxia telangiectasia (AT)
- chromosome 22q11.2 deletion syndrome (sometimes called "DiGeorge syndrome" (DGS))
- common variable immunodeficiency (CVID)
- SCID syndrome
- Wiskott-Aldrich syndrome (WAS)

Acquired Conditions That Can Lead to Lymphopenia
- infections such as human immunodeficiency virus (HIV), viral hepatitis, influenza, severe acute respiratory syndrome coronavirus 2 (SARS-CoV-2; the virus that causes COVID-19), tuberculosis (TB), pneumonia, sepsis, or malaria
- autoimmune disorders such as Sjögren syndrome, lupus, or rheumatoid arthritis (RA)
- blood cancer and other blood diseases, such as Hodgkin lymphoma (HL) and aplastic anemia (AA)
- some medical treatments, such as blood and bone marrow transplant, cancer treatment, steroid therapy, or major surgery
- drinking too much alcohol or poor nutrition (having a diet without enough protein or other nutrients)

SYMPTOMS OF LYMPHOPENIA

Lymphopenia symptoms can range from mild to serious and are correlated to the severity of the lymphopenia as well as its duration. People who have lymphopenia may have no symptoms at all. People who do not have enough lymphocytes may get infections more often. If you get colds or pneumonia often or a more unusual infection, your health-care provider may suspect that you have lymphopenia.

A low lymphocyte count alone may not cause any symptoms. Lymphopenia is usually found during a routine health checkup or when you are being tested for other diseases or conditions, such as HIV infection.

Lymphopenia can cause one of the following signs or symptoms:
- frequent infections, such as colds or pneumonia
- unusual infections caused by microbes, fungi, or parasites that rarely cause problems for people who have a healthy immune system
- long-lasting infections, such as tuberculosis
- missing or abnormal tonsils (small organs in the back of the throat)
- swollen lymph nodes
- skin conditions and abnormalities, such as alopecia (sudden hair loss), eczema (long-term itchy, red skin), pyoderma (bumps on the skin that turn into swollen, open sores), pale skin, jaundice (yellowing of the skin and eyes), small bruises, and sores in the mouth
- failure to thrive
- a spleen that is larger than normal that your health-care provider can feel in an exam

Your provider will do a physical exam and ask you about your symptoms to help diagnose lymphopenia. You will also likely need a blood test to confirm the diagnosis.

DIAGNOSIS OF LYMPHOPENIA

Your health-care provider will diagnose lymphopenia based on your medical and family health histories, a physical exam, and test results. Newborn screening may lead to early diagnosis of genetic diseases that can cause life-threatening lymphopenia.

A low lymphocyte count alone may not cause any symptoms. The condition is often found during a routine checkup or when your health-care provider tests you for other diseases or conditions. In other cases, your provider may order tests to diagnose lymphopenia after noticing that you have unusual infections, repeat infections, or infections that do not heal quickly.

Medical History and Physical Exam

Your provider will do a physical exam to look for signs of infection, such as fever. They may check your stomach for signs of a spleen that is larger than normal and your neck or armpits for signs of lymph nodes that are larger than normal.

Your provider will also look for symptoms of diseases and conditions that can affect your lymphocyte count, such as HIV and blood cancers.

Your provider may ask:

- about your risk of HIV infections, such as intravenous (IV) drug use, sexual partners, exposure to infectious blood or bodily fluids at work, or blood transfusions
- whether you have ever had cancer treatments such as radiation, chemotherapy, or immunotherapies
- whether you have ever been diagnosed with a blood disease or immune disorder or whether you have a family history of such illnesses
- about your diet and other lifestyle habits

CAN YOU PREVENT LYMPHOPENIA?

You may be able to prevent some types of lymphopenia by getting treatment for and managing medical conditions, following a healthy diet, and avoiding drinking too much alcohol.

There is no way to prevent lymphopenia that is caused by an inherited condition. You can take steps to manage your condition and lower your risk of complications such as infections.[3]

---

[3] "What Is Lymphopenia?" National Heart, Lung, and Blood Institute (NHLBI), May 31, 2022. Available online. URL: www.nhlbi.nih.gov/health/lymphopenia. Accessed May 12, 2023.

Section 18.4 | **Neutropenia**

WHAT IS NEUTROPENIA?

Neutropenia is a decrease in the number of white blood cells (WBCs). These cells are the body's main defense against infection. Neutropenia is common after receiving chemotherapy and increases your risk of infections.

WHY DOES CHEMOTHERAPY CAUSE NEUTROPENIA?

These cancer-fighting drugs work by killing fast-growing cells in the body—both good and bad. These drugs kill cancer cells, as well as healthy WBCs.

HOW DO YOU KNOW IF YOU HAVE NEUTROPENIA?

Your doctor or nurse will tell you. Because neutropenia is common after receiving chemotherapy, your doctor may draw some blood to look for neutropenia.

WHEN WILL YOU BE MOST LIKELY TO HAVE NEUTROPENIA?

Neutropenia often occurs between 7 and 12 days after you receive chemotherapy. This period can be different depending on the chemotherapy you get. Your doctor or nurse will let you know exactly when your WBC count is likely to be at its lowest. You should carefully watch for signs and symptoms of infection during this time.

HOW CAN YOU PREVENT NEUTROPENIA?

There is not much you can do to prevent neutropenia from occurring, but you can decrease your risk of getting an infection while your WBC count is low.

HOW CAN YOU PREVENT AN INFECTION?

In addition to receiving treatment from your doctor, the following suggestions can help prevent infections:
- Clean your hands frequently.
- Try to avoid crowded places and contact with people who are sick.

- Do not share food, drink cups, utensils, or other personal items, such as toothbrushes.
- Shower or bathe daily and use an unscented lotion to prevent your skin from becoming dry and cracked.
- Cook meat and eggs all the way through to kill any germs.
- Carefully wash raw fruits and vegetables.
- Protect your skin from direct contact with pet bodily waste (urine or feces) by wearing vinyl or household cleaning gloves when cleaning up after your pet. Wash your hands immediately afterward.
- Use gloves for gardening.
- Clean your teeth and gums with a soft toothbrush, and if your doctor or nurse recommends one, use a mouthwash to prevent mouth sores.
- Try and keep all your household surfaces clean.
- Get the seasonal flu shot as soon as it is available.

WHAT IF YOU HAVE TO GO TO THE EMERGENCY ROOM?

Cancer patients receiving chemotherapy should not sit in a waiting room for a long time. While you are receiving chemotherapy, fever may be a sign of infection. Infections can become serious very quickly. When you check in, tell them right away that you are getting chemotherapy and have a fever. This may be an indication of an infection.[4]

---

[4] "What You Need to Know Neutropenia and Risk for Infection," Centers for Disease Control and Prevention (CDC), October 20, 2011. Available online. URL: www.cdc.gov/cancer/preventinfections/pdf/neutropenia.pdf. Accessed June 6, 2023.

Part 4 | **Bleeding and Clotting Disorders**

Chapter 19 | **An Overview of Blood Clotting Disorders**

WHAT ARE BLOOD CLOTTING DISORDERS?

Blood clotting disorders are problems in the body's ability to control how the blood clots. Normally, blood clots form during an injury to prevent bleeding. If you have a clotting disorder, your blood may not clot enough, which can lead to too much bleeding, or your blood may form clots even without an injury.

Blood clotting disorders are sometimes called "coagulation disorders" or "thrombophilia." They are either inherited (meaning that you are born with the condition) or acquired (meaning you develop the condition as the result of another illness or injury). For example, antiphospholipid-antibody syndrome (APS) and disseminated intravascular coagulation (DIC) are types of acquired blood clotting disorders.

Blood clots can cause many health problems. Symptoms of blood clots depend on where in the body they form. Typically, they will form in the veins and appear in the legs or lungs. Blood clots in the legs can cause deep vein thrombosis (DVT). Blood clots in the lungs can cause a pulmonary embolism (PE). It is rare for blood clots to form in the arteries. When they do, they can lead to heart attack or stroke.

If you think you may have a blood clotting disorder, your doctor will ask about your family and medical history. They may also run tests to be sure of the diagnosis. If you have a blood clotting disorder, you may need medicine to stop the blood from clotting. Your doctor may also talk to you about ways to prevent blood clots and to stay healthy.

285

HOW DOES BLOOD CLOT?

When a blood vessel is injured, the damaged cells in the vessel wall send out chemical signals. These signals cause clots that slow or stop bleeding.

A blood clot forms through several steps (see Figure 19.1) :

- **The blood vessel narrows**. First, chemical signals cause the injured vessels to narrow to prevent more blood from leaking out.

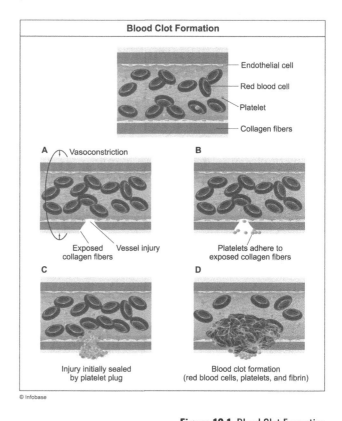

Figure 19.1. Blood Clot Formation

Infobase

- **Platelets travel to the site of the injury**. The chemical signals travel through your blood to the spleen, where many platelets are stored. The signals tell your spleen to release the platelets into your blood. Back at the injury site, the vessel walls become sticky and capture the platelets as they float past.

- **A platelet plug forms**. The platelets change shape and become stickier. This allows them to attach to the vessel wall and clump together into a plug.
- **The blood clot forms**. Clotting factors in your blood are normally turned off so that you do not form abnormal blood clots. When there is an injury, platelets release molecules into the blood that help turn on clotting factors. One important clotting factor is fibrin, a long, thin, and sticky protein. When it is turned on, it forms a mesh to hold the platelet plug in place. This is called a "fibrin clot." The mesh also traps red blood cells (RBCs) to form a blood clot. The platelets contract to pull the two sides of the damaged vessel closer together, so it is easier to repair.

Once the blood clot is formed, your body's immune system repairs the injury. At this point in the process, factors in your blood start to break down the blood clot.

If you do not have enough platelets or clotting factors in your blood, your blood will not be able to clot as well.

In other cases, your blood may clot too easily. Some conditions cause overactive clotting so that blood clots form in blood vessels throughout your body. Eventually, the platelets in your body are used up, which can then lead to bleeding. These conditions include the following:

- APS
- DIC
- thrombotic thrombocytopenic purpura (TTP)

TYPES OF BLOOD CLOTTING DISORDERS

Blood clotting disorders can either be inherited or acquired:

- **Inherited**. It means that your parents passed the gene for the disease onto you. Mutations, or changes in a certain gene, can make your blood more likely to form

clots. Some genetic changes are more common than others. Common genetic changes are not as likely to cause serious blood clots as the rarer genetic changes.
- **Acquired**. It means that you were not born with the disease, but you developed it due to another disease or condition.

Just because you have a blood clotting disorder does not mean that you will develop blood clots. But it does increase your chance of having blood clots throughout your lifetime.

Inherited Blood Clotting Disorders
Common inherited blood clotting disorders include the following:
- factor V Leiden mutation, which occurs in 5 percent of people of European descent
- prothrombin G20210A mutation (also called "factor II mutation"), which occurs in 2 percent of the population

Rare inherited blood clotting disorders include the following:
- deficiencies in blood clotting proteins called "protein C," "protein S," and "antithrombin"
- hyperhomocysteinemia
- sticky platelet syndrome

Acquired Blood Clotting Disorders
Examples of acquired blood clotting disorders include the following:
- **APS**. This is the most common acquired clotting disorder. APS is an autoimmune condition where the body makes antibodies that mistakenly attack cell molecules called "phospholipids." Higher levels of APS antibodies in the blood raise the risk of blood clots.
- **DIC**. This condition is caused by an infection (such as sepsis) or an injury.

CAUSES OF BLOOD CLOTTING DISORDERS
Blood clotting disorders occur when blood forms clots more often than it is supposed to. Your body maintains normal blood flow

because of a balance of molecules called "procoagulant factors" and "anticoagulant factors." Procoagulant factors help blood clots form, and anticoagulant factors prevent blood clots. Any imbalance of these factors can lead to a blood clotting disorder.

Many things can upset the balance of these factors.

Inherited blood disorders are caused by changes in the structures of your genes (called "mutations") before you are born.

Causes of acquired blood clotting disorders include the following:

- another condition, such as cancer, obesity, or an autoimmune disorder, such as lupus
- not moving for long periods of time, such as after surgery or if you are put on bed rest during pregnancy
- some medicines to treat cancer or bleeding disorders
- a vitamin deficiency in B_6, B_{12}, or folate that can cause high levels of an amino acid called "homocysteine"
- infection, such as sepsis, human immunodeficiency virus (HIV), or severe acute respiratory syndrome coronavirus 2 (SARS-CoV-2), the virus that causes coronavirus disease (COVID-19)

SYMPTOMS OF BLOOD CLOTTING DISORDERS

Blood clotting disorders that cause your blood to clot more than normal can be very serious. You may experience different symptoms depending on which part of your body is affected by the blood clot.

Symptoms can include the following:

- swollen and tender legs that are painful to the touch if you have blood clots that block blood flow to your leg veins (called "DVT")
- shortness of breath and chest pain if you have a blood clot that travels to the lungs (called a "PE")

Visit your doctor if you have these symptoms. DVT is not life-threatening, but it can lead to a life-threatening PE if not treated.

Less common, but just as serious, are blood clots that form in the arteries. These can lead to a heart attack or stroke.

You may have other symptoms, such as bruising easily or often or extreme tiredness if you have a bleeding disorder.

DIAGNOSIS OF BLOOD CLOTTING DISORDERS

To find out whether you have a blood clotting disorder, your doctor may ask you about:

- your medical history, including information about your symptoms, previous blood clots, autoimmune disorders, or miscarriages
- your family history, as blood clotting disorders often run in families

Your doctor may also do the following tests to find out whether you have a blood clotting disorder:

- Blood tests can help determine your blood's clotting process and balance of clotting factors. Sometimes, certain medicines can affect blood test results. Tell your doctor about all the over-the-counter (OTC) medicines you take.
- Genetic tests can tell you whether a relative has been diagnosed with a rare, inherited blood clotting disorder.

Your doctor may recommend that you visit a hematologist (a doctor who specializes in diagnosing and treating blood diseases and disorders) if you have frequent blood clots.

TREATMENT AND MANAGEMENT OF BLOOD CLOTTING DISORDERS

Some people with blood clotting disorders may never get blood clots and may not need treatment. Your doctor will consider your previous history of blood clots as well as your current risk factors to decide on a treatment plan.

How Are Blood Clotting Disorders Treated?

If you have a history of blood clots, your doctor may prescribe blood thinners. You may take blood thinner medicine by mouth (such as warfarin or aspirin) or as a shot (such as heparin). Side effects of warfarin and heparin include heavy bleeding, severe headaches, and dizziness. Warfarin can also interact with OTC medicines, such as cold or allergy medicines or ibuprofen.

Blood thinning medicine is all about balance. Your doctor will test your blood often to make sure the dose of medicine is correct, and your blood has the proper balance between bleeding and clotting.

A group of medicines called "direct oral anticoagulants" (DOACs) may be an alternative to warfarin or aspirin for some people, as they are safe and effective at preventing blood clots and do not require frequent blood testing. However, you may have to take more doses (twice daily compared to once a day for warfarin). DOACs are most often used in patients with low-risk, inherited blood clotting disorders (such as factor V Leiden and prothrombin G20210A). Talk to your doctor about whether DOACs may be right for you.

How Do Blood Clotting Disorders Affect Your Health?

It is important to know the causes and risk factors that may increase your chances of developing dangerous blood clots. It is important to get regular checkups and look out for the symptoms of blood clots. If left untreated, blood clots can cause serious problems, including the following:

- DVT, or a blood clot in the leg
- PE, or a blood clot that travels to the lung
- heart attack
- stroke

CAN BLOOD CLOTTING DISORDERS BE PREVENTED?

You cannot prevent blood clotting disorders that are inherited or acquired. Talk to your doctor about steps to help prevent blood clots if you are at risk.

Adopt Healthy Lifestyle Changes

- Choose healthy foods, such as fruits, vegetables, and whole grains, as a part of a heart-healthy eating plan.

- Be physically active to help your blood circulate and prevent the formation of blood clots.
- Quit smoking. Over time, smoking cigarettes can change the surface of the platelets in your blood and make them more likely to stick together and form blood clots.
- Manage stress to lower your chance of developing risk factors for blood clots, such as high blood pressure (HBP).

Avoid Certain Medicines

Some medicines increase your risk of blood clots, including hormone replacement therapy (HRT) for menopause and birth control pills with estrogen. Talk to your doctor about all the OTC medicines you take.

Talk to Your Doctor before Any Planned Surgeries

Blood clots can happen during surgery and while you are recovering from surgery. To prevent clotting, your doctor may give you blood thinners to take after the surgery or procedure.

Talk to Your Doctor If You Are Pregnant or Thinking of Becoming Pregnant

Some blood clotting disorders can be harmful to you or your pregnancy. Your doctor will go over the risks with you and provide a treatment plan for your specific circumstances.[1]

[1] "Blood Clotting Disorders," National Heart, Lung, and Blood Institute (NHLBI), March 24, 2022. Available online. URL: www.nhlbi.nih.gov/health/clotting-disorders. Accessed May 18, 2023.

Chapter 20 | Hemophilia

Chapter Contents

WHAT IS HEMOPHILIA?

Hemophilia is usually an inherited bleeding disorder in which the blood does not clot properly. This can lead to spontaneous bleeding as well as bleeding following injuries or surgery. Blood contains many proteins called "clotting factors" that can help stop bleeding. People with hemophilia have low levels of either factor VIII or factor IX.

The severity of hemophilia that a person has is determined by the amount of factors in the blood. The lower the amount of factors, the more likely it is that bleeding will occur, which can lead to serious health problems.

In rare cases, a person can develop hemophilia later in life. The majority of cases involve middle-aged or elderly people or young women who have recently given birth or are in the later stages of pregnancy. This condition often resolves with appropriate treatment.[1]

Hemophilia A affects 1 in 5,000 male births. About 400 babies are born with hemophilia A each year.

The exact number of people living with hemophilia in the United States is not known. Based on a recent study that used data collected on patients receiving care in federally funded hemophilia treatment centers (HTCs) during the period 2012–2018, as many as 33,000 males in the United States are living with the disorder.[2]

TYPES OF HEMOPHILIA

There are several different types of hemophilia. The following two are the most common:

- **Hemophilia A (classic hemophilia).** This type is caused by a lack or decrease of clotting factor VIII.
- **Hemophilia B (Christmas disease).** This type is caused by a lack or decrease of clotting factor IX.

[1] "What Is Hemophilia?" Centers for Disease Control and Prevention (CDC), August 1, 2022. Available online. URL: www.cdc.gov/ncbddd/hemophilia/facts.html. Accessed May 19, 2023.
[2] "Data & Statistics on Hemophilia," Centers for Disease Control and Prevention (CDC), August 1, 2022. Available online. URL: www.cdc.gov/ncbddd/hemophilia/data.html. Accessed May 19, 2023.

WHO IS AFFECTED BY HEMOPHILIA?

Hemophilia occurs in about 1 of every 5,000 male births. Based on a recent study that used data collected on patients receiving care in federally funded HTCs during the period 2012–2018, as many as 33,000 males in the United States are living with the disorder. Hemophilia A is about four times as common as hemophilia B, and about half of those affected have the severe form. Hemophilia affects people from all racial and ethnic groups.

CAUSES OF HEMOPHILIA

Hemophilia is caused by a mutation or change in one of the genes that provide instructions for making the clotting factor proteins needed to form a blood clot. This change or mutation can prevent the clotting protein from working properly or being missing altogether. These genes are located on the X chromosome. Males have one X and one Y chromosome (XY), and females have two X chromosomes (XX). Males inherit the X chromosome from their mothers and the Y chromosome from their fathers. Females inherit one X chromosome from each parent.

The X chromosome contains many genes that are not present on the Y chromosome. This means that males only have one copy of most of the genes on the X chromosome, whereas females have two copies. Thus, males can have a disease, such as hemophilia, if they inherit an affected X chromosome that has a mutation in either the factor VIII or factor IX gene. Females can also have hemophilia, but this is much rarer. In such cases, both X chromosomes are affected, or one is affected, and the other is missing or inactive. In these females, bleeding symptoms may be similar to males with hemophilia.

A female with one affected X chromosome is a "carrier" of hemophilia. Sometimes, a female who is a carrier can have symptoms of hemophilia. In addition, she can pass the affected X chromosome with the clotting factor gene mutation onto her children.

Even though hemophilia runs in families, some families have no prior history of family members with hemophilia. Sometimes, there are carrier females in the family but no affected boys, just by chance. However, about one-third of the time, the baby with hemophilia is the first one in the family to be affected by a mutation in the gene for the clotting factor.

Hemophilia can result in:

- bleeding within joints that can lead to chronic joint disease and pain
- bleeding in the head and sometimes in the brain, which can cause long-term problems such as seizures and paralysis
- death if the bleeding cannot be stopped or if it occurs in a vital organ such as the brain

SIGNS AND SYMPTOMS OF HEMOPHILIA

Common signs of hemophilia include the following:

- bleeding into the joints (often affecting the knees, elbows, and ankles)
- bleeding into the skin (which is bruising) or muscle and soft tissue, causing a buildup of blood in the area (called a "hematoma")
- bleeding of the mouth and gums and bleeding that is hard to stop after losing a tooth
- bleeding after circumcision (surgery performed on male babies to remove the hood of skin, called the "foreskin," covering the head of the penis)
- bleeding after having shots, such as vaccinations
- bleeding in the head of an infant after a difficult delivery
- blood in the urine or stool
- frequent and hard-to-stop nosebleeds

DIAGNOSIS OF HEMOPHILIA

Diagnosis includes screening tests and clotting factor tests. Screening tests are blood tests that show if the blood is clotting properly. Clotting factor tests, also called "factor assays," are required to diagnose a bleeding disorder. This blood test shows the type of hemophilia and the severity.

Families with a History of Hemophilia

Any family history of bleeding, such as following surgery or injury, or unexplained deaths among brothers, sisters, or other male relatives, such as maternal uncles, grandfathers, or cousins, should be discussed with a doctor to see if hemophilia was a cause. A doctor will often get a thorough family history to find out if a bleeding disorder exists in the family.

Many people who have or have had family members with hemophilia will ask that their baby boys get tested soon after birth. In the best of cases, testing for hemophilia is planned before the baby's delivery so that a sample of blood can be drawn from the umbilical cord (which connects the mother and baby before birth) immediately after birth and tested to determine the level of the clotting factors. Umbilical cord blood testing is better at finding low levels of factor VIII than it is at finding low levels of factor IX. This is because factor IX levels take more time to develop and are not at a normal level until a baby is at least six months of age. Therefore, a mildly low level of factor IX at birth does not necessarily mean that the baby has hemophilia B. A repeat test when the baby is older might be needed in some cases.

Families with No Previous History of Hemophilia

About one-third of babies who are diagnosed with hemophilia have no other family members with the disorder. A doctor might check for hemophilia in a newborn if:

- bleeding goes on for a long time after circumcision of the penis
- bleeding goes on for a long time after drawing blood and heel sticks (pricking the infant's heel to draw blood for newborn screening tests)
- bleeding in the head (scalp or brain) goes on after a difficult delivery or after using special devices or instruments to help deliver the baby (e.g., vacuum or forceps)
- unusual raised bruises or large numbers of bruises appear

If a child is not diagnosed with hemophilia during the newborn period, the family might notice unusual bruising once the child begins standing or crawling.

Those with severe hemophilia can have serious bleeding problems right away. Thus, they are often diagnosed during the first year of life. People with milder forms of hemophilia might not be diagnosed until later in life.

Screening Tests

Screening tests are blood tests that show if the blood is clotting properly. Types of screening tests are as follows.

COMPLETE BLOOD COUNT

This common test measures the amount of hemoglobin (the red pigment inside red blood cells (RBCs) that carries oxygen), the size and number of RBCs, and the number of different types of white blood cells (WBCs) and platelets found in the blood. The complete blood count (CBC) is normal in people with hemophilia. However, if a person with hemophilia has unusually heavy bleeding or bleeds for a long time, the hemoglobin and the RBC count can be low.

ACTIVATED PARTIAL THROMBOPLASTIN TIME TEST

This test measures how long it takes for blood to clot. It measures the clotting ability of factors VIII, IX, XI, and XII. If any of these clotting factors are too low, it takes longer than normal for the blood to clot. The results of this test will show a longer clotting time among people with hemophilia A or B.

PROTHROMBIN TIME TEST

This test also measures the time it takes for blood to clot. It primarily measures the clotting ability of factors I, II, V, VII, and X. If any of these factors are too low, it takes longer than normal for the blood to clot. The results of this test will be normal among most people with hemophilia A and B.

FIBRINOGEN TEST

This test also helps doctors assess a patient's ability to form a blood clot. This test is ordered either along with other blood clotting tests or when a patient has an abnormal PT or APTT test result or both. Fibrinogen is another name for clotting factor I.

Clotting Factor Tests

Clotting factor tests, also called "factor assays," are required to diagnose a bleeding disorder. This blood test shows the type of hemophilia and the severity (see Table 20.1). It is important to know the type and severity in order to create the best treatment plan.

Table 20.1. Type of Hemophilia and the Severity[3]

Severity	Levels of Factor VIII or IX in the Blood
Normal (person who does not have hemophilia)	50–100%
Mild hemophilia	Greater than 5% but less than 40%
Moderate hemophilia	1–5%
Severe hemophilia	Less than 1%

TREATMENT FOR HEMOPHILIA

The best way to treat hemophilia is to replace the missing blood clotting factor so that the blood can clot properly. This is typically done by injecting treatment products, called "clotting factor concentrates," into a person's vein. Clinicians typically prescribe treatment products for episodic care or prophylactic care. Episodic care is used to stop a patient's bleeding episodes; prophylactic care is used to prevent bleeding episodes from occurring. Nowadays, it is possible for people with hemophilia and their families to learn how to give their own clotting factor treatment products at home. Giving factor treatment products at home means that bleeds can be treated quicker, resulting in less serious bleeding and fewer side effects.[4]

---

[3] See footnote [1].
[4] "Treatment of Hemophilia," Centers for Disease Control and Prevention (CDC), August 8, 2022. Available online. URL: www.cdc.gov/ncbddd/hemophilia/treatment.html. Accessed May 19, 2023.

Section 20.2 | **Hemophilia in Women**

Hemophilia is caused by a problem in one of the genes that tell the body to make the clotting factors needed to form a blood clot. These genes are located on the X chromosome. All males have one X and one Y chromosome (XY), and all females have two X chromosomes (XX).

HEMOPHILIA CARRIERS

A female who inherits one affected X chromosome becomes a "carrier" of hemophilia. She can pass the affected gene on to her children. In addition, a female who is a carrier can sometimes have symptoms of hemophilia. In fact, some doctors describe these women as having mild hemophilia. Females who carry the hemophilia gene and have any symptoms of the disorder should be checked and cared for by a health-care provider.

PREGNANCY AND CHILDBIRTH

A woman who is a carrier of the hemophilia gene can have low factor VIII or factor IX levels and have symptoms of hemophilia. During pregnancy, the levels of protein factor VIII rise. This can make it difficult to determine the factor level and diagnose her carrier status if she has not already been diagnosed before pregnancy. Levels of factor IX do not increase during pregnancy.

It is important for the woman's health-care providers to be aware of her carrier status so that plans can be made for a safe delivery. If the woman is receiving care at a hemophilia treatment center (HTC), those doctors and nurses should be involved and work closely with the woman's doctor who is delivering the baby. Working together in this way will help the doctor who is delivering the baby take special safety measures to avoid injury to the child. These safety measures include not using forceps or a vacuum extractor to assist in the delivery of the baby, if possible.

If the mother is a hemophilia carrier, there is a chance that the baby will be born with hemophilia. In families with a known history of hemophilia or in those with a prenatal genetic diagnosis of hemophilia, one can plan special testing for hemophilia before the baby's delivery. Instead of a venipuncture, a sample of blood can be drawn from the umbilical cord (which connects the mother and baby before birth) and tested for clotting factor levels. In normal newborns, factor VIII levels are similar to adult normal values, and low levels indicate hemophilia. However, levels of factor IX, a vitamin K–dependent factor, may be low at birth and reach adult values by six months of age. Blood testing can also be done soon after a male baby is born. It is important to know as soon as possible after birth whether a baby has hemophilia so that special steps can be taken to prevent bleeding complications for the baby.

AFTER DELIVERY—THE MOTHER
Mothers who carry the hemophilia gene are at risk of serious bleeding after delivery. This is because the high levels of factor VIII during pregnancy fall back to lower levels after delivery. If the woman has low levels of factor IX, then she can bleed after delivery or surgery, such as a cesarean section (C-section). Some women have bleeding from the birth canal that lasts a long time. This is called "postpartum hemorrhage" and can require treatment to stop the bleeding.

AFTER DELIVERY—THE BABY
Testing for Hemophilia
Some babies should be tested for hemophilia soon after birth, including:
- babies born to families with a history of hemophilia
- babies whose mothers are carriers of hemophilia
- babies who have bleeding symptoms at birth

Cord blood can be used to test for clotting proteins. This should be repeated when the baby is six months of age to confirm the diagnosis of hemophilia.

Circumcision
Some parents choose to have their baby boys circumcised (removing the foreskin from the penis). Bleeding from circumcision is the

most common cause of bleeding among babies with hemophilia. It can occur days after the procedure is done and, for babies who have not been diagnosed already, often leads to the initial hemophilia diagnosis.

In a baby who may have hemophilia, avoid circumcision if possible. However, if circumcision is done, then a pediatric hematologist (a doctor who specializes in the blood) should be consulted before the procedure to ensure that the child receives proper treatment to prevent excessive bleeding.

Bleeding of the Head
The head is the second most common place of bleeding among babies affected by hemophilia. Because the head is squeezed when the baby goes through the birth canal, bleeding of the head can occur. Also, when forceps or a vacuum extractor is applied to the baby's head to assist with the delivery and help pull the baby out, bleeding can occur. Head bleeding can be in the scalp or into the brain, which is very serious. The signs and symptoms of bleeding into the brain in a newborn baby are very nonspecific and can be difficult to diagnose. Once it is diagnosed, bleeding in the head needs to be treated immediately with clotting factor concentrates. Without treatment to stop it, the bleeding can be life-threatening and can result in long-term brain damage.

Vaccines
All babies, including those with hemophilia, should get a vitamin K shot at birth, as well as other routine vaccines. All people with hemophilia should be vaccinated against hepatitis A and B. Pressure must be applied to the site of any shot, as well as to the site of heel sticks, to avoid bleeding among babies with hemophilia.[5]

[5] "Information on Hemophilia for Women," Centers for Disease Control and Prevention (CDC), August 8, 2022. Available online. URL: www.cdc.gov/ncbddd/hemophilia/women.html. Accessed May 19, 2023.

Section 20.3 | Living with Hemophilia

It is very important for you to take an active role in managing your own, or your child's, care. To make important decisions, you need to know about hemophilia, understand the treatment options, and then make the best possible choices for your health or the health of your child. If you do not understand any of the medical terms and concepts, ask your doctor to explain them. It will also help if you take notes and ask questions during doctor visits.

STEPS FOR LIVING

"Steps for Living" is an online program with information and resources for people with hemophilia and their families, as well as National Hemophilia Foundation and hemophilia treatment center (HTC) staff.

- **First step (for children eight years of age or younger).** It focuses on learning the basics of bleeding disorders, negotiating parent–provider relationships, and addressing childcare issues.
- **Next step (for children 9–15 years of age).** It provides information to families about working with schools (in areas such as legal rights, physical education classes, and field trips), gaining independence at home (e.g., transitioning to home infusions and self-infusions, setting limits, and deciding when to leave your child home alone), and making healthy decisions (for areas such as vacation and travel, organized sports, and nutrition).
- **Step up (for teens and young adults 16–25 years of age).** It covers topics such as talking about the disorder with others, higher education and job training, gaining independence, maintaining a healthy body, dating, and family life.
- **Step out (for adults 26 years of age and older).** It provides information to adults about adherence, aging health issues, living environments, workplace issues, financial health, and navigating the health-care system.

FIND GOOD MEDICAL CARE

Hemophilia is a complex disorder. Good quality medical care from doctors and nurses who know a lot about the disorder can help prevent some serious problems. Often, the best choice is a comprehensive HTC. An HTC provides care to address all issues related to the disorder, as well as education about the disorder. This care includes an annual comprehensive checkup. The team at an HTC consists of physicians (hematologists or blood specialists), nurses, social workers, physical therapists, and other health-care providers, all of whom are specialists in the care of people with bleeding disorders.

A study of 3,000 people with hemophilia by the Centers for Disease Control and Prevention (CDC) showed that those who used an HTC were 40 percent less likely to die of a hemophilia-related complication than those who did not receive care at such a treatment center. Similarly, people who used an HTC were 40 percent less likely to have to stay in a hospital for bleeding complications.

ENROLL IN COMMUNITY COUNTS

One of the major challenges facing researchers and scientists who work on rare disorders such as hemophilia is the lack of access to uniform health data. To address this issue and advance knowledge, the CDC supports and coordinates a project called "Community Counts." By participating in Community Counts, people with hemophilia can help advance knowledge in this area.

FIND A SUPPORT NETWORK

In the United States, you can contact the National Hemophilia Foundation or the Hemophilia Federation of America to get in touch with families in your area who have been affected by hemophilia. There are local chapters and associations in many areas of the country. By finding support within your community, you can learn more about resources available to meet the needs of families and people with hemophilia. Securing support and community resources can help increase your confidence in managing hemophilia, enhance your quality of life, and assist you in meeting the needs of family members. If you reside outside the United States, you can contact the World Federation of Hemophilia.

Blood Brotherhood

The Blood Brotherhood is a program from the Hemophilia Federation of America for adult men with hemophilia and von Willebrand disease (VWD). Blood Brotherhood provides several ways to connect with others:

- **Online forum**. The online forum is an Internet message board for adult men only. Register to participate in the Blood Brotherhood online forum.
- **Face-to-face meetings**. These meetings bring Blood Brothers together to connect and learn. Topic experts and activities are presented, addressing a variety of health and wellness issues.
- **National Blood Brotherhood calls and webinars**. Topic experts provide education and facilitate discussions and question-and-answer sessions around key topics that Blood Brotherhood members are asking about, such as financial health, retirement planning, and joint replacement.

BE PREPARED FOR AN EMERGENCY

It is important to develop an emergency plan before disaster strikes. It is especially important for people with bleeding disorders to have a plan in place in order to ensure that the same level of care is maintained in the event of a disaster. The CDC has developed a checklist to help you and your family be prepared.[6]

---

[6] "Information for People with Hemophilia," Centers for Disease Control and Prevention (CDC), August 25, 2022. Available online. URL: www.cdc.gov/ncbddd/hemophilia/people.html. May 19, 2023.

Section 20.4 | **Travel Safety Tips for Hemophilia**

Traveling with a bleeding disorder, such as hemophilia, can be stressful and challenging knowing that a bleed can happen at any time. Plan ahead to help manage bleeding episodes and medical emergencies that occur while away from home.

BEFORE YOU LEAVE FOR A TRIP
- Talk to your doctor about your travel plans to make sure you are in a healthy condition to travel.
- Ask your doctor if there are any recommended vaccinations based on your travel plans. Vaccinations, such as hepatitis A and B vaccines, are highly recommended for people with bleeding disorders.

WHAT TO PACK
Travel Letter
- Ask your doctor for a travel letter that describes your bleeding disorder and the medicine you take.
- Your travel letter will allow transportation security officials to make sure your medicine and medical supplies are allowed while traveling.
- If you are traveling internationally, consider having an additional copy of the travel letter written in the primary language spoken in the country you are visiting.

Medicine and Medical Supplies
- Medicine and medical supplies are exempt from airline baggage restrictions.
- Clearly label all medicine and medical supplies and pack them separately in a carry-on bag. If items are safely stored in your carry-on, you will be able to use your items at any time, and you will have your items with you in case your checked luggage is delayed or lost.

- If there are any items that should not be exposed to x-rays, request your items to be physically inspected by the transportation security official.
- Unexpected travel delays can happen. Pack extra amounts of medicine and supplies in the event that your return home is delayed.
- Pack the following medical supplies in your carry-on or in a bag you have with you at all times:
  - vials of factor medicine
  - diluent (This is a liquid used to form or thin a solution. Normal saline or sterile water are diluents that can be mixed with the factor powder.)
  - reconstitution device (This device is used to "reconstitute" or mix factor with a liquid (usually water), called a "diluent," before it can be infused or given to a person with hemophilia. The factor is stored in powdered form because it rapidly loses its power once mixed into a solution.)
  - syringes (needles)
  - alcohol and cotton pads
  - disinfectant (This product destroys bacteria or other harmful agents.)
  - containers to dispose of your used syringes (sharps)

A List of Hospitals

- Make a list of hospitals or hemophilia treatment centers (HTCs) and their contact information that are along your travel route.
- Use the HTC directory web page (www2a.cdc.gov/ncbddd/htcweb/WebUpdate.asp) for a list of HTCs in the United States. For a list of HTCs worldwide, use the World Federation of Hemophilia's Global Treatment Centre Directory at https://wfh.org/find-local-support/#HTCs.

Medical and Contact Information

- Keep a copy of your important medical and contact information with you.

- Consider wearing a medical ID emblem if traveling alone to help inform medical personnel if you become unconscious or unable to communicate during an emergency.[7]

Section 20.5 | Inhibitors and Hemophilia

WHAT ARE INHIBITORS?

People with hemophilia and those with von Willebrand disease (VWD) type 3 use treatment products called "clotting factor concentrates" ("factor"). These treatment products improve blood clotting, and they are used to stop or prevent a bleeding episode. Approximately 1 in 5 people with hemophilia A and about 3 in 100 people with hemophilia B will develop an antibody—called an "inhibitor"—to the treatment product (medicine). If you have hemophilia or VWD type 3, it is important to be tested for inhibitors once a year. When a person develops an inhibitor, the body stops accepting factor treatment product as a normal part of the blood. The body thinks factor is a foreign substance and tries to destroy it with an inhibitor. The inhibitor keeps the treatment from working, which makes it more difficult to stop a bleeding episode. People with hemophilia have a better quality of life today than ever before, but medical complications can still occur. Developing an inhibitor is one of the most serious and costly medical complications of a bleeding disorder because it becomes more difficult to treat bleeds. A person who develops an inhibitor will require special treatment until their body stops making inhibitors. Inhibitors most often appear during the first 50 times a person is treated with factor, but they can appear at any time.

[7] "Travel Safe with a Bleeding Disorder," Centers for Disease Control and Prevention (CDC), August 8, 2022. Available online. URL: www.cdc.gov/ncbddd/hemophilia/travel-safe.html. Accessed May 19, 2023.

COST OF TREATMENT FOR PEOPLE WITH INHIBITORS

Treatment for people with an inhibitor poses special challenges. The health-care costs associated with inhibitors can be staggering because of the amount and type of treatment product required to stop bleeding. Also, people with hemophilia who develop an inhibitor are twice as likely to be hospitalized for a bleeding complication, and they are at increased risk of death. The excess cost of care for each person with hemophilia and an inhibitor is over $800,000 per year, and based on the CDC's surveillance data, there are nearly 1,500 people living with an inhibitor in the United States.

RISK FACTORS AND CAUSES OF DEVELOPING INHIBITORS

All persons with hemophilia and VWD type 3 are at risk of developing an inhibitor. Scientists do not know exactly what causes inhibitors. Multiple research studies have shown that people with certain types of hemophilia gene mutations are more likely to develop an inhibitor. Hemophilia is caused by changes, called "mutations," within the genes that control normal blood clotting.

Some studies have found other characteristics that possibly play a role in increasing the risk of inhibitor development among people with hemophilia. These include the following:

- number of times one has used factor in their lifetime
- increased frequency and dose of treatment
- Black race or Hispanic ethnicity
- family history of inhibitors (other family members who have had inhibitors)

DIAGNOSIS OF INHIBITORS

Inhibitors are diagnosed with a blood test. The blood test measures if an inhibitor is present and the amount of inhibitor present (called an "inhibitor titer") in the blood. Inhibitor titers are measured in Nijmegen-Bethesda units (NBUs) if the lab test used was the Nijmegen-Bethesda assay (NBA) or Bethesda units (BU) if the lab test used was the Bethesda assay. A person with a high inhibitor titer has more inhibitor present in the blood compared to a person with a low inhibitor titer. Test results of 5.0 NBU/BU or lower are called "low titer inhibitors," whereas test results of greater than 5.0 NBU/BU are called "high titer inhibitors." People diagnosed with low titer inhibitors are more likely to have shorter and more successful inhibitor treatment than those with high titer inhibitors. For these reasons, it is important that all people with hemophilia or VWD type 3 who use factor get tested for inhibitors at least once a year. Eligible individuals can receive free inhibitor testing at federally funded HTCs through the Community Counts Registry for Bleeding Disorders Surveillance.

TREATMENT FOR INHIBITORS

Treatment for people who have an inhibitor is complex, and it remains one of the biggest challenges in the care of people with bleeding disorders. Some inhibitors, called "transient inhibitors," may disappear on their own without treatment. If possible, a person with an inhibitor should consider seeking care at an HTC. HTCs are specialized health-care centers that bring together a team of doctors (hematologists or blood specialists), nurses, and other health professionals experienced in treating people with bleeding disorders.

Some treatments for people with inhibitors include the following:

- **High-dose factor**. People with low titer inhibitors may be treated with higher amounts or increased frequency of factor to overcome the inhibitor and yet have enough leftovers to form a clot.
- **Bypassing agents**. Special blood products, called "bypassing agents," are used to treat bleeding episodes for people with high titer inhibitors. Instead of replacing the missing factor, they go around (or bypass) the factors that are blocked by the inhibitor to help the body form a normal clot. Close monitoring of people taking bypassing agents is important to make sure that their blood is not clotting too much or clotting in the wrong places in the body.
- **Products that mimic factor VIII**. This type of product works by replacing the function of factor VIII without being affected by inhibitors and can be used

to treat and prevent bleeding episodes in people with hemophilia A. This treatment product can be given by injection under the skin.

- **Immune tolerance induction (ITI) therapy.** The goal of ITI therapy is to stop the inhibitor from blocking factor in the blood and teach the body to accept factor as a normal part of blood. With ITI therapy, people receive large amounts of factor every day for many weeks or months.

All inhibitor treatment options require specialized medical expertise. Treatment can be costly, particularly bypassing agents and ITI. It is important that people who are being treated for inhibitors have their blood often tested to measure their inhibitor titers to be sure that the treatment is working. HTCs can serve a vital role in supporting patients who undergo intensive treatment regimens, such as ITI, for inhibitors.[8]

Section 20.6 | **Blood Safety and Hemophilia**

The safety of blood products is important for people with blood disorders such as hemophilia. Whether the need for blood is the result of an injury, a chronic medical need, or treatment of a blood disorder, blood and all of its components are quite literally essential parts of life.

Improvements in donor and blood screening have greatly reduced the risk of transmitting disease through blood and blood products. However, transfusion-related infections with known viruses continue to occur, and new and emerging viruses pose potential new threats to the safety of the blood supply. Therefore, monitoring the safety of blood and blood products in the people who use them is a key public health priority.

---

[8] "Inhibitors and Hemophilia," Centers for Disease Control and Prevention (CDC), August 8, 2022. Available online. URL: www.cdc.gov/ncbddd/hemophilia/inhibitors.html. Accessed June 1, 2023.

A PUBLIC HEALTH APPROACH

The availability of safe blood and blood products is an important public health issue. The Centers for Disease Control and Prevention (CDC) monitors blood product safety through the Registry for Bleeding Disorders Surveillance, a component of Community Counts.

Through the Registry for Bleeding Disorders Surveillance, the CDC monitors treatment-related complications in people who are more routinely exposed to blood and blood products. The CDC screens for blood-borne infections, such as hepatitis and human immunodeficiency virus (HIV; the virus that causes acquired immunodeficiency syndrome (AIDS)). Through this monitoring system, the CDC also documents potential risk factors for infectious diseases among people who have received blood products to treat bleeding episodes and identifies adverse reactions to blood products.

THE CDC'S SPECIMEN TRIAGE AND TRACKING TEAM LABORATORY

Blood samples from participating hemophilia treatment centers (HTCs) are sent to the CDC's Specimen Triage and Tracking Team (STATT) laboratory in Atlanta, Georgia. A portion of the blood sample is sent to the Division of Blood Disorders laboratory to test for infectious diseases. The remainder is frozen and stored at the serum bank for future blood safety studies or outbreak investigations.

For example, samples from the serum bank were used in 2004 to assess exposure to Parvovirus B19 (a virus that causes a common childhood illness) among young children with hemophilia who received clotting factor products made from donated blood. In that study, young children with hemophilia who had been treated with these products were more likely to have had the infection, suggesting that the virus was transmitted in the product. Since that time, additional steps have been taken in the manufacturing process of these products to reduce this type of risk.

BLOOD SAFETY COLLABORATIONS

The CDC collaborates with its federal partners in blood safety. The CDC works closely with the U.S. Food and Drug Administration

(FDA), which is responsible for regulating blood and blood products. The CDC participates in a variety of blood safety work groups across federal agencies, such as the U.S. Health and Human Services (HHS) Advisory Committee on Blood and Tissue Safety and Availability (ACBTSA), and work groups specific to pathogens, such as the Tickborne Working Group. In addition, the CDC, through the National Center for Emerging and Zoonotic Infectious Diseases (NCEZID), coordinates blood-related activities, including investigations, surveillance, research, policymaking, strategic planning, and communication for blood safety between divisions.[9]

---

[9] "Blood Safety and Hemophilia," Centers for Disease Control and Prevention (CDC), August 3, 2022. Available online. URL: www.cdc.gov/ncbddd/hemophilia/bloodsafety.html. Accessed May 19, 2023.

Chapter 21 | **Vitamin K Deficiency Bleeding**

WHAT IS VITAMIN K, AND WHY IS IT IMPORTANT?

Vitamin K is a substance that our body needs to form clots and stop bleeding. We get vitamin K from the food we eat. Some vitamin K is also made by the good bacteria that live in our intestines. Babies are born with very small amounts of vitamin K stored in their bodies, which can lead to serious bleeding problems if not supplemented.

WHAT IS VITAMIN K DEFICIENCY BLEEDING?

Vitamin K deficiency bleeding (VKDB) occurs when babies cannot stop bleeding because their blood does not have enough vitamin K to form a clot. The bleeding can occur anywhere on the inside or outside the body. When the bleeding occurs inside the body, it can be difficult to notice. Commonly, a baby with VKDB will bleed into his or her intestines or brain, which can lead to brain damage and even death. Infants who do not receive the vitamin K shot at birth can develop VKDB at any time up to six months of age.

WHY ARE BABIES MORE LIKELY TO HAVE VITAMIN K DEFICIENCY AND GET VITAMIN K DEFICIENCY BLEEDING?

All infants, regardless of sex, race, or ethnic background, are at higher risk for VKDB until they start eating regular foods, usually at the age of four to six months, and until the normal intestinal bacteria start making vitamin K. The following are the reasons for this:

- At birth, babies have very little vitamin K stored in their bodies because only small amounts pass to them through the placenta from their mothers.

315

- The good bacteria that produce vitamin K are not yet present in the newborn's intestines.
- Breast milk contains low amounts of vitamin K, so exclusively breastfed babies do not get enough vitamin K from breast milk alone.

WHAT MIGHT CAUSE BABIES TO BE DEFICIENT IN VITAMIN K AND HAVE BLEEDING PROBLEMS?

Some things can put infants at a higher risk of developing VKDB. Babies at greater risk include the following:

- **Babies who do not receive a vitamin K shot at birth**. The risk is even higher if they are exclusively breastfed.
- **Babies whose mothers used certain medications**. Medications such as isoniazid or medicines to treat seizures interfere with how the body uses vitamin K.
- **Babies who have liver disease**. Often, they cannot use the vitamin K their body stores.
- **Babies who have diarrhea, celiac disease, or cystic fibrosis (CF)**. These babies often have trouble absorbing vitamins, including vitamin K, from the foods they eat.

HOW OFTEN ARE BABIES AFFECTED WITH VITAMIN K DEFICIENCY BLEEDING?

Since babies can be affected until they are six months of age, health-care providers divide VKDB into three types: early, classical, and late (see Table 21.1):

- Early and classical VKDB are more common, occurring in 1 in 60 to 1 in 250 newborns, although the risk is much higher for early VKDB among those infants whose mothers used certain medications during the pregnancy.
- Late VKDB is rarer, occurring in 1 in 14,000 to 1 in 25,000 infants. Infants who do not receive a vitamin K shot at birth are 81 times more likely to develop late

VKDB than infants who do receive a vitamin K shot at birth.

Table 21.1. Characteristics of the Vitamin K Deficiency Bleeding (VKDB)

Type of VKDB	When It Occurs	Characteristics
Early-onset	within the first 24 hours after birth	• severe • mainly found in infants whose mothers used certain medications (such as medicines to treat seizures or isoniazid) that interfere with how the body uses vitamin K
Classic	2 days to 1 week after birth	• bruising • bleeding from the umbilical cord
Late-onset	1 week to 6 months after birth, most commonly 2–8 weeks after birth	• 30–60% of infants have bleeding within the brain • tends to occur in breastfed-only babies who have not received the vitamin K shot • warning bleeds are rare

WHAT THINGS SHOULD YOU LOOK FOR IN YOUR BABY IF YOU THINK HE OR SHE MIGHT HAVE VITAMIN K DEFICIENCY BLEEDING?

Babies with VKDB might develop any of the following signs:

- bruises, especially around the baby's head and face
- bleeding from the nose or umbilical cord
- skin color that is paler than before (For darker-skinned babies, the gums may appear pale.)
- white parts of your baby's eyes turning yellow
- stool that has blood in it and is black or dark and sticky (also called "tarry") or vomiting blood
- irritability, seizures, excessive sleepiness, or a lot of vomiting that may all be signs of bleeding in the brain

WHAT COULD YOU DO TO PREVENT YOUR BABY FROM GETTING VITAMIN K DEFICIENCY AND VITAMIN K DEFICIENCY BLEEDING?

The good news is that VKDB is easily prevented by giving babies a vitamin K shot into a muscle in the thigh. One shot given just after birth will protect your baby from VKDB. In order to ensure immediate bonding and contact between the newborn and mother, however, giving the vitamin K shot can be delayed up to six hours after birth.

IS THE VITAMIN K SHOT SAFE?

Yes. Many studies have shown that vitamin K is safe when given to newborns.[1]

---

[1] "Vitamin K Deficiency Bleeding," Centers for Disease Control and Prevention (CDC), February 10, 2023. Available online. URL: www.cdc.gov/ncbddd/vitamink/facts.html. Accessed June 2, 2023.

Chapter 22 | Immunoglobulin A Vasculitis

WHAT IS IMMUNOGLOBULIN A VASCULITIS?

Immunoglobulin A (IgA) vasculitis, formerly called "Henoch-Schönlein purpura" (HSP), is a disease that causes the antibody IgA to collect in small blood vessels, which then become inflamed and leak blood. Nearly all people with IgA vasculitis develop a red or purple rash. Some people with IgA vasculitis also develop problems with their gastrointestinal (GI) tract, joints, and kidneys because of inflamed blood vessels in the intestines, joints, and kidneys. In rare cases, the lungs, nervous system, or other organs may be affected.

HOW COMMON IS IMMUNOGLOBULIN A VASCULITIS?

Immunoglobulin A vasculitis is rare. The number of new cases of IgA vasculitis is approximately 3–27 cases per 100,000 in children and infants and fewer than 2 new cases per 100,000 in adults each year.

WHO IS MORE LIKELY TO DEVELOP IMMUNOGLOBULIN A VASCULITIS?

Immunoglobulin A vasculitis is most common in young children between the ages of four and seven, but people of all ages can be affected.

You may be more likely to develop IgA vasculitis if you have a family history of the disease.

ARE THERE LONG-TERM HEALTH PROBLEMS FROM IMMUNOGLOBULIN A VASCULITIS?

Most people recover from IgA vasculitis completely without treatment. The symptoms usually go away within a few weeks to months. The symptoms may return one or more times—usually within the first year—but typically go away again on their own.

The most common and serious long-term health problem caused by IgA vasculitis is chronic kidney disease (CKD). Severe kidney damage is rare, but if it does occur, it may require aggressive treatment. Adults are much more likely to develop CKD than children.

Women who have had IgA vasculitis and become pregnant are more likely to develop high blood pressure (HBP) and have protein in their urine during pregnancy. HBP in pregnancy causes health risks for the mother and baby. Pregnant women with a history of IgA vasculitis should be closely monitored by their health-care professionals.

WHAT CAUSES IMMUNOGLOBULIN A VASCULITIS?

Immunoglobulin A vasculitis occurs when your body's immune system attacks its own cells and organs. Researchers do not know what causes this unusual immune system response. However, many people have an infection of the upper respiratory tract—the nose, nasal cavity, pharynx, and larynx—before developing IgA vasculitis. IgA vasculitis has also been linked with the following:
- bacteria and viruses
- foods
- immunizations
- insect bites
- medicines

Certain genes may increase the risk for IgA vasculitis.

WHAT ARE THE SYMPTOMS OF IMMUNOGLOBULIN A VASCULITIS?

Some symptoms of IgA vasculitis are as follows:
- **Rash**. Leaking blood vessels cause a rash that looks like red or purple bruises or small red dots. The rash usually

appears on the legs and buttocks but may also appear on the arms, torso, and face. The rash is raised and does not disappear or turn pale when pressed. The rash is not painful and does not itch.

- **GI tract problems**. Abdominal pain can range from mild to severe, with nausea or vomiting. Blood may appear in the stool although the bleeding is usually not severe. In rare cases, more serious problems can occur, such as intussusception—a condition in which a section of the bowel folds into itself like a telescope, causing the bowel to become blocked.
- **Joint pain and swelling**. Pain and swelling often occur in the knees and ankles and sometimes occur in the elbows, wrists, and small joints of the fingers.
- **Kidney problems**. Hematuria—blood in the urine— is a common sign that IgA vasculitis has affected the kidneys. Proteinuria—large amounts of protein, including albumin, in the urine—and the development of HBP are signs of more severe kidney problems.
- **Other symptoms**. In some cases, boys with IgA vasculitis develop swelling of the testicles. Symptoms affecting the central nervous system (CNS), such as seizures, and lungs, such as pneumonia, have been seen in rare cases.

Rash, abdominal pain, joint pain, and swelling are often the first symptoms to appear, and they can occur in any order. Symptoms involving the kidneys rarely develop first.

HOW DO HEALTH-CARE PROFESSIONALS DIAGNOSE IMMUNOGLOBULIN A VASCULITIS?
Health-care professionals use your medical history, a physical exam, and lab tests to confirm your diagnosis of IgA vasculitis.

WHAT TESTS DO HEALTH-CARE PROFESSIONALS USE TO DIAGNOSE OR MONITOR IMMUNOGLOBULIN A VASCULITIS?
Your health-care professional may perform a skin or kidney biopsy, blood and urine tests, and sometimes an ultrasound of the kidneys

or abdomen to confirm the diagnosis and monitor your health. In some cases, a kidney biopsy may be used to assess and monitor the severity of the disease. Depending on the organs affected, your health-care professional may suggest other tests.

Skin Biopsy

Your health-care professional may obtain a skin biopsy to test for antibody deposits on your skin and confirm a diagnosis of IgA vasculitis. To do a skin biopsy, the health-care professional removes skin cells from your body to examine under a microscope. You will be given a local anesthetic, so you do not feel any pain.

Kidney Biopsy

You may also need a kidney biopsy. A kidney biopsy can confirm the diagnosis of IgA vasculitis and provide information on the amount of kidney damage. Your health-care professional will use the results of the kidney biopsy to help develop a treatment plan. The kidney biopsy is performed in a hospital with local anesthetic and, in some children, sedation.

Blood and Urine Tests

Your health-care professional may use blood and urine tests to check the health of your kidneys. A urine sample can be used to determine whether there is blood or protein in your urine, which is a sign that the IgA vasculitis is affecting your kidneys. A blood test can check how well your kidneys are working.

Ultrasound

Depending on your symptoms, your health-care professional may want you to have an ultrasound to check for GI or kidney problems.

Your health-care professional will monitor your symptoms to determine if they are getting better. You may continue to have blood and urine tests to check your kidney function for at least six months after most of your symptoms disappear. Your health-care professional will monitor you more closely if your tests show kidney damage, as this puts you at greater risk of developing CKD.

HOW DO HEALTH-CARE PROFESSIONALS TREAT IMMUNOGLOBULIN A VASCULITIS?

There is no specific treatment for IgA vasculitis. The disease usually goes away on its own. However, your health-care professional may suggest certain medicines to relieve symptoms, such as abdominal pain, joint pain, and swelling. If your kidneys are involved, the treatment goal will be to prevent CKD.

If you are taking a medicine that may have caused the IgA vasculitis, you will stop taking that medicine.

Treatments for Different Symptoms

- **Rash**. Your rash will usually go away without any specific treatment. In some people, the rash returns, but even the returning rash will go away without medicine.
- **GI tract problems**. To ease abdominal pain, your health-care professional may prescribe a corticosteroid—a medicine that lowers immune system activity and decreases swelling. In rare cases, when intussusception occurs, health-care professionals can correct the problem with a lower GI series, also called a "barium enema," that uses air or barium to gently push the telescoped part of the intestine into its proper position or correct the problem with surgery.
- **Joint pain and swelling**. Your health-care professional may prescribe a nonsteroidal anti-inflammatory drug (NSAID), such as ibuprofen, or a corticosteroid to ease joint pain and swelling. You should not take NSAIDs if you have decreased kidney function or you suspect your kidneys have been affected.
- **Kidney involvement**. In IgA vasculitis, the unusual activity of the immune system causes inflammation, which can lead to kidney damage. You may need to take a corticosteroid or other immunosuppressive medicine

to reduce inflammation, which can help prevent your immune system from causing more damage. If you have protein in your urine, your health-care professional may prescribe an angiotensin-converting enzyme (ACE) inhibitor or an angiotensin receptor blocker (ARB). ACE inhibitors and ARBs are blood pressure medicines that have been shown to reduce proteinuria and slow the progression of kidney disease.

- **Scrotum or testicles**. If you are experiencing pain in the scrotum or testicles, your health-care professional will recommend pain relief measures, including bed rest, applying ice or a cool pack, and placing a cushion under the scrotum to provide support.

HOW CAN YOU PREVENT IMMUNOGLOBULIN A VASCULITIS?

Experts have not yet found a way to prevent IgA vasculitis. If your kidneys have been affected by the disease, treatments may be available to help prevent serious kidney problems. Talk with your health-care professional about treatments and follow the treatment plan your health-care professional recommends.

HOW CAN YOUR DIET HELP PREVENT OR RELIEVE IMMUNOGLOBULIN A VASCULITIS?

Diet and nutrition have not been shown to play a role in causing or preventing IgA vasculitis.[1]

---

[1] "IgA Vasculitis," National Institute of Diabetes and Digestive and Kidney Diseases (NIDDK), April 2020. Available online. URL: www.niddk.nih.gov/health-information/kidney-disease/iga-vasculitis. Accessed May 19, 2023.

Chapter 23 | von Willebrand Disease

WHAT IS VON WILLEBRAND DISEASE?

von Willebrand disease (VWD) is a blood disorder in which the blood does not clot properly. Blood contains many proteins that help the blood clot when needed. One of these proteins is called "von Willebrand factor" (VWF). People with VWD have a low level of VWF in their blood, or the VWF protein does not work the way it should.

Normally, when a person is injured and starts to bleed, the VWF in the blood attaches to small blood cells called "platelets." This helps the platelets stick together, like glue, to form a clot at the site of injury and stop the bleeding. When a person has VWD, because the VWF does not work the way it should, the clot might take longer to form or form incorrectly, and bleeding might take longer to stop. This can lead to heavy, hard-to-stop bleeding. Although rare, the bleeding can be serious enough to damage joints or internal organs or even be life-threatening.

WHO IS AFFECTED BY VON WILLEBRAND DISEASE?

von Willebrand disease is the most common bleeding disorder, found in up to 1 percent of the U.S. population. This means that 3.2 million (or about 1 in every 100) people in the United States have the disease. Although VWD occurs among men and women equally, women are more likely to notice the symptoms because of heavy or abnormal bleeding during their menstrual periods and after childbirth. There are three major types of VWD: type 1, type 2, and type 3.

TYPES OF VON WILLEBRAND DISEASE

Type 1

This is the most common and mildest form of VWD, in which a person has lower-than-normal levels of VWF. A person with type 1 VWD may also have low levels of factor VIII, another type of blood-clotting protein. About 85 percent of people treated for VWD have type 1.

Type 2

With this type of VWD, although the body makes normal amounts of the VWF, the factor does not work the way it should. Type 2 is further broken down into four subtypes—2A, 2B, 2M, and 2N—depending on the specific problem with the person's VWF. Because the treatment is different for each type, it is important that a person know which subtype he or she has.

- **Type 2A**. The VWF is not the right size and does not help the platelets attach together in order to form a clot.
- **Type 2B**. The VWF attaches to platelets at the wrong time (when there is no injury). The body removes the platelets attached to VWF, causing a reduced amount of both platelets and VWF in the blood when needed to form a clot.
- **Type 2M**. The VWF does not attach to the platelets as it should, which decreases the platelets' ability to form a clot when an injury occurs.
- **Type 2N**. The VWF attaches to the platelets normally. However, the VWF does not attach to another protein, factor VIII, which is also needed for blood to clot. This causes the body to remove the factor VIII protein.

Type 3

This is the most severe form of VWD, in which a person has very little or no VWF and low levels of factor VIII. This is the rarest type of VWD. Only 3 percent of people with VWD have type 3.

CAUSES OF VON WILLEBRAND DISEASE

Most people who have VWD are born with it. It is almost always inherited, or passed down, from a parent to a child. VWD can be passed down from either the mother or the father, or both, to the child.

While rare, it is possible for a person to get VWD without a family history of the disease. This can happen if a spontaneous mutation occurs. That means there has been a change in the person's genes. Whether a child receives the affected gene from a parent or as a result of a mutation, once the child has it, the child can later pass it along to his or her children.

Also, it is rare, but possible, for a person to get or acquire VWD (they did not receive the affected gene from their parent or as a result of a mutation) later in life because of an underlying medical condition. This can happen when a person's own immune system (which controls the body's ability to fight germs and sickness) destroys his or her VWF, often as a result of the use of a medication or as a result of another disease. If VWD is acquired in this way, it cannot be passed along to any children.

SIGNS AND SYMPTOMS OF VON WILLEBRAND DISEASE
The major signs of VWD are as follows.

Frequent or Hard-to-Stop Nosebleeds
People with VWD might have nosebleeds that may include the following:
- starting without injury (spontaneous)
- occurring often, usually five times or more in a year
- lasting more than ten minutes
- needing packing (gauze placed in the nose) or cautery (a procedure to burn and seal blood vessels) to stop the bleeding

Easy Bruising
People with VWD might experience easy bruising that may include the following:
- occurring with very little or no trauma or injury
- being larger than the size of a quarter
- being not flat and having a raised lump

Heavy Menstrual Bleeding

Women with VWD might have heavy menstrual periods during which they experience:

- soaking through a pad or tampon every one to two hours (or more often) on the heaviest day(s)
- menstrual bleeding that lasts longer than seven days from the time bleeding starts until the time it ends
- flooding or gushing of blood
- passing blood clots (tissue) larger than the size of grapes or strawberries

A diagnosis of anemia (not having enough red blood cells (RBCs)) is made as a result of bleeding from heavy periods.

Longer than Normal Bleeding after Injury, Surgery, Childbirth, or Dental Work

People with VWD might have longer-than-normal bleeding after injury, surgery, or childbirth. This bleeding may be characterized in the following ways:

- After a cut to the skin, the bleeding lasts more than five minutes.
- Heavy or longer bleeding occurs after surgery. Bleeding sometimes stops but starts up again hours or days later.
- Heavy bleeding occurs during or after childbirth.

People with VWD might have longer-than-normal bleeding during or after dental work. The following are a few examples:

- Heavy bleeding occurs during or after dental surgery.
- The surgery site oozes blood longer than three hours after the surgery.
- The surgery site needs packing or cautery to stop the bleeding.

The amount of bleeding depends on the type and severity of VWD. Other common bleeding events include:

- blood in the stool (feces) from bleeding into the stomach or intestines

- blood in the urine from bleeding into the kidneys or bladder
- bleeding into joints or internal organs in severe cases (type 3 VWD)

DIAGNOSIS OF VON WILLEBRAND DISEASE

To find out if a person has VWD, the doctor will ask questions about personal and family histories of bleeding. The doctor will also check for unusual bruising or other signs of recent bleeding and order some blood tests to measure how the blood clots. The tests will provide information about the amount of clotting proteins present in the blood and if the clotting proteins are working properly. Because certain medications can cause bleeding, even among people without a bleeding disorder, the doctor will ask about recent or routine medications taken that could cause bleeding or make bleeding symptoms worse.

TREATMENTS FOR VON WILLEBRAND DISEASE

The type of treatment prescribed for VWD depends on the type and severity of the disease. For minor bleeds, treatment might not be needed.

The most commonly used types of treatment are as follows.

Desmopressin Acetate Injection

This medicine (DDAVP®) is injected into a vein to treat people with milder forms of VWD (mainly type 1). It works by making the body release more VWF into the blood. It also helps increase the level of factor VIII in the blood.

Desmopressin Acetate Nasal Spray

This high-strength nasal spray (Stimate®) is used to treat people with milder forms of VWD (mainly type 1). It works by making the body release more VWF into the blood.

Factor Replacement Therapy

Recombinant VWF (such as Vonvendi®) and medicines rich in VWF and factor VIII (e.g., Humate P®, Wilate®, Alphanate®, or Koate DVI®) are used to treat people with more severe forms of VWD or people with milder forms of VWD who do not respond well to the nasal spray. These medicines are injected into a vein in the arm to replace the missing factor in the blood.

Antifibrinolytic Drugs

These drugs (e.g., Amicar®, Lysteda®) are either injected or taken orally to help slow or prevent the breakdown of blood clots.

Birth Control Pills

Birth control pills can increase the levels of VWF and factor VIII in the blood and reduce menstrual blood loss. A doctor can prescribe these pills to women who have heavy menstrual bleeding.[1]

---

[1] "What Is von Willebrand Disease?" Centers for Disease Control and Prevention (CDC), December 30, 2022. Available online. URL: www.cdc.gov/ncbddd/vwd/facts.html. Accessed May 19, 2023.

Chapter 24 | **Factor Deficiencies**

Chapter Contents

Section 24.1 | Factor I Deficiency

Congenital afibrinogenemia is a bleeding disorder caused by impairment of the blood clotting process. Normally, blood clots protect the body after an injury by sealing off damaged blood vessels and preventing further blood loss. However, bleeding is uncontrolled in people with congenital afibrinogenemia. Newborns with this condition often experience prolonged bleeding from the umbilical cord stump after birth.

CAUSES OF FACTOR I DEFICIENCY

Congenital afibrinogenemia results from mutations in one of three genes: *FGA*, *FGB*, or *FGG*. Each of these genes provides instructions for making one part (subunit) of a protein called "fibrinogen." This protein is important for blood clot formation (coagulation), which is needed to stop excessive bleeding after injury. In response to injury, fibrinogen is converted to fibrin, the main protein in blood clots. Fibrin proteins attach to each other, forming a stable network that makes up the blood clot.

Congenital afibrinogenemia is caused by a complete absence of fibrinogen protein. Most *FGA*, *FGB*, and *FGG* gene mutations that cause this condition result in a premature stop signal in the instructions for making the respective protein. If any protein is made, it is nonfunctional. When any one subunit is missing, the fibrinogen protein is not assembled, which results in the absence of fibrin. Consequently, blood clots do not form in response to injury, leading to excessive bleeding seen in people with congenital afibrinogenemia.

SYMPTOMS OF FACTOR I DEFICIENCY

Nosebleeds (epistaxis) and bleeding from the gums or tongue are common and can occur after minor trauma or in the absence of injury (spontaneous bleeding). Some affected individuals experience bleeding into the spaces between joints (hemarthrosis) or the muscles (hematoma). Rarely, bleeding in the brain or other internal organs occurs, which can be fatal.

COMPLICATIONS OF FACTOR I DEFICIENCY

Women with congenital afibrinogenemia can have abnormally heavy menstrual bleeding (menorrhagia). Without proper treatment, women with this disorder may have difficulty carrying a pregnancy to term, resulting in repeated miscarriages.

FREQUENCY OF FACTOR I DEFICIENCY

Congenital afibrinogenemia is a rare condition that occurs in approximately 1 in 1 million newborns.

INHERITANCE OF FACTOR I DEFICIENCY

Congenital afibrinogenemia is inherited in an autosomal recessive pattern, which means both copies of the gene in each cell have mutations. The parents of an individual with an autosomal recessive condition each carry one copy of the mutated gene. The parents have about half the normal level of fibrinogen in their blood but typically do not show signs and symptoms of the condition.[1]

Section 24.2 | Factor II Deficiency

Prothrombin deficiency is a bleeding disorder that slows the blood clotting process.

CAUSES OF FACTOR II DEFICIENCY

Mutations in the *F2* gene cause prothrombin deficiency. The *F2* gene provides instructions for making the prothrombin protein (also called "coagulation factor II"), which plays a critical role in the formation of blood clots in response to injury. Prothrombin is the precursor to thrombin, a protein that initiates a series of chemical reactions to form a blood clot. After an injury, clots protect the

---

[1] MedlinePlus, "Congenital Afibrinogenemia," National Institutes of Health (NIH), September 1, 2014. Available online. URL: https://medlineplus.gov/genetics/condition/congenital-afibrinogenemia/. Accessed June 13, 2023.

body by sealing off damaged blood vessels and preventing further blood loss.

F2 gene mutations reduce the production of prothrombin in cells, which prevents clots from forming properly in response to injury. Problems with blood clotting can lead to excessive bleeding. Some mutations drastically reduce the activity of prothrombin and can lead to severe bleeding episodes. Other *F2* gene mutations allow for a moderate amount of prothrombin activity, typically resulting in mild bleeding episodes.

SYMPTOMS OF FACTOR II DEFICIENCY

People with this condition often experience prolonged bleeding following an injury, surgery, or having a tooth pulled. In severe cases of prothrombin deficiency, heavy bleeding occurs after minor trauma or even in the absence of injury (spontaneous bleeding). Women with prothrombin deficiency can have prolonged and sometimes abnormally heavy menstrual bleeding.

COMPLICATIONS OF FACTOR II DEFICIENCY

Serious complications can result from bleeding into the joints, muscles, brain, or other internal organs. Milder forms of prothrombin deficiency do not involve spontaneous bleeding, and the condition may only become apparent following surgery or a serious injury.

FREQUENCY OF FACTOR II DEFICIENCY

Prothrombin deficiency is very rare; it is estimated to affect 1 in 2 million people in the general population.

INHERITANCE OF FACTOR II DEFICIENCY

This condition is inherited in an autosomal recessive pattern, which means both copies of the gene in each cell have mutations. The parents of an individual with an autosomal recessive condition each carry one copy of the mutated gene, but they typically do not show signs and symptoms of the condition.[2]

---

[2] MedlinePlus, "Prothrombin Deficiency," National Institutes of Health (NIH), November 1, 2013. Available online. URL: https://medlineplus.gov/genetics/condition/prothrombin-deficiency/. Accessed June 13, 2023.

Section 24.3 | **Factor III Deficiency**

Hereditary antithrombin deficiency is a disorder of blood clotting. People with this condition are at higher-than-average risk of developing abnormal blood clots, particularly a type of clot that occurs in the deep veins of the legs. This type of clot is called a "deep vein thrombosis" (DVT). Affected individuals also have increased risk of developing a pulmonary embolism (PE), which is a clot that travels through the bloodstream and lodges in the lungs. In hereditary antithrombin deficiency, abnormal blood clots usually form only in veins although they may rarely occur in arteries.

CAUSES OF FACTOR III DEFICIENCY

Hereditary antithrombin deficiency is caused by mutations in the *SERPINC1* gene. This gene provides instructions for producing a protein called "antithrombin" (previously known as "antithrombin III"). This protein is found in the bloodstream and is important for controlling blood clotting. Antithrombin blocks the activity of proteins that promote blood clotting, especially a protein called "thrombin."

Most of the mutations that cause hereditary antithrombin deficiency change single protein building blocks (amino acids) in antithrombin, which disrupts its ability to control blood clotting. Individuals with this condition do not have enough functional antithrombin to inactivate clotting proteins, which results in increased risk of developing abnormal blood clots.

RISK FACTORS FOR FACTOR III DEFICIENCY

Some factors can increase the risk of abnormal blood clots in people with hereditary antithrombin deficiency. These factors include increasing age, surgery, or immobility. The combination of hereditary antithrombin deficiency and other inherited disorders of blood clotting can also influence risk. Women with hereditary antithrombin deficiency are at increased risk of developing an abnormal blood clot during pregnancy or soon after delivery. They may also have increased risk of pregnancy loss (miscarriage) or stillbirth.

WHO IS AT RISK OF DEVELOPING FACTOR III DEFICIENCY?

About half of people with hereditary antithrombin deficiency will develop at least one abnormal blood clot during their lifetime. These clots usually develop after adolescence.

FREQUENCY OF FACTOR III DEFICIENCY

Hereditary antithrombin deficiency is estimated to occur in about 1 in 2,000–3,000 individuals. Of people who have experienced an abnormal blood clot, about 1 in 20–200 has hereditary antithrombin deficiency.

INHERITANCE OF FACTOR III DEFICIENCY

Hereditary antithrombin deficiency is typically inherited in an autosomal dominant pattern, which means one altered copy of the *SERPINC1* gene in each cell is sufficient to cause the disorder. Inheriting two altered copies of this gene in each cell is usually incompatible with life; however, a few severely affected individuals have been reported with mutations in both copies of the *SERPINC1* gene in each cell.[3]

Section 24.4 | Factor V Deficiency

Factor V deficiency is a rare bleeding disorder.

CAUSES OF FACTOR V DEFICIENCY

Factor V deficiency is usually caused by mutations in the *F5* gene, which provides instructions for making a protein called "coagulation factor V." This protein plays a critical role in the coagulation

[3] MedlinePlus, "Hereditary Antithrombin Deficiency," National Institutes of Health (NIH), February 1, 2013. Available online. URL: https://medlineplus.gov/genetics/condition/hereditary-antithrombin-deficiency/. Accessed June 13, 2023.

system, which is a series of chemical reactions that form blood clots in response to injury. *F5* gene mutations that cause factor V deficiency prevent the production of functional coagulation factor V or severely reduce the amount of protein in the bloodstream. People with this condition typically have less than 10 percent of normal levels of coagulation factor V in their blood; the most severely affected individuals have less than 1 percent. A reduced amount of functional coagulation factor V prevents blood from clotting normally, causing episodes of abnormal bleeding that can be severe.

Very rarely, a form of factor V deficiency is caused by abnormal antibodies that recognize coagulation factor V. Antibodies normally attach (bind) to specific foreign particles and germs, marking them for destruction, but the antibodies in this form of factor V deficiency attack a normal human protein, leading to its inactivation. These cases are called "acquired factor V deficiency" and usually occur in individuals who have been treated with substances that stimulate the production of anti-factor V antibodies, such as bovine thrombin used during surgical procedures. There is no known genetic cause for this form of the condition.

SYMPTOMS OF FACTOR V DEFICIENCY

The signs and symptoms of this condition can begin at any age although the most severe cases are apparent in childhood. Factor V deficiency commonly causes nosebleeds, easy bruising, bleeding under the skin, bleeding of the gums, and prolonged or excessive bleeding following surgery, trauma, or childbirth. Women with factor V deficiency can have heavy or prolonged menstrual bleeding (menorrhagia). Bleeding into joint spaces (hemarthrosis) can also occur although it is rare.

COMPLICATIONS OF FACTOR V DEFICIENCY

Severely affected individuals have an increased risk of bleeding inside the skull (intracranial hemorrhage), in the lungs (pulmonary hemorrhage), or in the gastrointestinal tract, which can be life-threatening.

FREQUENCY OF FACTOR V DEFICIENCY

Factor V deficiency affects an estimated 1 in 1 million people. This condition is more common in countries such as Iran and southern India, where it occurs up to 10 times more frequently than in Western countries.

INHERITANCE OF FACTOR V DEFICIENCY

Factor V deficiency is inherited in an autosomal recessive pattern, which means both copies of the *F5* gene in each cell have mutations. Individuals with a mutation in a single copy of the *F5* gene have a reduced amount of coagulation factor V in their blood and can have mild bleeding problems although most have no related health effects.[4]

Section 24.5 | Factor V Leiden Thrombophilia

Factor V Leiden thrombophilia is an inherited disorder of blood clotting. Factor V Leiden is the name of a specific gene mutation that results in thrombophilia, which is an increased tendency to form abnormal blood clots that can block blood vessels.

People with factor V Leiden thrombophilia have higher-than-average risk of developing a type of blood clot called a "deep venous thrombosis." Deep venous thromboses occur most often in the legs although they can also occur in other parts of the body, including the brain, eyes, liver, and kidneys. Factor V Leiden thrombophilia also increases the risk that clots will break away from their original site and travel through the bloodstream. These clots can lodge in the lungs, where they are known as "pulmonary emboli." Although factor V Leiden thrombophilia increases the risk of blood clots, only about 10 percent of individuals with the factor V Leiden mutation ever develop abnormal clots.

---

[4] MedlinePlus, "Factor V deficiency," National Institutes of Health (NIH), May 1, 2013. Available online. URL: https://medlineplus.gov/genetics/condition/factor-v-deficiency. Accessed June 13, 2023.

CAUSES OF FACTOR V LEIDEN THROMBOPHILIA

A particular mutation in the *F5* gene causes factor V Leiden throm-bophilia. The *F5* gene provides instructions for making a protein called "coagulation factor V." This protein plays a critical role in the coagulation system, which is a series of chemical reactions that forms blood clots in response to injury.

The coagulation system is controlled by several proteins, includ-ing a protein called "activated protein C" (APC). APC normally inactivates coagulation factor V, which slows down the clotting process and prevents clots from growing too large. However, in people with factor V Leiden thrombophilia, coagulation factor V cannot be inactivated normally by APC. As a result, the clotting process remains active longer than usual, increasing the chance of developing abnormal blood clots.

RISK FACTORS OF FACTOR V LEIDEN THROMBOPHILIA

Some factors increase the risk of developing blood clots in people with factor V Leiden thrombophilia. These factors include increas-ing age, obesity, injury, surgery, smoking, pregnancy, and the use of oral contraceptives (birth control pills) or hormone replacement therapy (HRT).

WHO IS AT RISK OF DEVELOPING FACTOR V LEIDEN THROMBOPHILIA?

The risk of abnormal clots is also much higher in people who have a combination of the factor V Leiden mutation and another muta-tion in the *F5* gene. Additionally, the risk is increased in people who have the factor V Leiden mutation together with a mutation in another gene involved in the coagulation system.

COMPLICATIONS OF FACTOR V LEIDEN THROMBOPHILIA

The factor V Leiden mutation is associated with a slightly increased risk of pregnancy loss (miscarriage). Women with this mutation are two to three times more likely to have multiple (recurrent) mis-carriages or a pregnancy loss during the second or third trimester.

Some research suggests that the factor V Leiden mutation may also increase the risk of other complications during pregnancy, including pregnancy-induced high blood pressure (preeclampsia), slow fetal growth, and early separation of the placenta from the uterine wall (placental abruption). However, the association between the factor V Leiden mutation and these complications has not been confirmed. Most women with factor V Leiden thrombophilia have normal pregnancies.

FREQUENCY OF FACTOR V LEIDEN THROMBOPHILIA

Factor V Leiden is the most common inherited form of thrombophilia. Between 3 and 8 percent of people with European ancestry carry one copy of the factor V Leiden mutation in each cell, and about 1 in 5,000 people has two copies of the mutation. The mutation is less common in other populations.

INHERITANCE OF FACTOR V LEIDEN THROMBOPHILIA

The chance of developing an abnormal blood clot depends on whether a person has one or two copies of the factor V Leiden mutation in each cell. People who inherit two copies of the mutation, one from each parent, have a higher risk of developing a clot than people who inherit one copy of the mutation. Considering that about 1 in 1,000 people per year in the general population will develop an abnormal blood clot, the presence of one copy of the factor V Leiden mutation increases that risk to 3–8 in 1,000, and having two copies of the mutation may raise the risk to as high as 80 in 1,000.[5]

---

[5] MedlinePlus, "Factor V Leiden Thrombophilia," National Institutes of Health (NIH), August 1, 2010. Available online. URL: https://medlineplus.gov/genetics/condition/factor-v-leiden-thrombophilia. Accessed June 14, 2023.

Section 24.6 | Factor VII Deficiency

Factor VII deficiency is a rare bleeding disorder that varies in severity among affected individuals.

CAUSES OF FACTOR VII DEFICIENCY

The inherited form of factor VII deficiency, known as "congenital factor VII deficiency," is caused by mutations in the *F7* gene, which provides instructions for making a protein called "coagulation factor VII." This protein plays a critical role in the coagulation system, which is a series of chemical reactions that form blood clots in response to injury. These mutations reduce the amount of coagulation factor VII in the bloodstream. Such a reduction prevents blood from clotting normally, causing episodes of excessive bleeding. It is not known why some people with this condition have problems with thrombosis. Researchers also do not know what determines the severity of the condition; it does not appear to be related to the amount of coagulation factor VII in the bloodstream.

The noninherited form of the disorder, called "acquired factor VII deficiency," is less common than the congenital form. It can be caused by liver disease or by blood cell disorders, such as myeloma or aplastic anemia. Acquired factor VII deficiency can also be caused by certain drugs, such as medicines that prevent clotting, or by a deficiency of vitamin K.

SIGNS AND SYMPTOMS OF FACTOR VII DEFICIENCY

The signs and symptoms of this condition can begin at any age although the most severe cases are apparent in infancy. However, up to one-third of people with factor VII deficiency never have any bleeding problems. Factor VII deficiency commonly causes nosebleeds (epistaxis), bleeding of the gums, easy bruising, and prolonged or excessive bleeding following surgery or physical injury. Bleeding into joint spaces (hemarthrosis) and blood in the urine (hematuria) occasionally occur. Many women with factor VII deficiency have heavy or prolonged menstrual bleeding (menorrhagia).

COMPLICATIONS OF FACTOR VII DEFICIENCY

Severely affected individuals have an increased risk of bleeding inside the skull (intracranial hemorrhage) or in the GI tract, which can be life-threatening. Although factor VII deficiency is primarily associated with increased bleeding, some people with the condition have excessive blood clotting (thrombosis).

FREQUENCY OF FACTOR VII DEFICIENCY

Factor VII deficiency is estimated to affect 1 in 300,000 to 1 in 500,000 people. It is the most frequently occurring of a group of disorders classified as rare bleeding disorders.

INHERITANCE OF FACTOR VII DEFICIENCY

Congenital factor VII deficiency is inherited in an autosomal recessive pattern, which means both copies of the *F7* gene in each cell have mutations. The parents of an individual with an autosomal recessive condition each carry one copy of the mutated gene, but they typically do not show signs and symptoms of the condition.[6]

Section 24.7 | Factor VIII Deficiency

Hemophilia A is an inherited bleeding disorder in which the blood does not clot normally. People with hemophilia A will bleed more than normal after an injury, surgery, or dental procedure. This disorder can be severe, moderate, or mild. In severe cases, heavy bleeding occurs after a minor injury or even when there is no injury (spontaneous bleeding). Bleeding into the joints, muscles, brain, or organs can cause pain and other serious complications. In milder forms, there is no spontaneous bleeding, and the disorder might only be diagnosed after a surgery or serious injury.

---

[6] MedlinePlus, "Factor VII Deficiency," National Institutes of Health (NIH), October 1, 2016. Available online. URL: https://medlineplus.gov/genetics/condition/factor-vii-deficiency. Accessed June 14, 2023.

CAUSES OF HEMOPHILIA A

Hemophilia A is caused by having low levels of a protein called "factor VIII." Factor VIII is needed to form blood clots. The disorder is inherited in an X-linked recessive manner and is caused by changes in the *F8* gene.

WHO IS AT RISK OF DEVELOPING HEMOPHILIA A?

Hemophilia A mainly affects males.

WHEN DO SYMPTOMS OF HEMOPHILIA A BEGIN?

Symptoms of this disease may start to appear from birth to childhood.

SYMPTOMS OF HEMOPHILIA A

The following symptoms have been linked to hemophilia A:

- arthralgia (joint pain)
- bleeding with minor or no trauma
- reduced factor VIII activity (reduced activity of coagulation factor VIII, which is a cofactor in the intrinsic clotting cascade that is activated to factor VIIIa (a receptor for factors IXa and X) in the presence of minute quantities of thrombin)
- oral cavity bleeding
- spontaneous hematomas
- thromboembolism (the formation of a blood clot inside a blood vessel that subsequently travels through the bloodstream from the site where it formed to another location in the body, generally leading to vascular occlusion at the distant site)
- abnormality of the elbow
- gastrointestinal hemorrhage
- intramuscular hematoma (blood clots formed within muscle tissue following leakage of blood into the tissue)
- intraventricular hemorrhage (bleeding into the ventricles of the brain)

- joint hemorrhage
- intracranial hemorrhage (hemorrhage occurring within the skull)
- splenic rupture (a breach of the capsule of the spleen)

DIAGNOSIS OF HEMOPHILIA A

The diagnosis of hemophilia A is made through clinical symptoms and specific laboratory tests to measure the amount of clotting factors in the blood.

INHERITANCE OF HEMOPHILIA A

All individuals inherit two copies of most genes. The number of copies of a gene that need to have a disease-causing variant affects the way a disease is inherited. This disease is inherited in the X-linked recessive inheritance patterns.

X-Linked Recessive Inheritance

X-linked means the gene is located on the X chromosome, one of two sex chromosomes. Genes, like chromosomes, usually come in pairs. Recessive means that when there are two copies of the responsible gene, both copies must have a disease-causing change (pathogenic variant) in order for a person to have the disease. Mutation is an older term that is still sometimes used to mean a pathogenic variant.

Because women have two X chromosomes, a pathogenic variant for an X-lined recessive disease generally needs to occur in both copies of the gene to cause the disease. Because men have one X chromosome and thus only one copy of the gene, a pathogenic variant in their one copy is enough to cause the disease. Women who have a pathogenic variant in one copy of the gene are called "carriers." In rare cases, women carriers may experience mild-to-moderate symptoms, but most have no symptoms.

A woman who carries one X-linked gene variant has a 50 percent (one in two) chance of having a son with the disease and a 50 percent (one in two) chance of having a daughter who is a carrier. A man with an X-linked recessive disease cannot pass on the disease to his sons, but all of his daughters will be carriers. If a male child is the first person in a family with the disease, the pathogenic variant may have been inherited from the mother or may have occurred by chance for the first time in the child (de novo).[7]

Section 24.8 | Factor IX Deficiency

The *F9* gene provides instructions for making a protein called "coagulation factor IX." Coagulation factors are a group of related proteins that are essential for the formation of blood clots. After an injury, clots protect the body by sealing off damaged blood vessels and preventing further blood loss.

Coagulation factor IX is made in the liver. This protein circulates in the bloodstream in an inactive form until an injury that damages blood vessels occurs. In response to injury, coagulation factor IX is activated by another coagulation factor called "factor XIa." The active protein (coagulation factor IXa) interacts with coagulation factor VIII and other molecules. These interactions set off a chain of additional chemical reactions that form a blood clot.

HEALTH CONDITIONS RELATED TO GENETIC CHANGES
Hemophilia

Mutations in the *F9* gene cause a type of hemophilia called "hemophilia B." More than 900 alterations in this gene have been identified. The most common mutations change single DNA building blocks (base pairs) in the gene. A small percentage of mutations delete or insert multiple base pairs or rearrange segments of DNA within the gene.

---

[7] Genetic and Rare Diseases Information Center (GARD), "Hemophilia A," National Center for Advancing Translational Sciences (NCATS), February 2023. Available online. URL: https://rarediseases.info.nih.gov/diseases/6591/hemophilia-a. Accessed June 14, 2023.

Factor Deficiencies

Mutations in the *F9* gene lead to the production of an abnormal version of coagulation factor IX or reduce the amount of this protein. The altered or missing protein cannot participate effectively in the blood clotting process. As a result, blood clots cannot form properly in response to injury. These problems with blood clotting lead to excessive bleeding that can be difficult to control.

Mutations that completely eliminate the activity of coagulation factor IX result in severe hemophilia. Mutations that reduce but do not eliminate the protein's activity usually cause mild or moderate hemophilia.

Several mutations near the beginning of the *F9* gene sequence cause an unusual form of hemophilia known as "hemophilia B Leyden." People with these mutations are born with very low levels of functional coagulation factor IX, but hormonal changes cause the levels of this protein to increase gradually during puberty. As a result, adults with hemophilia B Leyden rarely experience episodes of abnormal bleeding.

Other Disorders

Several rare mutations in the *F9* gene cause an increased sensitivity (hypersensitivity) to a drug called "warfarin." This medication is an anticoagulant, which means it is used to prevent the formation or growth of abnormal blood clots. Warfarin works by reducing the amount of active factor IX and three other coagulation proteins.

The mutations responsible for warfarin hypersensitivity each change a single base pair in the *F9* gene. These mutations do not cause hemophilia B, and people with these genetic changes only have bleeding problems if they are treated with warfarin. Warfarin reduces the amount of coagulation factor IX to very low levels in these individuals, which prevents the blood from clotting normally and can lead to recurrent, severe bleeding problems. To avoid these complications, people with warfarin hypersensitivity can be treated with other anticoagulant medications.[8]

---

[8] MedlinePlus, "*F9* Gene," National Institutes of Health (NIH), May 1, 2010. Available online. URL: https://medlineplus.gov/genetics/gene/f9. Accessed June 14, 2023.

Section 24.9 | **Factor X Deficiency**

Factor X deficiency is a rare disorder that affects the blood's ability to clot. The severity of the disorder and the associated signs and symptoms can vary significantly from person to person. Common features of factor X deficiency may include easy bruising, frequent nosebleeds, bleeding gums, blood in the urine, and prolonged bleeding after minor injuries. Women with factor X deficiency may also experience heavy menstrual bleeding and may have an increased risk for first-trimester miscarriages.

Acquired (noninherited) factor X deficiency, which is the most common form of the disorder, generally occurs in people with no family history of the disorder. Acquired factor X deficiency has a variety of causes, including liver disease, vitamin K deficiency, exposure to certain medications that affect clotting, and certain types of cancer. The inherited form of factor X deficiency (also called "congenital factor X deficiency") is caused by changes in the *F10* gene and is inherited in an autosomal recessive manner.

CAUSES OF FACTOR X DEFICIENCY

Factor X deficiency is a genetic disease, which means that it is caused by one or more genes not working correctly. Disease-causing variants, or differences, in the *F10* genes are known to cause this disease.

WHEN DO SYMPTOMS OF FACTOR X DEFICIENCY BEGIN?

Symptoms of this disease may start to appear at any time in life.

SYMPTOMS OF FACTOR X DEFICIENCY

The following symptoms have been linked to factor X deficiency:
- **Prolonged prothrombin time (PT).** Increased time to coagulation in the PT test, which is a measure of the extrinsic pathway of coagulation. The results of the PT test are often expressed in terms of the international

normalized ratio (INR), which is calculated as a ratio of the patient's PT to a control PT standardized for the potency of the thromboplastin reagent developed by the World Health Organization (WHO) using the formula: INR is equal to patient PT divided by control PT.

- **Reduced factor X activity**. Reduced activity of coagulation factor X. The extrinsic and intrinsic pathways converge at factor X. The extrinsic pathway activates factor X by means of d factor VII with its cofactor, tissue factor. The intrinsic pathway activates factor X by means of the tenase complex (Ca^{2+} and factors VIIIa, IXa, and X) on the surface of activated platelets. Factor Xa, in turn, activates prothrombin (factor II) to thrombin (factor IIa).
- **Prolonged bleeding after dental extraction**. Prolonged bleeding postdental extraction that is sufficient to require medical intervention.
- **Prolonged bleeding after surgery**. Bleeding that persists longer than the normal time following a surgical procedure.
- **Epistaxis**. Nosebleed that refers to a hemorrhage localized in the nose.
- **Gingival bleeding**. Hemorrhage affecting the gingiva.
- **Abnormal umbilical stump bleeding**. Abnormal bleeding of the umbilical stump following separation of the cord at approximately 7–10 days after birth.
- **Antepartum hemorrhage**. Significant maternal hemorrhage/bleeding in the second half of pregnancy and prior to the birth of the baby.
- **Bruising susceptibility**. An ecchymosis (bruise) refers to skin discoloration caused by the escape of blood into the tissues from ruptured blood vessels. This term refers to an abnormally increased susceptibility to bruising. The corresponding phenotypic abnormality is generally elicited on medical history as a report of frequent ecchymoses or bruising without adequate trauma.

- **Gastrointestinal hemorrhage**. Hemorrhage affecting the gastrointestinal (GI) tract.
- **Intramuscular hematoma**. Blood clots formed within muscle tissue following leakage of blood into the tissue.
- **Joint hemorrhage**. Hemorrhage occurring within a joint.
- **Menorrhagia**. Prolonged and excessive menses at regular intervals in excess of 80 mL or lasting longer than seven days.
- **Oral cavity bleeding**. Recurrent or excessive bleeding from the mouth.
- **Postpartum hemorrhage**. Significant maternal hemorrhage/blood loss following delivery of a child.
- **Spontaneous hematomas**. Spontaneous development of hematomas (hematoma) or bruises without significant trauma.
- **Hemoperitoneum**. Accumulation of blood in the peritoneal cavity owing to internal hemorrhage.
- **Subarachnoid hemorrhage**. Hemorrhage occurring between the arachnoid mater and the pia mater.

DIAGNOSIS OF FACTOR X DEFICIENCY

Factor X deficiency can be diagnosed based on the symptoms and through laboratory tests to measure clotting time.

INHERITANCE

All individuals inherit two copies of most genes. The number of copies of a gene that need to have a disease-causing variant affects the way a disease is inherited. This disease is inherited in the autosomal recessive inheritance pattern.

Autosomal Recessive Inheritance

Autosomal means the gene is located on any chromosome except the X or Y chromosomes (sex chromosomes). Genes, like chromosomes, usually come in pairs. Recessive means that both copies of the responsible gene must have a disease-causing change (pathogenic variant) in order for a person to have the disease. Mutation is an older term that is still sometimes used to mean a pathogenic variant.

A person who has an autosomal recessive disease receives a gene with a pathogenic variant from each of their parents. Each parent is a carrier that means they have a pathogenic variant in only one copy of the gene. Carriers of an autosomal recessive disease usually do not have any symptoms of the disease. When two carriers of an autosomal recessive disease have children, there is a 25 percent (one in four) chance of having a child who has the disease.[9]

Section 24.10 | Factor XI Deficiency

Factor XI deficiency is a disorder that can cause abnormal bleeding due to a shortage (deficiency) of the factor XI protein, which is involved in blood clotting. This condition is classified as either partial or severe based on the degree of deficiency of the factor XI protein. However, regardless of the severity of the protein deficiency, most affected individuals have relatively mild bleeding problems, and some people with this disorder have few symptoms.

CAUSES OF FACTOR XI DEFICIENCY

Most cases of factor XI deficiency are caused by mutations in the *F11* gene, which provides instructions for making the factor XI protein. This protein plays a role in the coagulation cascade, which is a series of chemical reactions that forms blood clots in response to injury. After an injury, clots seal off blood vessels to stop bleeding and trigger blood vessel repair.

Mutations in the *F11* gene result in a shortage (deficiency) of functional factor XI. This deficiency impairs the coagulation

---

[9] Genetic and Rare Diseases Information Center (GARD), "Congenital Factor X Deficiency," National Center for Advancing Translational Sciences (NCATS), February 2023. Available online. URL: https://rarediseases.info.nih.gov/diseases/6404/factor-x-deficiency. Accessed June 14, 2023.

cascade, slowing the process of blood clotting and leading to the bleeding problems associated with this disorder. The amount of functional factor XI remaining varies depending on the particular mutation and whether one or both copies of the *F11* gene in each cell have mutations. However, the severity of the bleeding problems in affected individuals does not necessarily correspond to the amount of factor XI in the bloodstream and can vary even within the same family. Other genetic and environmental factors likely play a role in determining the severity of this condition.

Some cases of factor XI deficiency are not caused by *F11* gene mutations. In these cases, the condition is called "acquired factor XI deficiency." It can be caused by other disorders, such as conditions in which the immune system malfunctions and attacks the factor XI protein. Because factor XI is made primarily by cells in the liver, acquired factor XI deficiency can also occur as the result of severe liver disease or receiving a transplanted liver from an affected individual. In addition, approximately 25 percent of people with another disorder called "Noonan syndrome" have factor XI deficiency.

SYMPTOMS OF FACTOR XI DEFICIENCY

The most common feature of factor XI deficiency is prolonged bleeding after trauma or surgery, especially involving the inside of the mouth and nose (oral and nasal cavities) or the urinary tract. If the bleeding is left untreated after surgery, solid swellings consisting of congealed blood (hematomas) can develop in the surgical area.

Other signs and symptoms of this disorder can include frequent nosebleeds, easy bruising, bleeding under the skin, and bleeding of the gums. Women with this disorder can have heavy or prolonged menstrual bleeding (menorrhagia) or prolonged bleeding after childbirth. In contrast to some other bleeding disorders, spontaneous bleeding into the urine (hematuria), GI tract, or skull cavity is not common in factor XI deficiency although it can occur in severely affected individuals. Bleeding into the muscles or joints, which can cause long-term disability in other bleeding disorders, generally does not occur in this condition.

FREQUENCY OF FACTOR XI DEFICIENCY

Factor XI deficiency is estimated to affect approximately 1 in 1 million people worldwide. The severe deficiency disorder is much more common in people with central and eastern European (Ashkenazi) Jewish ancestry, occurring in about 1 in 450 individuals in that population. Researchers suggest that the actual prevalence of factor XI deficiency may be higher than reported because mild cases of the disorder often do not come to medical attention.

INHERITANCE OF FACTOR XI DEFICIENCY

Severe factor XI deficiency is passed down in an autosomal recessive pattern, which means both copies of the *F11* gene in each cell have mutations. The parents of these individuals each carry one copy of the mutated gene and have partial factor XI deficiency; they rarely show severe signs and symptoms of the condition.

In some families, this condition is inherited in an autosomal dominant pattern, which means one copy of the altered *F11* gene in each cell is sufficient to cause the disorder. In these cases, an affected person has one parent with the condition.

The acquired form of factor XI deficiency is not inherited and does not run in families.[10]

Section 24.11 | Factor XII Deficiency

The *F12* gene provides instructions for making a protein called "coagulation factor XII." Coagulation factors are a group of related proteins that are essential for normal blood clotting (coagulation). After an injury, clots protect the body by sealing off damaged blood vessels and preventing further blood loss. Factor XII circulates in the bloodstream in an inactive form until it is activated, usually by coming in contact with damaged blood vessel walls. Upon

---

[10] MedlinePlus, "Factor XI deficiency," National National Institutes of Health (NIH), August 1, 2018. Available online. URL: https://medlineplus.gov/genetics/condition/factor-xi-deficiency. Accessed June 14, 2023.

activation, factor XII interacts with coagulation factor XI. This interaction sets off a chain of additional chemical reactions that form a blood clot.

Factor XII also plays a role in stimulating inflammation, a normal body response to infection, irritation, or other injury. When factor XII is activated, it also interacts with a protein called "plasma prekallikrein." This interaction initiates a series of chemical reactions that lead to the release of a protein called "bradykinin." Bradykinin promotes inflammation by increasing the permeability of blood vessel walls, allowing more fluids to leak into body tissues. This leakage causes the swelling that accompanies inflammation.

HEALTH CONDITIONS RELATED TO GENETIC CHANGES
Hereditary Angioedema

At least two mutations in the *F12* gene are associated with hereditary angioedema type III. These mutations change single protein building blocks (amino acids) in factor XII, which increases the activity of the protein. As a result, more bradykinin is produced, which allows additional fluids to leak through blood vessel walls. The accumulation of fluids in body tissues leads to episodes of swelling in people with hereditary angioedema type III.

Other Disorders

Approximately 20 mutations in the *F12* gene that cause factor XII deficiency have been identified. Factor XII deficiency is an inherited condition characterized by a shortage of factor XII in the blood. Individuals with this condition usually do not experience abnormal bleeding or other symptoms. Factor XII deficiency is typically discovered during routine blood testing because reduced levels of factor XII cause the blood to take longer to clot in a test tube. Most of the mutations that cause factor XII deficiency change single amino acids, which alters the structure of factor XII. It remains unclear why individuals with factor XII deficiency do not experience abnormal bleeding like those with deficiencies of other coagulation factors.[11]

[11] MedlinePlus, "*F12* Gene," National Institutes of Health (NIH), April 1, 2009. Available online. URL: https://medlineplus.gov/genetics/condition/factor-xi-deficiency. Accessed June 14, 2023.

Section 24.12 | **Factor XIII Deficiency**

Factor XIII deficiency is a rare bleeding disorder. Researchers have identified an inherited form and a less severe form that is acquired during a person's lifetime.

CAUSES OF FACTOR XIII DEFICIENCY

Inherited factor XIII deficiency results from mutations in the *F13A1* gene or, less commonly, the *F13B* gene. These genes provide instructions for making the two parts (subunits) of a protein called "factor XIII." This protein plays a critical role in the coagulation cascade, which is a series of chemical reactions that forms blood clots in response to injury. After an injury, clots seal off blood vessels to stop bleeding and trigger blood vessel repair. Factor XIII acts at the end of the cascade to strengthen and stabilize newly formed clots, preventing further blood loss.

Mutations in the *F13A1* or *F13B* gene significantly reduce the amount of functional factor XIII available to participate in blood clotting. In most people with the inherited form of the condition, factor XIII levels in the bloodstream are less than 5 percent of normal. A loss of this protein's activity weakens blood clots, preventing the clots from stopping blood loss effectively.

The acquired form of factor XIII deficiency results when the production of factor XIII is reduced or when the body uses factor XIII faster than cells can replace it. Acquired factor XIII deficiency is generally mild because levels of factor XIII in the bloodstream are 20–70 percent of normal; levels above 10 percent of normal are usually adequate to prevent spontaneous bleeding episodes.

Acquired factor XIII deficiency can be caused by disorders including an inflammatory disease of the liver called "hepatitis," scarring of the liver (cirrhosis), inflammatory bowel disease, overwhelming bacterial infections (sepsis), and several types of cancer. Acquired factor XIII deficiency can also be caused by abnormal activation of the immune system, which produces specialized proteins called "autoantibodies" that attack and disable the factor XIII protein. The production of autoantibodies against factor XIII is sometimes associated with immune system diseases such as systemic lupus erythematosus and rheumatoid arthritis. In other cases, the trigger for autoantibody production is unknown.

RISK FACTORS OF FACTOR XIII DEFICIENCY

Inherited factor XIII deficiency also increases the risk of spontaneous bleeding inside the skull (intracranial hemorrhage), which is the leading cause of death in people with this condition.

Acquired factor XIII deficiency becomes apparent later in life. People with the acquired form are less likely to have severe or life-threatening episodes of abnormal bleeding than those with the inherited form.

SYMPTOMS OF FACTOR XIII DEFICIENCY

Signs and symptoms of inherited factor XIII deficiency begin soon after birth, usually with abnormal bleeding from the umbilical cord stump. If the condition is not treated, affected individuals may have episodes of excessive and prolonged bleeding that can be life-threatening. Abnormal bleeding can occur after surgery or minor trauma. The condition can also cause spontaneous bleeding into the joints or muscles, leading to pain and disability. Women with inherited factor XIII deficiency tend to have heavy or prolonged menstrual bleeding (menorrhagia) and may experience recurrent pregnancy losses (miscarriages). Other signs and symptoms of inherited factor XIII deficiency include nosebleeds, bleeding of the gums, easy bruising, problems with wound healing, bleeding after surgery, and abnormal scar formation.

FREQUENCY OF FACTOR XIII DEFICIENCY

Inherited factor XIII deficiency affects one to three per million people worldwide. Researchers suspect that mild factor XIII deficiency, including the acquired form of the disorder, is underdiagnosed because many affected people never have a major episode of abnormal bleeding that would lead to a diagnosis.

INHERITANCE OF FACTOR XIII DEFICIENCY

Inherited factor XIII deficiency is considered to have an autosomal recessive pattern of inheritance, which means that it results when both copies of either the *F13A1* gene or the *F13B* gene in each cell have mutations.

Some people, including parents of individuals with factor XIII deficiency, carry a single mutated copy of the *F13A1* or *F13B* gene in each cell. These mutation carriers have a reduced amount of factor XIII in their bloodstream (20–60% of normal), and they may experience abnormal bleeding after surgery, dental work, or major trauma. However, most people who carry one mutated copy of the *F13A1* or *F13B* gene do not have abnormal bleeding episodes under normal circumstances, and so they never come to medical attention.

The acquired form of factor XIII deficiency is not inherited and does not run in families.[12]

[12] MedlinePlus, "Factor XIII Deficiency," National Institutes of Health (NIH), January 1, 2019. Available online. URL: https://medlineplus.gov/genetics/condition/factor-xiii-deficiency. Accessed June 14, 2023.

Chapter 25 | **Hereditary Hemorrhagic Telangiectasia**

WHAT IS HEREDITARY HEMORRHAGIC TELANGIECTASIA?

Hereditary hemorrhagic telangiectasia (HHT) is a disorder in which some blood vessels do not develop properly. A person with HHT may form blood vessels without the capillaries (tiny blood vessels that pass blood from arteries to veins) that are usually present between arteries and veins. The space between an artery and a vein is often fragile and can burst and bleed much more easily than other blood vessels. Men, women, and children from all racial and ethnic groups can be affected by HHT and experience the problems associated with this disorder, some of which are serious and potentially life-threatening. Fortunately, if HHT is discovered early, effective treatments are available. However, there is no cure for HHT.

CAUSES OF HEREDITARY HEMORRHAGIC TELANGIECTASIA

Hereditary hemorrhagic telangiectasia is a genetic disorder. Each person with HHT has one gene that is altered (mutated), which causes HHT, as well as one normal gene. It takes only one mutant gene to cause HHT. When someone with HHT has children, each child has a 50 percent chance of receiving the mutant gene from his or her parent and, therefore, having HHT as well. Each child also has a 50 percent chance of receiving the normal gene and not being affected by HHT. At least five different genes can cause HHT, three of which are known.

SIGNS OF HEREDITARY HEMORRHAGIC TELANGIECTASIA

Nosebleeds are the most common sign of HHT, resulting from small abnormal blood vessels within the inside layer of the nose. Abnormal blood vessels in the skin can appear on the hands, fingertips, face, lips, lining of the mouth, and nose as delicate red or purplish spots that lighten briefly when touched. Bleeding within the stomach or intestines is another possible indicator of HHT that occurs because of abnormal blood vessels lining the digestive tract. Additional signs of HHT include abnormal artery-vein connections within the brain, lungs, and liver, which often do not display any warning signs before rupturing.

DIAGNOSIS OF HEREDITARY HEMORRHAGIC TELANGIECTASIA

Hereditary hemorrhagic telangiectasia can be diagnosed by performing genetic testing. Genetic testing can detect a gene mutation in about three-fourths of families with signs of HHT, which, if found, can establish the diagnosis of HHT in individuals and families who are unsure about whether they have HHT. HHT can also be diagnosed by using clinical criteria (presence of signs and a history of signs in a parent, sibling, or child).

COMPLICATIONS AND TREATMENTS OF HEREDITARY HEMORRHAGIC TELANGIECTASIA

The complications of HHT can vary widely, even among people affected by HHT in the same family. Complications and treatment of HHT depend on the parts of the body that are affected by this disorder. Treatment may include controlling bleeding and anemia and preventing complications from abnormal artery–vein connections in the lungs and brain.[1]

---

[1] "Facts about Hereditary Hemorrhagic Telangiectasia (HHT)," Centers for Disease Control and Prevention (CDC), April 28, 2023. Available online. URL: www.cdc.gov/ncbddd/hht/index.html. Accessed June 5, 2023.

Chapter 26 | **Bruises and Excessive Bleeding**

BRUISES

A bruise is a mark on your skin caused by blood trapped under the surface. It happens when an injury crushes small blood vessels but does not break the skin. Those vessels break open and leak blood under the skin.

Bruises are often painful and swollen. You can get skin, muscle, and bone bruises. Bone bruises are the most serious.

It can take months for a bruise to fade, but most last about two weeks. They start off a reddish color and then turn bluish-purple and greenish-yellow before returning to normal. To reduce bruising, ice the injured area and elevate it above your heart. See your health-care provider if you seem to bruise for no reason or if the bruise appears to be infected.[1]

THE WHAT, WHY, AND HOW OF BRUISES

Many things can cause a bruise: minor injuries, falls, and small collisions. While bruises may hurt, they are usually harmless. But, sometimes, they might be a sign of a deeper problem.

If you bump part of your body hard enough, you can break tiny blood vessels under your skin. But, if you do not break the skin, the blood has nowhere to go. It gets trapped under the skin's surface, causing a bruise.

---

[1] MedlinePlus, "Bruises," National Institutes of Health (NIH), November 14, 2016. Available online. URL: https://medlineplus.gov/bruises.html. Accessed May 19, 2023.

When you first get a bruise, the newly trapped blood makes it look pink or red. Over the next few weeks, the body naturally breaks down the blood and absorbs it. So, as the bruise fades, it changes colors. This is part of the normal healing process. Some bruises can take weeks or months to heal.

What can contribute to bruising? Some people bruise more easily than others, says Dr. José López, an expert on bleeding disorders at Bloodworks Northwest Research Institute. This can be influenced by many things, including your genes. Other factors, such as diet, can also affect how easily you bruise. For example, deficiencies in vitamin C or K can make you bruise more easily.

Some people may just be more prone to bumping into things. And skin naturally becomes thinner and bruises more easily as you age.

You can take steps to make your home safer from minor bumps and falls. Keep walkways clear of clutter and furniture. Good lighting can also help you avoid bumping into things.

Bruises may be painful, but they are usually not dangerous. If a bruise does hurt, an over-the-counter (OTC) painkiller may help. But some drugs used to treat pain, such as aspirin or ibuprofen, can actually increase the tendency to bruise, Dr. López explains.

Putting ice on the affected area for a few minutes at a time can help reduce swelling. Wrap the ice in a clean towel to avoid irritating the skin.

If you notice a change in where or how often you are bruising, consider talking with a health-care professional. "If bruising becomes really common, if it is not provoked, or if there is a change in your bruising patterns, get it checked out," Dr. López says.

These can be signs that bleeding is happening inside the body when it should not. Others include a rash made of tiny bruises called "purpura." Or tiny, pinpoint-sized red spots called "petechiae."

Excessive bruising can be triggered by many things. Examples include liver problems caused by heavy drinking or certain types of cancer. It can also be a sign of a rare problem such as an inherited bleeding disorder. If you notice someone has bruises regularly, it may suggest serious problems in their home, such as domestic violence.

Medications can also be a cause of excessive bruising. Almost any medication has the potential to change the way platelets work in the body, Dr. López says. Platelets are tiny, disc-shaped cells that play an important role in helping your blood clot. "They're one of the things that stop you from bleeding," says Dr. López. Let your health-care provider know if you notice bruising soon after taking a new drug.

Bruises may be a sign of a serious problem, but in most cases, they are harmless.[2]

BLEEDING AND BRUISING (THROMBOCYTOPENIA) AND CANCER TREATMENT

Some cancer treatments, such as chemotherapy and targeted therapy, can increase your risk of bleeding and bruising. These treatments can lower the number of platelets in the blood. Platelets are the cells that help your blood clot and stop bleeding. When your platelet count is low, you may bruise or bleed a lot or very easily and have tiny purple or red spots on your skin. This condition is called "thrombocytopenia." It is important to tell your doctor or nurse if you notice any of these changes.

Call your doctor or nurse if you have more serious problems, such as:
- bleeding that does not stop after a few minutes; bleeding from your mouth, your nose, or when you vomit; bleeding from your vagina when you are not having your period (menstruation); urine that is red or pink; stools that are black or bloody; or bleeding during your period that is heavier or lasts longer than normal
- head or vision changes such as bad headaches or changes in how well you see or feeling confused or very sleepy

Ways to Manage Bleeding and Bruising
Steps to take if you are at increased risk of bleeding and bruising:
- **Avoid certain medicines**. Many OTC medicines contain aspirin or ibuprofen, which can increase your

[2] *NIH News in Health*, "Bruising Questions," National Institutes of Health (NIH), January 2022. Available online. URL: https://newsinhealth.nih.gov/2022/01/bruising-questions. Accessed May 19, 2023.

risk of bleeding. When in doubt, be sure to check the label. Get a list of medicines and products from your health-care team that you should avoid taking. You may also be advised to limit or avoid alcohol if your platelet count is low.

- **Take extra care to prevent bleeding**. Brush your teeth gently with a very soft toothbrush. Wear shoes, even when you are inside. Be extra careful when using sharp objects. Use an electric shaver, not a razor. Use lotion and a lip balm to prevent dry, chapped skin and lips. Tell your doctor or nurse if you are constipated or notice bleeding from your rectum.
- **Care for bleeding or bruising**. If you start to bleed, press down firmly on the area with a clean cloth. Keep pressing until the bleeding stops. If you bruise, put ice on the area.

Talking with Your Health-Care Team about Bleeding and Bruising

Prepare for your visit by making a list of questions to ask your health-care provider. Consider adding the following questions to your list:

- What steps can I take to prevent bleeding or bruising?
- How long should I wait for the bleeding to stop before I call you or go to the emergency room?
- Do I need to limit or avoid things that could increase my risk of bleeding, such as alcohol or sexual activity?
- What medicines, vitamins, or herbs should I avoid? Could I get a list from you of medicines to avoid?[3]

---

[3] "Bleeding and Bruising (Thrombocytopenia) and Cancer Treatment," National Cancer Institute (NCI), December 29, 2022. Available online. URL: www.cancer.gov/about-cancer/treatment/side-effects/bleeding-bruising. Accessed May 19, 2023.

Chapter 27 |
Antiphospholipid Syndrome

WHAT IS ANTIPHOSPHOLIPID SYNDROME?

Antiphospholipid syndrome (APS) is an autoimmune disorder that causes abnormal blood clots to form. Autoimmune disorders occur when your body's immune system makes antibodies that attack and damage your own tissues or cells.

Normally, antibodies protect your body from viruses or bacteria, but in APS, antibodies attack the body's healthy cells. High levels of APS antibodies raise the risk of blood clots. The specific antibodies in APS are called "antiphospholipids" because they attack and damage parts of cells called "phospholipids." The damage increases the chance that blood clots will form in both veins and arteries.

WHAT ARE THE RISK FACTORS OF ANTIPHOSPHOLIPID SYNDROME?

Your family history and genes, other medical conditions, medicines, procedures, or lifestyle factors may raise your risk of APS. These factors may raise your risk of APS antibodies, trigger blood clotting in APS, or both. APS can also affect people of any age.

Other common risk factors include the following:
- **Sex**. APS is more common in women than men.
- **Family history**. APS may sometimes run in families.
- **Diagnosis of another autoimmune disorder**.
  APS is most common in people who have lupus.

In fact, 20–30 percent of people with lupus have antiphospholipid antibodies. Of those, about one in three develop blood clots in their arteries or veins.

- **Bacterial or viral infections**. Human immunodeficiency virus (HIV), hepatitis C, and the bacteria that causes Lyme disease can increase your risk of making APS antibodies or triggering APS.

WHAT ARE THE SYMPTOMS OF ANTIPHOSPHOLIPID SYNDROME?

High levels of APS antibodies in the blood raise the risk of health problems, but some people will never develop blood clots.

Symptoms of abnormal blood clotting include the following:
- chest pain and shortness of breath
- nausea (feeling sick to your stomach)
- pain, redness, warmth, and swelling in the arms or legs
- speech changes
- upper body discomfort in the arms, back, neck, and jaw

Less common symptoms of APS include the following:
- a lacy-looking red rash on wrists and knees
- chronic (ongoing) headaches
- heart valve problems
- memory loss

HOW WILL YOUR DOCTOR DIAGNOSE ANTIPHOSPHOLIPID SYNDROME?

Your doctor will talk to you about your medical history and may do blood tests. The blood tests look for the three APS antibodies in your blood: anticardiolipin, beta-2 glycoprotein I (β2GPI), and lupus anticoagulant.

To be diagnosed with APS, you must have APS antibodies and a history of health problems related to the disorder. You will likely see a hematologist, who is a doctor who specializes in blood disorders.

HOW IS ANTIPHOSPHOLIPID SYNDROME TREATED?

Currently, APS has no cure. However, medicines can help prevent health problems caused by the condition. The goals of treatment are to prevent blood clots from forming and keep existing clots from getting larger.

Your doctor may prescribe blood thinner medicine, such as warfarin, heparin, or aspirin. Your doctor will know which medicine is best for you.

Going to the doctor and getting treatment is important for people with APS. If left untreated, APS can cause life-threatening blood clots that can lead to a heart attack or stroke.

Untreated APS in pregnancy can result in a higher risk of miscarriages and preeclampsia (high blood pressure (HBP) during pregnancy).[1]

[1] "Antiphospholipid Syndrome (APS)," National Heart, Lung, and Blood Institute (NHLBI), March 24, 2022. Available online. URL: www.nhlbi.nih.gov/health/antiphospholipid-syndrome. Accessed May 16, 2023.

Chapter 28 | **Disseminated Intravascular Coagulation**

WHAT IS DISSEMINATED INTRAVASCULAR COAGULATION?

Disseminated intravascular coagulation (DIC) is a rare but serious condition that causes abnormal blood clotting throughout the body's blood vessels. You may develop DIC if you have an infection or injury that affects the body's normal blood clotting process.

DIC progresses through two stages: overactive clotting followed by bleeding.

- **Stage one**. Overactive clotting leads to blood clots throughout the blood vessels. The clots can reduce or block blood flow, which can damage organs.
- **Stage two**. As DIC progresses, the overactive clotting uses up platelets and clotting factors that help the blood to clot. Without these platelets and clotting factors, DIC leads to bleeding just beneath the skin, in the nose or mouth, or deep inside the body.

WHAT CAUSES DISSEMINATED INTRAVASCULAR COAGULATION?

Disseminated intravascular coagulation is usually caused by inflammation from an infection, injury, or illness. Some common causes are as follows:

- **Sepsis**. This is a body-wide response to infection that causes inflammation. Sepsis is the most common risk factor for DIC.
- **Major damage to organs or tissues**. This may be caused by cirrhosis of the liver, pancreatitis, severe injury, burns, or major surgery.

- **Severe immune reactions**. Your body may overreact because of a failed blood transfusion, rejection of an organ transplant, or a toxin such as snake venom.
- **Serious pregnancy-related problems**. These include the placenta separating from the uterus before delivery, amniotic fluid entering the bloodstream, or serious bleeding during or after delivery.
- **Cancer**. Various types of leukemia can result in DIC.

DIC is a rare complication of COVID-19. People who develop DIC are more likely to have severe complications, such as organ failure, that can often be life-threatening.

WHAT ARE THE SYMPTOMS OF DISSEMINATED INTRAVASCULAR COAGULATION?
If you think you might have DIC, watch for the following symptoms:
- bleeding at wound sites or from the nose, gums, or mouth
- blood in the stool or urine
- bruising in small dots or larger patches on the body
- chest pain
- pain, redness, warmth, and swelling of the leg

HOW IS DISSEMINATED INTRAVASCULAR COAGULATION DIAGNOSED?
Your doctor will diagnose DIC based on your medical history, a physical exam, and tests. Your doctor will also look for the cause of DIC because it does not occur on its own.

Medical History and Physical Exam
To help diagnose DIC, your doctor will ask about any medical conditions or recent events, such as illness or an injury, that could cause or be a risk factor for DIC. Your doctor will do a physical exam to look for symptoms of blood clots, bleeding, or a condition that could cause DIC or a complication of DIC.

Blood Tests

If your doctor suspects DIC, they may do several blood tests. Based on the results of your blood tests, your doctor may use a scoring system to diagnose DIC. The higher the score, the more likely it is that you have DIC. To make a diagnosis, your doctor may repeat some tests and watch your condition over time.

Tests for Other Medical Conditions

Your doctor may suggest other tests or procedures to find out whether a different condition is causing your symptoms. These tests may include the following:

- **ADAMTS13 testing**. This is to check blood levels and activity of this protein, which can be low in a condition called "thrombotic thrombocytopenic purpura" (TTP).
- **Liver biopsy and liver function tests**. These tests are to check for cirrhosis or chronic liver disease, which may have symptoms like DIC.

HOW IS DISSEMINATED INTRAVASCULAR COAGULATION TREATED?
Treatment

Treatment for DIC depends on your symptoms and how serious they are. The main goals of treatment for DIC are to control clotting and bleeding and to treat the underlying cause. DIC may go away once the underlying cause is treated. In the meantime, your doctor may use medicines or procedures to help stop the bleeding.

Medicines

Your doctor may use anticoagulants, also called "blood thinners," to reduce blood clotting. They can be given as a pill, as an injection, or through an IV. Possible side effects include bleeding, especially if you are taking other medicines that also thin your blood, such as aspirin.

Procedures and Therapies

Common treatment options include the following:

- clotting factor replacement therapy
- plasma transfusion
- platelet transfusion

Without treatment, DIC can lead to complications caused by overactive clotting or from the bleeding that follows. These complications can be life-threatening and may include the following:

- acute respiratory distress syndrome (ARDS)
- bleeding in the gastrointestinal (GI) tract
- heart attack
- shock
- stroke
- venous thromboembolism (VTE)[1]

---

[1] "Disseminated Intravascular Coagulation (DIC)," National Heart, Lung, and Blood Institute (NHLBI), March 24, 2022. Available online. URL: www.nhlbi.nih.gov/health/disseminated-intravascular-coagulation. Accessed May 19, 2023.

Chapter 29 | Hypercoagulation Disorders

Chapter Contents

Section 29.1 | Excessive Blood Clotting

WHAT IS A BLOOD CLOT?

A blood clot is a mass of blood that forms when platelets, proteins, and cells in the blood stick together. When you get hurt, your body forms a blood clot to stop the bleeding. After the bleeding stops and healing takes place, your body usually breaks down and removes the blood clot.

WHAT IS EXCESSIVE BLOOD CLOTTING?

Sometimes, the blood clots form where they should not; your body makes too many blood clots or abnormal blood clots; or the blood clots do not break down as they should. These blood clots can be dangerous and may cause other health problems.

Blood clots can form in, or travel to, the blood vessels in the limbs, lungs, brain, heart, and kidneys.

TYPES OF EXCESSIVE BLOOD CLOTTING

The types of problems blood clots can cause will depend on where they are:

- **Deep vein thrombosis (DVT)**. DVT is a blood clot in a deep vein, usually in the lower leg, thigh, or pelvis. It can block a vein and cause damage to your leg.
- **Pulmonary embolism (PE)**. A PE can happen when a DVT breaks off and travels through the bloodstream to the lungs. It can damage your lungs and prevent your other organs from getting enough oxygen.
- **Cerebral venous sinus thrombosis (CVST)**. CVST is a rare blood clot in the venous sinuses in your brain. Normally, the venous sinuses drain blood from your brain. CVST blocks the blood from draining and can cause a hemorrhagic stroke.
- **Blood clots in other parts of the body**. Such clots can cause problems such as an ischemic stroke, a heart attack, kidney problems, kidney failure, and pregnancy-related problems.

WHO IS AT RISK OF EXCESSIVE BLOOD CLOTTING?

The following factors can raise the risk of excessive blood clotting:

- atherosclerosis
- atrial fibrillation (AF)
- cancer and cancer treatments
- certain genetic disorders
- certain surgeries
- coronavirus disease 2019 (COVID-19)
- diabetes
- family history of blood clots
- overweight and obesity
- pregnancy and giving birth
- serious injuries
- some medicines, including birth control pills
- smoking
- staying in one position for a long time, such as being in the hospital or taking a long car or plane ride

WHAT ARE THE SYMPTOMS OF EXCESSIVE BLOOD CLOTTING?

The symptoms of blood clots can be different depending on where the blood clot is:

- **In the abdomen**. You may experience abdominal pain, nausea, and vomiting.
- **In an arm or leg**. There will be sudden or gradual pain, swelling, tenderness, and warmth.
- **In the lungs**. Shortness of breath, pain with deep breathing, rapid breathing, and increased heart rate will be the symptoms.
- **In the brain**. You may have symptoms such as trouble speaking, vision problems, seizures, weakness on one side of the body, and sudden severe headache.
- **In the heart**. You will have chest pain, sweating, shortness of breath, and pain in the left arm.

HOW IS EXCESSIVE BLOOD CLOTTING DIAGNOSED?

Your health-care provider may diagnose excessive blood clotting in one or more of the following ways:

- a physical exam
- a medical history
- blood tests, including a D-dimer test
- imaging tests, such as:
  - ultrasound
  - x-rays of the veins (venography) or blood vessels (angiography) that are taken after you get an injection of special dye. The dye shows up on the x-ray and allows the provider to see how the blood flows.
  - computed tomography (CT) Scan

WHAT ARE THE TREATMENTS FOR EXCESSIVE BLOOD CLOTTING?

Treatments for excessive blood clotting depend on where the blood clot is located and how severe it is. Treatments may include the following:

- blood thinners
- other medicines, including thrombolytics (Thrombolytics are medicines that dissolve blood clots. They are usually used when the blood clots are severe.)
- surgery and other procedures to remove the blood clots

CAN EXCESSIVE BLOOD CLOTTING BE PREVENTED?

You may be able to prevent excessive blood clotting by:

- moving around as soon as possible after having been confined to your bed, such as after surgery, illness, or injury
- getting up and moving around every few hours when you have to sit for long periods of time, for example, if you are on a long flight or car trip
- regular physical activity
- not smoking
- staying at a healthy weight

Some people at high risk may need to take blood thinners to prevent excessive blood clotting.[1]

Section 29.2 | Deep Vein Thrombosis

WHAT IS DEEP VEIN THROMBOSIS?
Deep vein thrombosis (DVT) is an underdiagnosed and serious but preventable medical condition that occurs when a blood clot forms in a deep vein. These clots usually develop in the lower leg, thigh, or pelvis, but they can also occur in the arm.

It is important to know about DVT because it can happen to anybody and can cause serious illness, disability, and, in some cases, death. The good news is that DVT is preventable and treatable if discovered early.

RISK FACTORS FOR DEEP VEIN THROMBOSIS
Almost anyone can have DVT. However, certain factors can increase the chance of having this condition. The chance increases even more for someone who has more than one of the following factors at the same time.

The following is a list of factors that increase the risk of developing DVT:
- injury to a vein, often caused by:
  - fractures
  - severe muscle injury
  - major surgery (particularly involving the abdomen, pelvis, hip, or legs)
- slow blood flow, often caused by:
  - confinement to bed (e.g., due to a medical condition or after surgery)
  - limited movement (e.g., a cast on a leg to help heal an injured bone)

[1] MedlinePlus, "Blood Clots," National Institutes of Health (NIH), April 21, 2021. Available online. URL: https://medlineplus.gov/bloodclots.html. Accessed May 19, 2023.

- sitting for a long time, especially with crossed legs
- paralysis
- increased estrogen, often caused by:
  - birth control pills
  - hormone replacement therapy (HRT), sometimes used after menopause
  - pregnancy, for up to three months after giving birth
- certain chronic medical illnesses, such as:
  - heart disease
  - lung disease
  - cancer and its treatment
  - inflammatory bowel disease (IBD; Crohn's disease or ulcerative colitis (UC))
- other factors that increase the risk of DVT, including:
  - previous DVT or PE
  - family history of DVT or PE
  - age (Risk increases as age increases.)
  - obesity
  - a catheter located in a central vein
  - inherited clotting disorders

SYMPTOMS OF DEEP VEIN THROMBOSIS

About half of people with DVT have no symptoms at all. The following are the most common symptoms of DVT that occur in the affected part of the body:

- swelling
- pain
- tenderness
- redness of the skin

If you have any of these symptoms, you should see your doctor as soon as possible.

COMPLICATIONS OF DEEP VEIN THROMBOSIS

The most serious complication of DVT happens when a part of the clot breaks off and travels through the bloodstream to the lungs, causing a blockage called "pulmonary embolism" (PE). If the clot is small and with appropriate treatment, people can recover from PE. However, there could be some damage to the lungs. If the clot is large, it can stop blood from reaching the lungs and is fatal.

In addition, one-third to one-half of people who have DVT will have long-term complications caused by the damage the clot does to the valves in the vein, called "postthrombotic syndrome" (PTS). People with PTS have symptoms such as swelling, pain, discoloration, and, in severe cases, scaling or ulcers in the affected part of the body. In some cases, the symptoms can be so severe that a person becomes disabled.

For some people, DVT and PE can become chronic illnesses; about 30 percent of people who have had DVT or PE are at risk for another episode.

DIAGNOSIS OF DEEP VEIN THROMBOSIS
The diagnosis of DVT requires special tests that can only be performed by a doctor. That is why it is important for you to seek medical care if you experience any of the symptoms of DVT.

TREATMENTS FOR DEEP VEIN THROMBOSIS
Medication is used to prevent and treat DVT. Compression stockings (also called "graduated compression stockings") are sometimes recommended to prevent DVT and relieve pain and swelling. These might need to be worn for two years or more after having DVT. In severe cases, the clot might need to be removed surgically.

PREVENTION OF DEEP VEIN THROMBOSIS
The following tips can help prevent DVT:
- Move around as soon as possible after having been confined to bed, such as after surgery, illness, or injury.
- If you are at risk of DVT, talk to your doctor about the following:
  - graduated compression stockings (sometimes called "medical compression stockings")

- medication (anticoagulants) to prevent DVT
- When sitting for long periods of time, such as when traveling for more than four hours, do the following:
  - Get up and walk around every one to two hours.
  - Exercise your legs while you are sitting by:
    - raising and lowering your heels while keeping your toes on the floor
    - raising and lowering your toes while keeping your heels on the floor
    - tightening and releasing your leg muscles
  - Wear loose-fitting clothes.
- You can reduce your risk by maintaining a healthy weight, avoiding a sedentary lifestyle, and following your doctor's recommendations based on your individual risk factors.[2]

Section 29.3 | Pulmonary Embolism

WHAT IS A PULMONARY EMBOLISM?

A pulmonary embolism (PE) is a sudden blockage in a lung artery. It usually happens when a blood clot breaks loose and travels through the bloodstream to the lungs. PE is a serious condition that can cause:

- permanent damage to the lungs
- low oxygen levels in your blood
- damage to other organs in your body from not getting enough oxygen

PE can be life-threatening, especially if a clot is large or if there are many clots.

---

[2] "Venous Thromboembolism (Blood Clots)," Centers for Disease Control and Prevention (CDC), June 9, 2022. Available online. URL: www.cdc.gov/ncbddd/dvt/facts.html. Accessed May 19, 2023.

WHAT CAUSES A PULMONARY EMBOLISM?

The cause is usually a blood clot in the leg called a "deep vein thrombosis" (DVT) that breaks loose and travels through the bloodstream to the lungs.

WHO IS AT RISK FOR A PULMONARY EMBOLISM?

Anyone can get a PE, but certain things, including the following, can raise your risk of PE:

- having surgery, especially joint replacement surgery
- certain medical conditions, including the following:
  - cancers
  - heart diseases
  - lung diseases
  - a broken hip or leg bone or other trauma
- having hormone-based medicines, such as birth control pills or hormone replacement therapy (HRT)
- being pregnant and having childbirth (The risk is highest for about six weeks after childbirth.)
- not moving for long periods, such as being on bed rest, having a cast, or taking a long plane flight
- getting older, especially after age 40
- family history and certain genetic changes that increase your risk of blood clots
- having obesity

WHAT ARE THE SYMPTOMS OF A PULMONARY EMBOLISM?

Half the people who have PE have no symptoms. If you do have symptoms, they can include shortness of breath, chest pain, or coughing up blood. Symptoms of a blood clot include warmth, swelling, pain, tenderness, and redness of the leg.

HOW IS A PULMONARY EMBOLISM DIAGNOSED?

It can be difficult to diagnose PE. To make a diagnosis, your health-care provider will:

- take your medical history
- ask about your symptoms and risk factors for PE

- do a physical exam
- run some tests, including various imaging tests and possibly some blood tests

WHAT ARE THE TREATMENTS FOR A PULMONARY EMBOLISM?

If you have PE, you need medical treatment right away. The goal of treatment is to break up clots and help keep other clots from forming. Treatment options include medicines and procedures.

Medicines

- Anticoagulants, or blood thinners, keep blood clots from getting larger and stop new clots from forming. You might get them as an injection, a pill, or through an intravenous (IV). They can cause bleeding, especially if you are taking other medicines that also thin your blood, such as aspirin.
- Thrombolytics are medicines to dissolve blood clots. You may get them if you have large clots that cause severe symptoms or other serious complications. Thrombolytics can cause sudden bleeding, so they are used if your PE is serious and may be life-threatening.

Procedures

- Catheter-assisted thrombus removal uses a flexible tube to reach a blood clot in your lung. Your health-care provider can insert a tool in the tube to break up the clot or to deliver medicine through the tube. Usually, you will get medicine to put you to sleep for this procedure.
- A vena cava filter may be used in some people who cannot take blood thinners. Your health-care provider inserts a filter inside a large vein called the "vena cava." The filter catches blood clots before they travel to the lungs, which prevents PE. But the filter does not stop new blood clots from forming.

CAN PULMONARY EMBOLISM BE PREVENTED?

Preventing new blood clots can prevent PE. Prevention may include the following:

- continuing to take blood thinners and getting regular checkups with your provider to make sure that the dosage of your medicines is working to prevent blood clots but not causing bleeding
- practicing heart-healthy lifestyle changes, such as heart-healthy eating, exercise, and quitting smoking
- using compression stockings to prevent DVT
- moving your legs when sitting for long periods of time (such as on long trips)
- moving around as soon as possible after surgery or being confined to a bed[3]

---

[3] MedlinePlus, "Pulmonary Embolism," National Institutes of Health (NIH), June 8, 2020. Available online. URL: https://medlineplus.gov/pulmonaryembolism.html. Accessed May 19, 2023.

Chapter 30 |
Thrombocytopenia

Chapter Contents

Section 30.1 | Thrombocytopenia: An Overview

Thrombocytopenia is a condition that occurs when the platelet count in your blood is too low. Platelets are tiny blood cells that are made in the bone marrow from larger cells. When you are injured, platelets stick together to form a plug to seal your wound. This plug is called a "blood clot." Platelets are also called "thrombocytes" because a blood clot is also called a "thrombus."

A normal platelet count in adults ranges from 150,000 to 450,000 platelets per microliter of blood. A platelet count of less than 150,000 platelets per microliter is lower than normal. When you have a low platelet count, you may have trouble stopping bleeding. Bleeding can happen inside your body, underneath your skin, or from the surface of your skin. You may not have serious bleeding until your platelet count is very low.

Thrombocytopenia can be life-threatening, especially if you have serious bleeding or bleeding in your brain. Early treatment can help you avoid serious complications.

WHAT CAUSES THROMBOCYTOPENIA?

Thrombocytopenia can be inherited or acquired. "Inherited" means your parents pass the gene for the condition to you. "Acquired" means you are not born with the condition, but you develop it later. Sometimes, the cause of thrombocytopenia is not known.

You may have a low platelet count for the following reasons:
- Your body's bone marrow does not make enough platelets.
- Your bone marrow makes enough platelets, but your body destroys them or uses them up.
- Your spleen holds on to too many platelets. The spleen is an organ in your abdomen. It normally stores about one-third of the body's platelets. It also helps your body fight infection.

The following factors can raise your risk of thrombocytopenia:
- **Environment**. Exposure to toxic chemicals—such as pesticides, arsenic, and benzene—can slow the production of platelets.

- **Lifestyle habits**. Alcohol slows the production of platelets. Drinking too much alcohol can cause your platelet count to drop for a short time. This is more common in people who have low levels of vitamin B_{12} or folate.
- **Medicines**. Some medicines can slow the production of platelets. Also, a reaction to medicine can confuse your body and cause it to destroy its platelets.
- **Other medical conditions**. Examples of health problems that can reduce your platelet count are as follows:
  - Aplastic anemia is a rare, serious blood disorder that develops when the bone marrow stops making enough new blood cells.
  - Autoimmune diseases, such as immune thrombocytopenia (ITP), lupus, and rheumatoid arthritis (RA), can cause your immune system to attack and destroy your platelets by mistake.
  - Cancer, such as leukemia or lymphoma, can damage your bone marrow and destroy blood stem cells. When stem cells are damaged, they do not grow into healthy blood cells. Cancer treatments, such as radiation and chemotherapy, also destroy the stem cells.
  - Conditions that cause blood clots, such as thrombotic thrombocytopenic purpura (TTP) and disseminated intravascular coagulation (DIC), can cause your body to use up all your platelets. This leads to a low platelet count.
  - Infections from bacteria and viruses can lower your platelet count for a while.
  - A spleen that is larger than normal may remove or store too many platelets, and you may not have enough platelets in your blood.
- **Pregnancy**. Some pregnant women develop mild thrombocytopenia when they are close to delivery. The exact cause is not known.
- **Surgery**. Platelets can be destroyed when they pass through artificial heart valves, blood vessel grafts, or machines and tubing used for blood transfusions or bypass surgery.

WHAT ARE THE SYMPTOMS OF THROMBOCYTOPENIA?

Bleeding causes the main symptoms of thrombocytopenia. Symptoms can appear suddenly or over time. Mild thrombocytopenia often has no symptoms. Many times, it is found during a routine blood test. Signs of bleeding may include the following:

- bleeding that lasts a long time, even from small injuries
- petechiae, which are small, flat red spots under the skin caused by blood leaking from blood vessels
- purpura, which is bleeding in your skin that can cause red, purple, or brownish-yellow spots
- nosebleeds or bleeding from your gums
- blood in your urine or stool, which can appear as red blood or as a dark, tarry color
- heavy menstrual bleeding

HOW IS THROMBOCYTOPENIA DIAGNOSED?

To diagnose thrombocytopenia, your provider will ask about your medical and family history. They will also ask about your symptoms and do a physical exam to look for signs of bleeding.

Your provider may order one or more of the following blood tests:

- **Complete blood count (CBC)**. This test measures the levels of platelets and other blood cells in your blood.
- **Blood smear**. For this test, some of your blood is put on a slide. A microscope is used to look at your platelets.
- **Bone marrow tests**. These tests check whether your bone marrow is healthy.

HOW IS THROMBOCYTOPENIA TREATED?

Treatment for thrombocytopenia depends on what caused it and whether you have any symptoms. If you have mild thrombocytopenia, you may not need treatment. A fully normal platelet count is not necessary to prevent serious bleeding, even with serious cuts or accidents.

If you have serious bleeding or a high risk of complications, you may need medicines or procedures. Also, you will need to treat the condition that is causing the low platelet count.

If a reaction to a medicine is causing a low platelet count, your provider may prescribe another medicine. Most people recover after the initial medicine has been stopped. For heparin-induced thrombocytopenia (HIT), stopping the heparin is not enough. Often, you will need another medicine to prevent blood clotting.

If your immune system is causing a low platelet count, your provider may prescribe medicines to suppress the immune system.

Medicines

Corticosteroids, such as prednisone, are commonly used to treat a low platelet count. These medicines (steroids for short) help increase your platelet count.

You may need medicines such as eltrombopag and romiplostim to help your body make more platelets. Medicines such as immuno-globulins and rituximab can help stop your immune system from destroying your platelets.

Other Procedures

If medicines do not work, you may need one of the following procedures:

- Blood or platelet transfusions are used to treat people who are bleeding heavily or are at a high risk of bleeding. During this procedure, a needle is used to insert an intravenous (IV) line into one of your blood vessels. Through this line, you receive healthy blood or platelets. If you have HIT, a platelet transfusion can raise your risk of blood clots.
- Surgery to remove your spleen (splenectomy) can help increase the platelet count in your blood. Your spleen stores platelets. Possible complications include bleeding, infection, and abnormal blood clots.[1]

---

[1] "Thrombocytopenia," National Heart, Lung, and Blood Institute (NHLBI), March 24, 2022. Available online. URL: www.nhlbi.nih.gov/health/thrombocytopenia. Accessed May 19, 2023.

Section 30.2 | Immune Thrombocytopenic Purpura

Immune thrombocytopenic purpura (ITP), also called "immune thrombocytopenia," is a disorder characterized by a blood abnormality called "thrombocytopenia," which is a shortage of blood cells called "platelets" that are needed for normal blood clotting.

CAUSES OF IMMUNE THROMBOCYTOPENIC PURPURA

The genetic cause of immune thrombocytopenia is unclear. This condition occurs when the body's own immune system malfunctions and attacks the body's tissues and organs (autoimmunity). Normally, the immune system produces proteins called "antibodies," which attach to specific foreign particles and germs, marking them for destruction. In ITP, the immune system abnormally destroys platelets and makes fewer platelets than normal. People with immune thrombocytopenia produce antibodies that attack normal platelets. The platelets are destroyed and eliminated from the body, resulting in a shortage of these cells in affected individuals. Some of these antibodies also affect the cells in the bone marrow that produce platelets (known as "megakaryocytes"), which leads to a decrease in platelet production, further reducing the number of platelets in the blood.

In some people with immune thrombocytopenia, the abnormal immune reactions may coincide with an infection by certain viruses or bacteria. Exposure to these foreign invaders may trigger the body to fight the infection, but the immune system also mistakenly attacks platelets.

Genetic variations (polymorphisms) in a few genes have been found in some people with immune thrombocytopenia and may increase the risk of abnormal immune reactions. However, the contribution of these genetic changes to the development of immune thrombocytopenia is unclear.

When the condition is due to the targeted destruction of platelets by the body's own immune cells, it is known as "primary immune thrombocytopenia." Immune thrombocytopenia following bacterial or viral infection is considered primary because the infection triggers a platelet-specific immune reaction, typically without any other signs or symptoms. However, immune thrombocytopenia can be a feature of other immune disorders, such as common variable immune deficiency, which occurs when the immune system has a decreased ability to protect the body against foreign invaders, or other autoimmune disorders, such as systemic lupus erythematosus (SLE). Immune thrombocytopenia can also occur with other blood disorders, including a form of cancer of the blood-forming tissue known as "chronic lymphocytic leukemia," and human immunode-ficiency virus (HIV) infection. When immune thrombocytopenia is a feature of other disorders, the condition is known as "secondary immune thrombocytopenia."

SYMPTOMS OF IMMUNE THROMBOCYTOPENIC PURPURA

Immune thrombocytopenic purpura may not cause any symptoms. However, ITP can cause bleeding that is hard to stop. This bleeding can be inside your body, underneath your skin, or from your skin.

Signs of bleeding may include the following:
- petechiae, which are small, flat red spots under the skin caused by blood leaking from blood vessels
- purpura, which is bleeding in your skin that can cause red, purple, or brownish-yellow spots
- clotted or partially clotted blood under your skin (called a "hematoma") that looks or feels like a lump
- nosebleeds (epistaxis) or bleeding from your gums
- blood in your urine or stool
- heavy menstrual bleeding
- extreme tiredness

COMPLICATIONS OF IMMUNE THROMBOCYTOPENIC PURPURA

In severe cases, individuals may have gastrointestinal (GI) bleeding or blood in the urine or stool or heavy and prolonged menstrual bleeding (menorrhagia). In very rare instances, bleeding inside the skull (intracranial hemorrhage) can occur, which can be life-threatening. A greater reduction in platelet numbers is often asso-ciated with more frequent bleeding episodes and an increased risk of severe bleeding.

WHEN DOES IMMUNE THROMBOCYTOPENIC PURPURA DEVELOP?

While ITP can be diagnosed at any age, there are two periods when the condition is most likely to develop: early childhood and late adulthood. In children, the reduction in platelets is often sudden, but platelet levels usually return to normal levels within weeks to months. ITP in children is often preceded by a minor infection, such as an upper respiratory infection, but the relationship between the infection and ITP is not clear. In adults, the development of ITP is usually gradual, and the condition tends to persist throughout life.

FREQUENCY OF IMMUNE THROMBOCYTOPENIC PURPURA

The incidence of ITP is approximately 4 per 100,000 children and 3 per 100,000 adults. In adults with ITP, women are affected more often than men.

It is likely that this condition is underdiagnosed because those with mild signs and symptoms often do not seek medical attention.

INHERITANCE OF IMMUNE THROMBOCYTOPENIC PURPURA

Immune thrombocytopenia and other autoimmune disorders can run in families, but the inheritance pattern is usually unknown. People with a first-degree relative (such as a parent or sibling) with immune thrombocytopenia likely have an increased risk of developing the disorder themselves.[2]

DIAGNOSIS OF IMMUNE THROMBOCYTOPENIC PURPURA

To diagnose ITP, your provider will ask about your medical and family history. They will also ask about your symptoms and do a physical exam to look for signs of bleeding.

Your provider may order one or more of the following blood tests:

- **Complete blood count (CBC).** This test measures your platelet count and the number of other blood cells in your blood.

---

[2] MedlinePlus, "Immune Thrombocytopenia," National Institutes of Health (NIH), June 1, 2017. Available online. URL: https://medlineplus.gov/genetics/condition/immune-thrombocytopenia. Accessed May 19, 2023.

- **Blood smear**. For this test, some of your blood is put on a slide. A microscope is used to look at your platelets.
- **Bone marrow tests**. These tests check whether your bone marrow is healthy. You may need this test to confirm that you have ITP and not another platelet disorder, especially if your treatment is not working.

You may also have a blood test to check for the antibodies that attack platelets.

If you are at risk for HIV, hepatitis C, or *Heliobacter pylori*, your provider may screen you for these infections, which might be linked to ITP.

TREATMENT FOR IMMUNE THROMBOCYTOPENIC PURPURA

For most children and adults, ITP is not a serious condition. Acute ITP in children often goes away on its own within a few weeks or months and does not return. For a small number of children, ITP does not go away on its own, and the child may need treatment.

Chronic ITP varies from person to person and can last for many years. Even people who have serious types of chronic ITP can live for decades. Most people who have chronic ITP can stop treatment at some point and maintain a safe platelet count.

Treatment depends on your platelet count and whether you have any symptoms. In mild cases, you may not need any treatment, and your provider will monitor your condition to make sure that your platelet count does not become too low. If you need treatment, your treatment plan may include medicines and procedures. If your ITP was caused by an infection, treating the infection may help increase your platelet count and lower your risk of bleeding problems.

Medicines

Medicines are often used as the first treatment for both children and adults.

Corticosteroids, such as prednisone and dexamethasone, are commonly used to treat ITP. These medicines help increase your platelet count. However, steroids have many side effects. Some people relapse (get worse) when treatment ends.

Other medicines used to raise the platelet count include the following:

- eltrombopag
- immune globulin
- rituximab
- romiplostim

Removal of Your Spleen

Doctors can surgically remove your spleen (splenectomy) if necessary. The spleen is an organ in your upper left abdomen. It makes antibodies that help fight infections. In ITP, these antibodies destroy platelets by mistake.

Removing your spleen may raise your risk of infections. Before you have the surgery, your doctor may give you vaccines to help prevent infections. They will explain what steps you can take to help avoid infections and what symptoms to watch for.

Platelet Transfusions

Some people who have ITP with serious bleeding may need to have a platelet transfusion. This is done in a hospital. Some people will need platelet transfusions before having surgery.

For a platelet transfusion, donor platelets from a blood bank are injected into your bloodstream. This increases your platelet count for a short time.[3]

---

[3] "Platelet Disorders—Immune Thrombocytopenia (ITP)," National Heart, Lung, and Blood Institute (NHLBI), March 24, 2022. Available online. URL: www.nhlbi.nih.gov/health/immune-thrombocytopenia. Accessed May 19, 2023.

Section 30.3 | **Thrombotic Thrombocytopenic Purpura**

Thrombotic thrombocytopenic purpura (TTP) is a rare, life-threatening blood disorder. In TTP, blood clots form in small blood vessels throughout your body. The clots can limit or block the flow of blood to your organs, such as your brain, kidneys, and heart. This can prevent your organs from working properly and can damage your organs.

The increased clotting that occurs in TTP also uses up your platelets. Platelets are tiny blood cells that help form blood clots. These cell fragments stick together to seal small cuts and breaks in your blood vessels to stop bleeding. When your platelets are used up, you do not have enough platelets to form blood clots when necessary. This may cause bleeding and bruising.

"Thrombotic" refers to the blood clots that form; "thrombocytopenic" means the blood has a lower-than-normal platelet count; and "purpura" refers to purple bruises caused by bleeding under your skin.

TTP usually occurs suddenly and lasts for days or weeks, but it can continue for months. TTP can also cause red blood cells (RBCs) to break apart faster than your body can replace them. This leads to a rare form of anemia called "hemolytic anemia."

TTP can be fatal. Without treatment, it can cause long-term problems, such as brain damage or a stroke.

CAUSES OF THROMBOTIC THROMBOCYTOPENIC PURPURA

Thrombotic thrombocytopenic purpura occurs when you do not have the right amount of an enzyme (a type of protein in your blood) called "ADAMTS13." This enzyme controls how your blood clots. If you do not have enough ADAMTS13, your body makes too many blood clots.

TTP can be inherited or acquired. "Inherited" means that your parents passed the gene for the disease on to you. In inherited TTP, the *ADAMTS13* gene is faulty. Mutations, or changes, in the *ADAMTS13* gene can cause your body to make an ADAMTS13 enzyme that does not work properly. If you inherit TTP, you are born with two copies of the faulty gene—one from each parent. Most often, the parents each have one copy of the faulty gene but have no signs or symptoms of TTP. "Acquired" means that you were not born with the disease, but you developed it due to another disease or condition. In acquired TTP, the *ADAMTS13* gene is not faulty. Instead, your body makes antibodies (proteins) that stop the ADAMTS13 enzyme from working properly.

RISK FACTORS OF THROMBOTIC THROMBOCYTOPENIC PURPURA

The following factors can raise your risk of TTP:

- **Age**. Acquired TTP mostly occurs in adults, but it can affect children. Inherited TTP mainly affects newborns and children.
- **Other medical conditions**. Cancer, human immunodeficiency virus (HIV), lupus, and infections can cause TTP. Obesity and pregnancy can also raise your risk.
- **Race and ethnicity**. Acquired TTP more often occurs in African Americans than in other racial groups.
- **Sex**. Acquired TTP more often occurs in women than in men.
- **Some medical procedures**. Surgery and blood and marrow stem cell transplants can raise your risk of TTP.
- **Some medicines**. Chemotherapy, ticlopidine, clopidogrel, cyclosporine A, and hormone therapy can cause TTP.

Quinine, which is a substance often found in tonic water and nutritional health products, can also raise your risk.

SYMPTOMS OF THROMBOTIC THROMBOCYTOPENIC PURPURA

The symptoms of TTP may happen suddenly. Most people who have inherited TTP begin to have symptoms soon after birth. However, some do not have symptoms until they are adults.

The symptoms of TTP are caused by blood clots, a low platelet count, and damaged RBCs. Your symptoms may include:

- petechiae, which are small, flat red spots under the skin caused by blood leaking from blood vessels
- purpura, which is bleeding in your skin that can cause red, purple, or brownish-yellow spots
- paleness or jaundice (a yellowish color of the skin or whites of the eyes)
- extreme tiredness
- a fever
- a fast heart rate or shortness of breath
- headache, speech changes, confusion, coma, stroke, or seizure
- a low amount of urine, or protein or blood in your urine
- feeling sick to your stomach (nausea), vomiting, and diarrhea

DIAGNOSIS OF THROMBOTIC THROMBOCYTOPENIC PURPURA

To diagnose TTP, your provider will ask about your medical and family history. They will ask about your symptoms and do a physical exam to look for signs of TTP.

Your provider may order one or more of the following blood tests:

- **ADAMTS13 assay**. A lack of activity in the ADAMTS13 enzyme causes TTP. For this test, a sample of blood is drawn from a vein, usually in your arm. The blood is sent to a special lab to test for the enzyme's activity.
- **Bilirubin test**. When RBCs die, they release a protein called "hemoglobin" into your bloodstream. The body breaks down hemoglobin into a compound called "bilirubin." If you have TTP, your bilirubin level may be high because your body is breaking down RBCs faster than normal.
- **Blood smear**. For this test, some of your blood is put on a slide. A microscope is used to look at your blood

cells. If you have TTP, your RBCs will look torn and broken.

- **Bone marrow tests**. These tests check whether your bone marrow is healthy.
- **Complete blood count (CBC)**. This test measures the levels of RBCs, white blood cells (WBCs), and platelets in your blood.
- **Coombs test**. This blood test is used to find out whether TTP is causing hemolytic anemia. In TTP, hemolytic anemia develops because RBCs are broken into pieces as they try to squeeze around blood clots. When TTP is the cause of hemolytic anemia, the Coombs test is negative. The test is positive if antibodies (proteins) are destroying your RBCs.
- **Kidney function tests and urine tests**. These tests show whether your kidneys are working well. If you have TTP, you may have blood or protein in your urine. Also, your blood creatinine level may be high. Creatinine is a blood product that is normally removed by the kidneys.
- **Lactate dehydrogenase (LDH) test**. This blood test measures a protein called "LDH." Hemolytic anemia causes RBCs to break down and release LDH into the blood. LDH is also released from tissues that are injured by blood clots because of TTP.

TREATMENT OF THROMBOTIC THROMBOCYTOPENIC PURPURA

Thrombotic thrombocytopenic purpura can cause life-threatening complications if it is not treated right away. Plasma treatments and medicines are the most common ways to treat TTP. If these treatments do not work, you may need surgery. Treatments are done in a hospital.

Plasma Treatments

- **Therapeutic plasma exchange (plasmapheresis)**. It is used to treat acquired TTP. In this procedure, the liquid part of your blood (plasma) is replaced with donor plasma using a machine that collects the cells in the blood. It removes antibodies (proteins) in your blood that damage your ADAMTS13 enzyme. Plasma exchange also replaces the ADAMTS13 enzyme. You will get this treatment daily until any organ problems have gone away, your platelet count is stable, and damage to your RBCs has stopped.

- **Plasma infusion**. It is used to treat inherited TTP. For this treatment, donor plasma is given through an intravenous (IV) line inserted into a vein. This is done to replace the missing or faulty ADAMTS13 enzyme.

Plasma treatments usually continue until the results of your blood tests and symptoms improve. This can take days or weeks, depending on your condition. You will stay in the hospital while you recover.

Medicines

Corticosteroids, such as prednisone, are commonly used together with plasma treatments. These medicines (steroids, for short) can slow or stop your body from forming antibodies against the ADAMTS13 enzyme. The steroids used to treat TTP are different from the illegal steroids that some athletes take to enhance performance. Corticosteroids are not habit-forming, even if you take them for many years.

Other medicines used to treat TTP include rituximab, vincristine, cyclophosphamide, and cyclosporine A.

Surgery to Remove Your Spleen

The spleen is an organ in your upper left abdomen. Your spleen makes the antibodies that block ADAMTS13 enzyme activity. Removing your spleen stops your body from making these antibodies. This surgery is used to treat TTP if other treatments do not work for you.

WHAT HEALTH PROBLEMS CAN THROMBOTIC THROMBOCYTOPENIC PURPURA CAUSE?

Some people fully recover from TTP. However, relapses (flare-ups) are common. They can happen in people who have acquired and inherited TTP. If you have frequent relapses, you may need ongoing treatment.

Without treatment, TTP can cause frequent blood clots. These blood clots can block blood flow to your organs and cause complications, including the following:

- a stroke
- brain damage
- coma
- problems with your kidneys
- reduced blood flow to your digestive system, which may cause diarrhea, pain in your abdomen, and other digestive problems
- reduced blood flow to your heart, which may cause a heart attack
- seizures[4]

---

[4] "Thrombotic Thrombocytopenic Purpura (TTP)," National Heart, Lung, and Blood Institute (NHLBI), March 24, 2022. Available online. URL: www.nhlbi.nih.gov/health/thrombotic-thrombocytopenic-purpura. Accessed May 19, 2023.

Part 5 | **Circulatory Disorders**

Chapter 31 | **Blood Pressure Disorders**

Chapter Contents

WHAT IS HYPERTENSION?

High blood pressure (HBP) is a common disease in which blood flows through blood vessels, or arteries, at higher-than-normal pressures. Blood pressure is the force of blood pushing against the walls of your arteries as the heart pumps blood. HBP, sometimes called "hypertension," is when this force against the artery walls is too high. Your doctor may diagnose you with HBP if you have consistent HBP readings.

To control or lower HBP, your doctor may recommend that you adopt heart-healthy lifestyle changes—such as heart-healthy eating patterns, including the Dietary Approaches to Stop Hypertension (DASH) eating plan—alone or with medicines. Controlling or lowering blood pressure can also help prevent or delay HBP complications, such as chronic kidney disease (CKD), heart attack, heart failure, stroke, and possibly vascular dementia.

CAUSES OF HYPERTENSION

Eating too much sodium and having certain medical conditions can cause HBP. Taking certain medicines, including birth control pills (BCPs) or over-the-counter (OTC) cold relief medicines, can also make blood pressure rise.

Eating Too Much Sodium

Unhealthy eating patterns, particularly eating too much sodium, are common causes of HBP in the United States. Healthy lifestyle changes can help prevent or treat HBP.

Other Medical Conditions

Other medical conditions change the way your body controls fluids, sodium, and hormones in your blood. Other medical causes of HBP include:
- certain tumors
- CKD

- being overweight or obese
- sleep apnea
- thyroid problems

RISK FACTORS FOR HYPERTENSION

There are many risk factors for HBP. Some risk factors, such as unhealthy lifestyle habits, can be changed. Other risk factors, such as age, family history and genetics, race and ethnicity, and sex, cannot be changed. Healthy lifestyle changes can decrease your risk of developing HBP.

Age

Blood pressure tends to increase with age. Our blood vessels naturally thicken and stiffen over time. These changes increase the risk for HBP.

However, the risk of HBP is increasing for children and teens, possibly due to the rise in the number of children and teens who are overweight or obese.

Family History and Genetics

HBP often runs in families. Much of the understanding of the body systems involved in HBP has come from genetic studies. Research has identified many gene variations associated with small increases in the risk of developing HBP. Research suggests that certain deoxyribonucleic acid (DNA) changes during fetal development may also lead to the development of HBP later in life.

Unhealthy Lifestyle Habits

Unhealthy lifestyle habits can increase the risk of HBP. These habits include:
- unhealthy eating patterns, such as eating too much sodium
- drinking too much alcohol
- being physically inactive

Race or Ethnicity

HBP is more common in African American adults than in White, Hispanic, or Asian adults. Compared with other racial or ethnic groups, African Americans tend to have higher average blood pressure numbers and get HBP earlier in life.

Sex

Before the age of 55, men are more likely than women to develop HBP. After the age of 55, women are more likely than men to develop HBP.

SIGNS, SYMPTOMS, AND COMPLICATIONS OF HYPERTENSION

It is important to have regular blood pressure readings taken and to know your numbers because HBP does not usually cause symptoms until serious complications occur. Undiagnosed or uncontrolled HBP can cause the following complications:

- aneurysms
- CKD
- eye damage
- heart attack
- heart failure
- peripheral artery disease (PAD)
- stroke
- vascular dementia

SCREENING AND PREVENTION OF HYPERTENSION

Everyone three years of age or older should have their blood pressure checked by a health-care provider at least once a year. Your doctor will use a blood pressure test to see if you have consistent HBP readings. Even small increases in systolic blood pressure can weaken and damage your blood vessels. Your doctor will recommend heart-healthy lifestyle changes to help control your blood pressure and prevent you from developing HBP.

Screening for Consistently High Blood Pressure Readings

Your doctor will use a blood pressure test to see if you have higher-than-normal blood pressure readings. The reading is made up of two numbers, with the systolic number above the diastolic number. These numbers are measures of pressure in millimeters of mercury (mm Hg).

Your blood pressure is considered high when you have consistent systolic readings of 140 mm Hg or higher or diastolic readings of 90 mm Hg or higher. Based on research, your doctor may also consider you to have HBP if you are an adult or a child 13 years of age or older who has consistent systolic readings of 130–139 mm Hg or diastolic readings of 80–89 mm Hg and you have other cardiovascular risk factors.

For children younger than 13 years of age, blood pressure readings are compared to readings common for children of the same age, sex, and height.

Talk to your doctor if your blood pressure readings are consistently higher than normal.

A blood pressure test is easy and painless, and it can be done in a doctor's office or clinic. A health-care provider will use a gauge, stethoscope, or electronic sensor and a blood pressure cuff to measure your blood pressure. To prepare, take the following steps:

- Do not exercise, drink coffee, or smoke cigarettes for 30 minutes before the test.
- Go to the bathroom before the test.
- For at least five minutes before the test, sit in a chair and relax.
- Make sure your feet are flat on the floor.
- Do not talk while you are relaxing or during the test.
- Uncover your arm for the cuff.
- Rest your arm on a table, so it is supported and at the level of your heart.

If it is the first time your provider has measured your blood pressure, you may have readings taken on both arms.

Even after taking these steps, your blood pressure reading may not be accurate for other reasons, including the following:

- **You are excited or nervous**. The phrase "white coat hypertension" refers to blood pressure readings that are only high when taken in a doctor's office compared with readings taken in other places. Doctors can detect this type of HBP by reviewing readings from the office and from other places.
- **Your blood pressure tends to be lower when measured at the doctor's office**. This is called "masked HBP." When this happens, your doctor will have difficulty detecting HBP.
- **The wrong blood pressure cuff was used**. Your readings can appear different if the cuff is too small or too large. It is important for your health-care team to track your readings over time and ensure the correct pressure cuff is used for your sex and age.

Your doctor may run additional tests to confirm an initial reading. To gather more information about your blood pressure, your doctor may recommend wearing a blood pressure monitor to record readings over 24 hours. Your doctor may also teach you how to take blood pressure readings at home.

Healthy Lifestyle Changes to Prevent High Blood Pressure

Healthy lifestyle changes can help prevent HBP from developing. Healthy lifestyle changes include choosing heart-healthy eating patterns, such as the DASH eating plan; being physically active; aiming for a healthy weight; quitting smoking; and managing stress.[1]

---

[1] "High Blood Pressure," National Heart, Lung, and Blood Institute (NHLBI), March 24, 2022. Available online. URL: www.nhlbi.nih.gov/health/high-blood-pressure. Accessed May 30, 2023.

Section 31.2 | **Pulmonary Hypertension**

WHAT IS PULMONARY HYPERTENSION?

Pulmonary hypertension is a condition that affects the blood vessels in the lungs. It develops when the blood pressure in your lungs is higher than normal. About 1 percent of people globally have pulmonary hypertension.

Pulmonary hypertension makes the heart work harder than normal to pump blood into the lungs. This can damage the heart and cause symptoms such as shortness of breath, chest pain, and light-headedness.

Pulmonary hypertension can develop on its own or be caused by another disease or condition. There are five different groups of pulmonary hypertension:

- **Group 1**. Pulmonary arterial hypertension (PAH).
- **Group 2**. Pulmonary hypertension due to left-sided heart disease.
- **Group 3**. Pulmonary hypertension due to lung disease and/or hypoxia.
- **Group 4**. Pulmonary hypertension due to pulmonary artery obstructions, including chronic thromboembolic pulmonary hypertension (CTEPH).
- **Group 5**. Pulmonary hypertension with unknown and/or multiple causes.

Over 50 percent of pulmonary arterial hypertension cases worldwide have no known cause. In the United States, the most common type of pulmonary hypertension is caused by left-sided heart disease, such as left heart failure. Several other medical conditions and environmental factors can raise your likelihood of developing pulmonary hypertension. Your health-care provider will consider your symptoms and health history before conducting tests to diagnose pulmonary hypertension.

Treatments for pulmonary hypertension will depend on the cause of the condition. Many times, there is no cure for pulmonary hypertension, but your provider can work with you to manage the symptoms. This may include medicine or healthy lifestyle changes.

WHAT CAUSES PULMONARY HYPERTENSION?

The cause of pulmonary hypertension is not always clear. Certain medical conditions can damage, change, or block the blood vessels of the pulmonary arteries, which can lead to pulmonary hypertension.

Some examples of medical conditions include the following:

- left heart diseases, such as left heart failure, which may be caused by HBP throughout your body, or coronary heart disease
- other heart and blood vessel diseases, such as congenital (inherited) heart defects
- lung diseases, such as chronic obstructive pulmonary disease (COPD), interstitial lung disease, emphysema, or sleep apnea
- other medical conditions, such as liver disease, sickle cell disease (SCD), blood clots in the lungs, or connective tissue disorders, including scleroderma

WHAT RAISES THE RISK OF PULMONARY HYPERTENSION?

Several factors can increase your risk of developing pulmonary hypertension that include the following:

- **Age**. Pulmonary hypertension can occur at any age, but your risk increases as you get older. The condition is usually diagnosed between ages 30 and 60.
- **Environment**. You may be at an increased risk of pulmonary hypertension if you have or are exposed to asbestos or certain infections caused by parasites.
- **Family history and genetics**. Certain genetic disorders, such as Down syndrome, congenital heart disease, and Gaucher disease, can increase your risk of pulmonary hypertension. A family history of blood clots also increases your risk.
- **Lifestyle habits**. Unhealthy lifestyle habits, such as smoking and illegal drug use, can raise your risk of developing pulmonary hypertension.

- **Medicine**. Some prescribed medicines used to treat cancer and depression may increase your risk of pulmonary hypertension.
- **Sex**. Pulmonary hypertension is more common in women than in men. Pulmonary hypertension with certain types of heart failure is also more common in women.

SYMPTOMS OF PULMONARY HYPERTENSION

Symptoms of pulmonary hypertension are sometimes hard to recognize. People may have symptoms for years before being diagnosed. This is because many symptoms of pulmonary hypertension are also symptoms of other medical conditions.

Some symptoms of pulmonary hypertension include the following:

- chest pain
- coughing that is dry or produces blood
- shortness of breath
- dizziness that may lead to fainting
- nausea and vomiting
- hoarseness
- fatigue
- swelling of the abdomen, legs, or feet
- weakness
- wheezing, which is a whistling sound when you breathe out

Symptoms can get worse over time. For example, in the early stages of pulmonary hypertension, you may only have shortness of breath with exercise. As the disease progresses, shortness of breath will occur more often.

When to Call 911

If you experience chest pain and shortness of breath, seek emergency medical care. This may be a sign of a heart attack or a blood clot in your lungs (pulmonary embolism).

DIAGNOSIS OF PULMONARY HYPERTENSION

To diagnose pulmonary hypertension, your doctor may ask you questions about your medical history and do a physical exam. Based on your symptoms and risk factors, your doctor may refer you to a lung specialist (pulmonologist) or a heart and blood vessel specialist (cardiologist). Your doctor will diagnose you with pulmonary hypertension if tests show higher-than-normal pressure in the arteries of the lungs (pulmonary arteries).

Medical History and Physical Exam

Your doctor may ask you about any symptoms you have been experiencing and any risk factors, such as other medical conditions you have.

Your doctor will also perform a physical exam to look for signs that may help diagnose your condition. As part of this exam, your doctor may do the following:

- Check whether the oxygen levels in your blood are low. This may be done by pulse oximetry, in which a probe is placed on your finger to check your oxygen levels.
- Feel your liver to see if it is larger than normal.
- Listen to your heart to see if there are changes in how it sounds and also to find out if your heartbeat is faster than normal or irregular or if you have a new heart murmur.
- Listen to your lungs for sounds that could be caused by heart failure or interstitial lung disease.
- Look at the veins in your neck to see if they are larger than normal.
- Look for swelling in your abdomen and legs that may be caused by fluid buildup.
- Measure your blood pressure.

Diagnostic Tests

There are many tests that doctors can use to tell if you have pulmonary hypertension. The most common tests to measure the pressure in your pulmonary arteries are cardiac catheterization and echocardiography. Normal pressure in the pulmonary arteries is between 11 and 20 mm Hg. If the pressure is too high, you may have pulmonary hypertension. A pressure of 25 mm Hg or greater measured by cardiac catheterization or 35–40 mm Hg or greater on echocardiography suggests pulmonary hypertension.

Other tests may include the following:

- Blood tests look for blood clots, stress on the heart, or anemia.
- Heart imaging tests, such as cardiac magnetic resonance imaging (MRI), take detailed pictures of the structure and functioning of the heart and surrounding blood vessels.
- Lung imaging tests, such as chest x-ray, look at the size and shape of the heart and surrounding blood vessels, including the pulmonary arteries.
- Electrocardiogram (ECG or EKG) looks for changes in the electrical activity of your heart. This can help detect if certain parts of the heart are damaged or working too hard. In pulmonary hypertension, the heart can become overworked due to damage or changes in the pulmonary arteries.

Test for Other Medical Conditions

Your doctor may order additional tests to see whether another condition or medicine may be causing your pulmonary hypertension. Doctors can use this information to develop your treatment plan.

CAN YOU PREVENT PULMONARY HYPERTENSION?

Prevention is not always possible since the cause of pulmonary hypertension is not always clear. Your doctor may suggest a preventative screening if you have a known risk factor or medical condition that causes pulmonary hypertension. Your doctor may also recommend prevention strategies to help you lower your risk of developing pulmonary hypertension.[2]

---

[2] "Pulmonary Hypertension," National Heart, Lung, and Blood Institute (NHLBI), May 1, 2023. Available online. URL: www.nhlbi.nih.gov/health/pulmonary-hypertension. Accessed May 22, 2023.

Section 31.3 | **Preeclampsia and Eclampsia**

Preeclampsia and eclampsia are part of the spectrum of high blood pressure (HBP), or hypertensive, disorders that can occur during pregnancy.

At the mild end of the spectrum is gestational hypertension, which occurs when a woman who previously had normal blood pressure develops HBP when she is more than 20 weeks pregnant, and her blood pressure returns to normal within 12 weeks after delivery. This problem usually occurs without other symptoms. In many cases, gestational hypertension does not harm the mother or fetus. Severe gestational hypertension, however, may be associated with preterm birth and infants who are small for their age at birth. Some women who have gestational hypertension later develop preeclampsia.

Preeclampsia is similar to gestational hypertension because it also involves HBP at or after 20 weeks of pregnancy in a woman whose blood pressure was normal before pregnancy. But preeclampsia can also include blood pressure at or greater than 140/90 mm Hg, increased swelling, and protein in the urine. The condition can be serious and is a leading cause of preterm birth (before 37 weeks of pregnancy). If it is severe enough to affect brain function, causing seizures or coma, it is called "eclampsia."

A serious complication of hypertensive disorders in pregnancy is HELLP syndrome, a situation in which a pregnant woman with preeclampsia or eclampsia suffers damage to the liver and blood cells. The letters in the name HELLP stand for the following problems:

- H—hemolysis, in which oxygen-carrying red blood cells break down
- EL—elevated liver enzymes, showing damage to the liver
- LP—low platelet count, meaning that the cells responsible for stopping bleeding are low

Postpartum preeclampsia describes preeclampsia that develops after the baby is delivered, usually between 48 hours and six weeks after delivery. Symptoms can include HBP, severe headache, visual changes, upper abdominal pain, and nausea or vomiting. Postpartum preeclampsia can occur regardless of whether a woman has HBP or preeclampsia during pregnancy.

Postpartum eclampsia refers to seizures that occur between 48 and 72 hours after delivery. Symptoms also include HBP and difficulty breathing. About one-third of eclampsia cases occur after delivery, and nearly half of those are more than 48 hours after the birth.

Postpartum preeclampsia and eclampsia can be serious and, if not treated quickly, may result in death.

WHAT CAUSES PREECLAMPSIA AND ECLAMPSIA?

The causes of preeclampsia and eclampsia are not known. These disorders previously were believed to be caused by a toxin called "toxemia" in the blood, but health-care providers now know that is not true. Nevertheless, preeclampsia is sometimes still referred to as "toxemia."

To learn more about preeclampsia and eclampsia, scientists are investigating many factors that could contribute to the development and progression of these diseases, including:
- placental abnormalities, such as insufficient blood flow
- genetic factors
- environmental exposures
- nutritional factors
- maternal immunology and autoimmune disorders
- cardiovascular and inflammatory changes
- hormonal imbalances

WHAT ARE THE RISKS OF PREECLAMPSIA AND ECLAMPSIA TO THE MOTHER?
Risks during Pregnancy

Preeclampsia during pregnancy is mild in the majority of cases. However, a woman can progress from mild to severe preeclampsia or to full eclampsia very quickly, even in a matter of days. Both preeclampsia and eclampsia can cause serious health problems for the mother and infant.

Women with preeclampsia are at increased risk for damage to the kidneys, liver, brain, and other organ and blood systems. Preeclampsia may also affect the placenta. The condition could lead to a separation of the placenta from the uterus (referred to as "placental abruption"), preterm birth, and pregnancy loss or stillbirth. In some cases, preeclampsia can lead to organ failure or stroke.

In severe cases, preeclampsia can develop into eclampsia, which includes seizures. Seizures in eclampsia may cause a woman to lose consciousness and twitch uncontrollably. If the fetus is not delivered, these conditions can cause the death of the mother and/or the fetus.

Although most pregnant women in developed countries survive preeclampsia, it is still a major cause of illness and death globally. According to the World Health Organization (WHO), preeclampsia and eclampsia cause 14 percent of maternal deaths each year, or about 50,000–75,000 women worldwide.

Risks after Pregnancy

In uncomplicated preeclampsia, the mother's HBP and other symptoms usually go back to normal within six weeks of the infant's birth. However, studies have shown that women who had preeclampsia are four times more likely than women who did not have preeclampsia to later develop hypertension (HBP) and are twice as likely to later develop ischemic heart disease (reduced blood supply to the heart muscle, which can cause heart attacks), a blood clot in a vein, and stroke.

Less commonly, mothers who had preeclampsia can experience permanent damage to their organs, such as their kidneys and liver. They can also experience fluid in the lungs. In the days following birth, women with preeclampsia remain at an increased risk for developing eclampsia and seizures.

In some women, preeclampsia develops between 48 hours and six weeks after they deliver their baby—a condition called "postpartum preeclampsia." Postpartum preeclampsia can occur in women who had preeclampsia during pregnancy and among those who did not. One study found that slightly more than one-half of women who had postpartum preeclampsia did not have preeclampsia during pregnancy. If a woman has seizures within 72 hours of delivery, she may have postpartum eclampsia. It is important to recognize and treat postpartum preeclampsia and eclampsia because the risk of complications may be higher than if the conditions had occurred during pregnancy. Postpartum preeclampsia and eclampsia can progress very quickly if not treated and may lead to stroke or death.

WHAT ARE THE RISKS OF PREECLAMPSIA AND ECLAMPSIA TO THE FETUS?

Preeclampsia may be related to problems with the placenta early in the pregnancy. Such problems pose risks to the fetus, including:

- lack of oxygen and nutrients, which can impair fetal growth
- preterm birth
- stillbirth if placental abruption leads to heavy bleeding in the mother
- infant death

Stillbirths are more likely to occur when the mother has a more severe form of preeclampsia, including HELLP syndrome.

Infants whose mothers had preeclampsia are also at increased risk for later problems, even if they were born at full term (39 weeks of pregnancy). Infants born preterm due to preeclampsia face a higher risk of some long-term health issues, mostly related to being born early, including learning disorders, cerebral palsy, epilepsy, deafness, and blindness. Infants born preterm may also have to be hospitalized for a long time after birth and may be smaller than infants born full-term. Infants who experience poor growth in the uterus may later be at a higher risk of diabetes, congestive heart failure, and HBP.

HOW MANY WOMEN ARE AFFECTED BY OR AT RISK OF PREECLAMPSIA?

Although preeclampsia occurs primarily in first pregnancies, a woman who had preeclampsia in a previous pregnancy is seven times more likely to develop preeclampsia in a later pregnancy.

Other factors that can increase a woman's risk include:

- chronic HBP or kidney disease before pregnancy
- HBP or preeclampsia in an earlier pregnancy
- women who are overweight or obese
- women older than 40 years of age
- multiple gestation (being pregnant with more than one fetus)
- women who have had preeclampsia before (Non-White women are more likely than White women to develop preeclampsia again in a later pregnancy.)

According to the World Health Organization (WHO), among women who have had preeclampsia, about 20–40 percent of their daughters and 11–37 percent of their sisters will also get the disorder.

Preeclampsia is also more common among women who have histories of certain health conditions, such as migraines, diabetes, rheumatoid arthritis (RA), lupus, scleroderma, urinary tract infections (UTIs), gum disease, polycystic ovary syndrome (PCOS), multiple sclerosis (MS), gestational diabetes, and sickle cell disease (SCD).

Preeclampsia is also more common in pregnancies resulting from egg donation, donor insemination, or in vitro fertilization (IVF).

The U.S. Preventive Services Task Force (USPSTF) recommends that women who are at high risk for preeclampsia take low-dose aspirin starting after 12 weeks of pregnancy to prevent preeclampsia. Women who are pregnant or who are thinking about getting pregnant should talk with their health-care provider about preeclampsia risk and ways to reduce the risk.

WHAT ARE THE SYMPTOMS OF PREECLAMPSIA AND ECLAMPSIA AND HEMOLYSIS, ELEVATED LIVER ENZYMES, LOW PLATELET COUNT SYNDROME?
Preeclampsia
Possible symptoms of preeclampsia include:

- HBP
- too much protein in the urine

- swelling in a woman's face and hands (A woman's feet might swell too, but swollen feet are common during pregnancy and may not signal a problem.)
- systemic problems, such as headache, blurred vision, and right upper quadrant abdominal pain

Eclampsia
The following symptoms are cause for immediate concern:
- seizures
- severe headache
- vision problems, such as temporary blindness
- abdominal pain, especially in the upper right area of the belly
- nausea and vomiting
- smaller urine output or not urinating very often

Hemolysis, Elevated Liver Enzymes, Low Platelet Count Syndrome
HELLP syndrome can lead to serious complications, including liver failure and death.

A pregnant woman with HELLP syndrome might bleed or bruise easily and/or experience abdominal pain, nausea or vomiting, headache, or extreme fatigue. Although most women who develop HELLP syndrome already have HBP and preeclampsia, sometimes, the syndrome is the first sign. In addition, HELLP syndrome can occur without a woman having either HBP or protein in her urine.[3]

[3] "Preeclampsia and Eclampsia," *Eunice Kennedy Shriver* National Institute of Child Health and Human Development (NICHD), November 19, 2018. Available online. URL: www.nichd.nih.gov/health/topics/preeclampsia/conditioninfo. Accessed June 6, 2023.

Section 31.4 | **Hypotension**

WHAT IS HYPOTENSION?

Hypotension is abnormally low blood pressure. Sometimes, blood pressure that is too low can also cause problems.

Blood pressure is the force of your blood pushing against the walls of your arteries. Each time your heart beats, it pumps out blood into the arteries. Your blood pressure is highest when your heart beats, pumping the blood. This is called "systolic pressure." When your heart is at rest, between beats, your blood pressure falls. This is the "diastolic pressure." Your blood pressure reading uses these two numbers. Usually, they are written one above or before the other, such as 120/80. If your blood pressure reading is 90/60 or lower, you have low blood pressure.

Some people have low blood pressure all the time. They have no symptoms, and their low readings are normal for them. In other people, blood pressure drops below normal because of a medical condition or certain medicines. Some people may have symptoms of low blood pressure when standing up too quickly. Low blood pressure is a problem only if it causes dizziness, fainting, or, in extreme cases, shock.[4]

CAUSES OF HYPOTENSION

Conditions or factors that disrupt the body's ability to control blood pressure cause hypotension. The different types of hypotension have different causes.

Orthostatic Hypotension

Orthostatic hypotension has many causes. Sometimes, two or more factors combine to cause this type of low blood pressure.

Dehydration is the most common cause of orthostatic hypotension. Dehydration occurs if the body loses more water than it takes in.

[4] MedlinePlus, "Low Blood Pressure," National Institutes of Health (NIH), January 28, 2019. Available online. URL: https://medlineplus.gov/lowbloodpressure.html#summary. Accessed June 7, 2023.

You may become dehydrated if you do not drink enough fluids or if you sweat a lot during physical activity. Fever, vomiting, and severe diarrhea can also cause dehydration.

Orthostatic hypotension may also occur during pregnancy, but it usually goes away after birth.

Because an older body does not manage changes in blood pressure as well as a younger body, getting older can also lead to this type of hypotension.

Postprandial hypotension (a type of orthostatic hypotension) mostly affects older adults. Postprandial hypotension is a sudden drop in blood pressure after a meal.

Certain medical conditions can raise your risk of orthostatic hypotension, including:

- heart conditions, such as heart attack, heart valve disease, bradycardia (a very low heart rate), and heart failure (These conditions prevent the heart from pumping enough blood to the body.)
- anemia
- severe infections
- endocrine conditions, such as thyroid disorders, Addison disease, low blood sugar, and diabetes
- central nervous system (CNS) disorders, such as Parkinson disease (PD)
- pulmonary embolism (PE)

Some medicines for HBP and heart disease can raise your risk of orthostatic hypotension. These medicines include:

- diuretics, also called "water pills"
- calcium channel blockers
- angiotensin-converting enzyme (ACE) inhibitors
- angiotensin II receptor blockers (ARBs)
- nitrates
- beta-blockers

Medicines for conditions such as anxiety, depression, erectile dysfunction (ED), and CNS disorders can also increase your risk of orthostatic hypotension.

Other substances, when taken with HBP medicines, can also lead to orthostatic hypotension. These substances include alcohol, barbiturates, and some prescription and over-the-counter (OTC) medicines.

Finally, other factors or conditions that can trigger orthostatic hypotension include being out in the heat or being immobile for a long time. Immobile means you cannot move around very much.

Neurally Mediated Hypotension

Neurally mediated hypotension (NMH) occurs when the brain and heart do not communicate with each other properly.

For example, when you stand for a long time, blood begins to pool in your legs. This causes your blood pressure to drop. In NMH, the body mistakenly tells the brain that blood pressure is high. In response, the brain slows the heart rate. This makes blood pressure drop even more, causing dizziness and other symptoms.

Severe Hypotension Linked to Shock

Many factors and conditions can cause severe hypotension linked to shock. Some of these factors can also cause orthostatic hypotension. In shock, though, blood pressure drops very low and does not return to normal on its own.

A major decrease in the heart's ability to pump blood can also cause shock. This is known as "cardiogenic shock."

A heart attack, PE, or an ongoing arrhythmia that disrupts heart function can cause this type of shock.

A sudden and extreme relaxation of the arteries linked to a drop in blood pressure can also cause shock. This is known as "vasodilatory shock." It can occur due to:
- a severe head injury
- a reaction to certain medicines
- liver failure
- poisoning
- a severe allergic reaction (called "anaphylactic shock")

What Causes Low Blood Pressure?

Many systems of the body, including organs, hormones, and nerves, regulate blood pressure. For example, the autonomic nervous system sends the "fight-or-flight" signal that, depending on the situation, tells the heart and other systems in the body to increase or decrease blood pressure. Problems with the autonomic nervous system, such as in PD, can cause low blood pressure.

Other causes of low blood pressure include the following:
- blood loss from an injury that causes a sudden drop in blood pressure
- dehydration
- diabetes
- heart problems such as arrhythmias (irregular heartbeat)
- medicines to treat HBP, depression, or PD
- pregnancy

Older adults also have a higher risk for symptoms of low blood pressure, such as falling, fainting, or dizziness upon standing up or after a meal. Older adults are more likely to develop low blood pressure as a side effect of medicines taken to control HBP.

RISK FACTORS FOR HYPOTENSION

Hypotension can affect people of all ages. However, people in certain age groups are more likely to have certain types of hypotension.

Older adults are more likely to have orthostatic and postprandial hypotension. Children and young adults are more likely to have NMH.

People who take certain medicines—such as diuretics or other HBP medicines—are at an increased risk for hypotension. Certain conditions also increase the risk of hypotension. Examples include CNS disorders (such as PD) and some heart conditions.

Other risk factors for hypotension include being immobile for long periods, being out in the heat for a long time, and pregnancy. Hypotension during pregnancy is normal and usually goes away after birth.

SIGNS, SYMPTOMS, AND COMPLICATIONS OF HYPOTENSION
Orthostatic Hypotension and Neurally Mediated Hypotension
The signs and symptoms of orthostatic hypotension and NMH are similar. They include:
- dizziness or light-headedness
- blurry vision
- confusion
- weakness
- fatigue (feeling tired)
- nausea (feeling sick to your stomach)

Orthostatic hypotension may happen within a few seconds or minutes of standing up after you have been sitting or lying down.

You may feel that you are going to faint, or you may actually faint. These signs and symptoms go away if you sit or lie down for a few minutes until your blood pressure adjusts to normal.

The signs and symptoms of NMH occur after standing for a long time or in response to an unpleasant, upsetting, or scary situation. The drop in blood pressure with NMH does not last long and often goes away after sitting down.

Severe Hypotension Linked to Shock
In shock, not enough blood and oxygen flow to the body's major organs, including the brain. The early signs and symptoms of reduced blood flow to the brain include light-headedness, sleepiness, and confusion.

In the earliest stages of shock, it may be hard to detect any signs or symptoms. In older people, the first symptom may only be confusion.

Over time, as shock worsens, a person will not be able to sit up without passing out. If the shock continues, the person will lose consciousness. Shock is often fatal if not treated right away.

Other signs and symptoms of shock vary, depending on what is causing the shock. When low blood volume (e.g., from major blood loss) or poor pumping action in the heart (e.g., from heart failure) causes shock:
- the skin becomes cold and sweaty (It often looks blue or pale. If pressed, the color returns to normal more

slowly than usual. A bluish network of lines appears under the skin.)
- the pulse becomes weak and rapid
- the person begins to breathe very quickly

When extreme relaxation of blood vessels causes shock (such as in vasodilatory shock), a person feels warm and flushed at first. Later, the skin becomes cold and sweaty, and the person feels very sleepy.

Shock is an emergency and must be treated right away. If a person has signs or symptoms of shock, call 911.

What Should You Do If You Have Symptoms?

Sitting down may relieve the symptoms. If your blood pressure drops too low, your body's vital organs do not get enough oxygen and nutrients. When this happens, low blood pressure can lead to shock, which requires immediate medical attention. Signs of shock include cold and sweaty skin, rapid breathing, a blue skin tone, or a weak and rapid pulse. Call 911 if you notice signs of shock in yourself or someone else.

Talk to your doctor about your symptoms. Your doctor will use a blood pressure test to diagnose low blood pressure. Other tests may include blood, urine, or imaging tests and a tilt table test if you faint often.

HOW IS HYPOTENSION TREATED?

You may not need treatment for low blood pressure. Depending on your symptoms, treatment may include drinking more fluids to prevent dehydration, taking medicines to raise your blood pressure, or adjusting medicines that cause low blood pressure.

Your doctor may talk to you about lifestyle changes, including changing what and how you eat and how you sit and stand up. Your doctor may also recommend compression stockings if you stand for long periods.[5]

---

[5] "Hypotension," National Heart, Lung, and Blood Institute (NHLBI), March 24, 2022. Available online. URL: www.nhlbi.nih.gov/health/low-blood-pressure. Accessed June 7, 2023.

Section 31.5 | **Shock**

Shock happens when not enough blood and oxygen can get to your organs and tissues. It causes very low blood pressure and may be life-threatening. It often happens along with a serious injury.

There are several kinds of shock. Hypovolemic shock happens when you lose a lot of blood or fluids. Causes include internal or external bleeding, dehydration, burns, and severe vomiting and/or diarrhea. Septic shock is caused by infections in the bloodstream. A severe allergic reaction can cause anaphylactic shock. An insect bite or sting might cause it. Cardiogenic shock happens when the heart cannot pump blood effectively. This may happen after a heart attack. Neurogenic shock is caused by damage to the nervous system.

Symptoms of shock include:

- confusion or lack of alertness
- loss of consciousness
- sudden and ongoing rapid heartbeat
- sweating
- pale skin
- a weak pulse
- rapid breathing
- decreased or no urine output
- cool hands and feet

Shock is a life-threatening medical emergency, and it is important to get help right away. Treatment for shock depends on the cause.[6]

ANAPHYLACTIC SHOCK

Anaphylaxis is a serious allergic reaction. It can begin very quickly, and symptoms may be life-threatening. The most common causes are reactions to foods (especially peanuts), medications, and

---

[6] MedlinePlus, "Shock," National Institutes of Health (NIH), October 11, 2016. Available online. URL: https://medlineplus.gov/shock.html. Accessed May 19, 2023.

stinging insects. Other causes include exercise and exposure to latex. Sometimes, no cause can be found.

It can affect many organs, including:

- skin—itching, hives, redness, swelling
- nose—sneezing, stuffy nose, runny nose
- mouth—itching, swelling of the lips or tongue
- throat—itching, tightness, trouble swallowing, swelling of the back of the throat
- chest—shortness of breath, coughing, wheezing, chest pain or tightness
- heart—weak pulse, passing out, shock
- gastrointestinal (GI) tract—vomiting, diarrhea, cramps
- nervous system—dizziness or fainting

If someone is having a serious allergic reaction, call 911. If an auto-injector is available, give the person the injection right away.[7]

CARDIOGENIC SHOCK

Cardiogenic shock, also known as "cardiac shock," happens when your heart cannot pump enough blood and oxygen to the brain and other vital organs. This is a life-threatening emergency. It is treatable if diagnosed right away, so it is important to know the warning signs.

Without oxygen-rich blood reaching the brain and other vital organs, your blood pressure drops, and your pulse slows. You may have symptoms such as confusion, sweating, and rapid breathing. You may also lose consciousness.

Most often, the cause of cardiogenic shock is a serious heart attack. Other health problems that may lead to cardiogenic shock include heart failure, which happens when the heart cannot pump enough blood to meet the body's needs; chest injuries; and blood clots in the lungs.

Treatment focuses on getting blood flowing properly and protecting organs from damage. Some people may need a heart

---

[7] MedlinePlus, "Anaphylaxis," National Institutes of Health (NIH), September 21, 2016. Available online. URL: https://medlineplus.gov/anaphylaxis.html. Accessed May 19, 2023.

transplant or a permanently implanted device to help keep blood flowing to the heart. If not treated quickly, cardiogenic shock can be fatal or lead to organ failure or brain injury.[8]

STREPTOCOCCAL TOXIC SHOCK SYNDROME

Streptococcal toxic shock syndrome (STSS) is a rare but serious bacterial infection. STSS can develop very quickly into low blood pressure, multiple organ failure, and even death.

Bacteria called "group A *Streptococcus*" (group A strep) can cause STSS when they spread into deep tissues and the bloodstream.[9]

Section 31.6 | Syncope

WHAT IS SYNCOPE?

Syncope is used to describe a loss of consciousness for a short period of time. It can happen when there is a sudden change in the blood flow to the brain. Syncope is usually called "fainting" or "passing out."

There are different types of syncope; they depend on the part of the body affected or the cause of blood flow changes. Syncope can also be a symptom of heart disease or other heart problems. It may also show a higher risk for some neurological conditions such as neuropathy.[10]

---

[8] "Cardiogenic Shock," National Heart, Lung, and Blood Institute (NHLBI), March 24, 2022. Available online. URL: www.nhlbi.nih.gov/health/cardiogenic-shock. Accessed May 19, 2023.
[9] "Group A Streptococcal (GAS) Disease," Centers for Disease Control and Prevention (CDC), June 27, 2022. Available online. URL: www.cdc.gov/groupastrep/diseases-public/streptococcal-toxic-shock-syndrome.html. Accessed May 19, 2023.
[10] "Syncope," National Institute of Neurological Disorders and Stroke (NINDS), January 20, 2023. Available online. URL: www.ninds.nih.gov/health-information/disorders/syncope. Accessed May 19, 2023.

WHAT CAUSES SYNCOPE?

Fainting usually happens when your blood pressure drops suddenly, causing a decrease in blood flow to your brain. It is more common in older people. Some causes of fainting include:

- heat or dehydration
- emotional distress
- standing up too quickly
- certain medicines
- drop in blood sugar
- heart problems[11]

SYMPTOMS OF SYNCOPE

The symptoms of syncope that usually happen before someone loses consciousness include the following:

- feeling dizzy
- feeling light-headed
- feeling like they have to vomit
- having an unclear vision or blacking out
- having cold or clammy skin

People who experience syncope may pass out for a minute or two. They will slowly come back to normal. Syncope can happen in healthy people. It affects people of all ages but happens most often in older adults.

The first thing to look for is that the person is still breathing after they faint. The individual should lie down for 10–15 minutes, if they can, in a cool, quiet area. If this is not possible, they should sit up with their head between their knees. Sipping on cold water can also help. People tend to recover within a few minutes to a few hours.

Treatment focuses on finding out the causes and trying to avoid passing out. When you start to feel symptoms, the following are a few things you can do to help prevent fainting:

- Make a fist.
- Cross your legs.

---

[11] MedlinePlus, "Fainting," National Institutes of Health (NIH), August 4, 2016. Available online. URL: https://medlineplus.gov/fainting.html. Accessed May 19, 2023.

- Squeeze your thighs together.
- Tighten the muscles in your arms.

Syncope can be life-threatening if it is not treated the right way.

HOW COULD YOU OR YOUR LOVED ONE HELP IMPROVE CARE FOR PEOPLE WITH SYNCOPE?

Consider participating in a clinical trial, so clinicians and scientists can learn more about syncope and related conditions. Clinical research uses human volunteers to help researchers learn more about a disorder and perhaps find better ways to detect, treat, or prevent disease safely.

All types of volunteers are needed—those who are healthy or may have an illness or disease—of all different ages, sexes, races, and ethnicities to ensure that study results apply to as many people as possible and that treatments will be safe and effective for everyone who will use them.[12]

---

[12] See footnote [10].

Chapter 32 |
Atherosclerosis

Atherosclerosis is a common condition that develops when a sticky substance called "plaque" builds up inside your artery. Disease linked to atherosclerosis is the leading cause of death in the United States. About half of Americans between ages 45 and 84 have atherosclerosis and do not know it.

Atherosclerosis develops slowly as cholesterol, fat, blood cells, and other substances in your blood form plaque. When the plaque builds up, it causes your arteries to narrow (see Figure 32.1). This reduces the supply of oxygen-rich blood to tissues of vital organs in the body.

Atherosclerosis can affect most of the arteries in the body, including arteries in the heart, brain, arms, legs, pelvis, and kidneys. It has different names based on which arteries are affected.

- **Coronary artery disease (CAD)**. CAD is plaque buildup in the arteries of your heart.
- **Peripheral artery disease (PAD)**. PAD most often is plaque buildup in the arteries of the legs, but it can also build up in your arms or pelvis.
- **Carotid artery disease**. This is plaque buildup in the neck arteries. It reduces blood flow to the brain.
- **Renal artery stenosis**. This is plaque buildup in the arteries that supply blood to your kidneys.
- **Vertebral artery disease**. This is atherosclerosis in the arteries that supply blood to the back of the brain. This area of the brain controls body functions that are needed to keep you alive.
- **Mesenteric artery ischemia**. This is plaque buildup in the arteries that supply the intestines with blood.

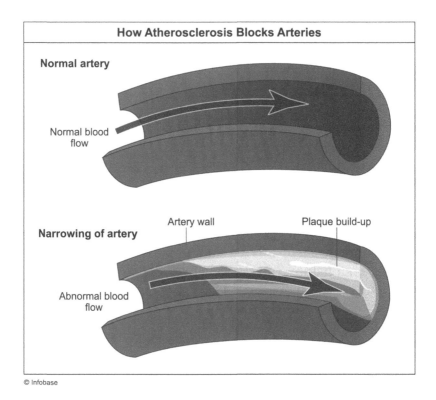

Figure 32.1. How Atherosclerosis Blocks Arteries

Infobase

Reduced blood flow can lead to symptoms such as angina. If a plaque bursts, a blood clot may form that may block the artery completely or travel to other parts of the body. Blockages, either complete or incomplete, can cause complications, including heart attack, stroke, vascular dementia, erectile dysfunction (ED), or limb loss. Atherosclerosis can cause death and disability.

Plaque often starts to build up during childhood and gets worse with age. Risk factors include unhealthy cholesterol levels, unhealthy lifestyle habits, and your gene.

The good news is that most people can prevent or delay the initiation and progression of atherosclerosis by following steps for heart-healthy living.

CAUSES AND RISK FACTORS FOR ATHEROSCLEROSIS

Risk factors are conditions or habits that make a person more likely to develop a disease. Nearly half of Americans have high blood pressure (HBP) or unhealthy cholesterol levels, or they smoke. These are key risk factors that can trigger the start of plaque buildup.

What Causes Atherosclerosis?

Plaque buildup in the arteries starts with damage to the arteries. Risk factors such as unhealthy lifestyle habits, medical conditions, or genes can lead to this damage.

Inflammatory cells travel to the damaged areas of the artery and release chemical signals. The signals cause cholesterol and cell waste to collect at the damaged spots. This buildup attracts white blood cells (WBCs) that eat the cholesterol and clump together, forming plaque. The artery narrows as the plaque grows, reducing the flow of oxygen-rich blood to the limbs and organs. Over time, the plaque can break and flow into the bloodstream. This may lead to the formation of blood clots, which can block blood flow. If this happens, nearby tissue cannot get enough oxygen and may die.

What Raises the Risk of Atherosclerosis?

The risk factors for plaque buildup are often linked. For example, smoking and a lack of regular physical activity raise your risk of unhealthy levels of cholesterol, which can lead to plaque buildup.

Other common risk factors for plaque buildup are listed below.

- **HBP**. Over time, HBP can damage artery walls, allowing plaque to build up.
- **Diabetes**. High blood sugar can damage the inner layers of the arteries, causing plaque buildup.
- **Metabolic syndrome**. High levels of cholesterol and triglycerides in your blood increase your risk.
- **Unhealthy diet**. Eating a lot of foods high in saturated fats can increase your cholesterol levels.
- **Family history**. Your gene may increase your risk, especially if you have a common inherited cholesterol disorder called "familial hypercholesterolemia."

- **Inflammatory diseases**. When you have conditions such as rheumatoid arthritis (RA) and psoriasis, high levels of inflammation can end up irritating your blood vessels, which can lead to plaque buildup.
- **Older age**. For most people, plaque buildup starts in childhood and gets worse as they get older. In men, the risk increases after age 45. In women, the risk increases after age 55. The risk for women is even higher if they have endometriosis or polycystic ovary syndrome (PCOS) or if they have gestational diabetes or preeclampsia during pregnancy.

What Should You Do If You Have Risk Factors?

Talk with your health-care team about your heart health. Together, you can set up a plan to reduce your risk, monitor your health, and manage your risk factors to delay or prevent disease caused by atherosclerosis. Starting treatment early is the key to preventing symptoms.

SYMPTOMS OF ATHEROSCLEROSIS

Early stages of atherosclerosis often do not develop with symptoms. Symptoms may first appear when you are under physical or emotional stress—times when the body needs more oxygen.

Atherosclerosis leads to poor oxygen-rich blood supply, as well as symptoms that can affect your quality of life (QOL). Symptoms depend on which arteries are affected and how much blood flow is blocked.

- Chest pain (angina), cold sweats, dizziness, extreme tiredness, heart palpitations (feeling that your heart is racing), shortness of breath, nausea, and weakness are all symptoms of coronary heart disease.
- Pain, aching, heaviness, and cramping in the legs when walking or climbing stairs are the main symptoms of PAD. The symptoms also go away after rest.
- Problems with thinking and memory, weakness or numbness on one side of the body or face, and vision

trouble are all early symptoms of vertebral artery disease. Transient ischemic attack (TIA), commonly called a "ministroke," is a more serious symptom.

- Severe pain following meals, weight loss, and diarrhea are symptoms of mesenteric artery ischemia of the intestines.
- ED is an early warning sign that a man may be at higher risk for atherosclerosis and its complications. If you have ED, talk with your health-care team about your risk of plaque buildup.

You may not notice other symptoms until plaque buildup causes serious problems. Seeing your doctor regularly is important, as they may be able to find plaque buildup before it gets serious. For example:

- Plaque buildup in the arteries of the neck (carotid artery disease) can cause a bruit. This is a whooshing sound that your doctor hears when using a stethoscope. Severe symptoms of a bruit include a TIA.
- Using a stethoscope, doctors may hear a bruit in your belly, which is an early sign of plaque buildup in the arteries that deliver blood to the kidneys (renal artery stenosis). As the disease worsens, it can cause HBP, extreme tiredness, loss of appetite, nausea (feeling sick to the stomach), swelling in the hands or feet, and itchiness or numbness.

Talk to your doctor about your symptoms and whether you have risk factors for atherosclerosis.

DIAGNOSIS OF ATHEROSCLEROSIS

To diagnose atherosclerosis, your doctor will check the results of blood tests, imaging procedures, and other tests and also ask about your medical and family history. A physical exam helps detect symptoms.

Screening Tests

Beginning at age 20, your doctor will regularly check to see if you have risk factors for plaque buildup in the arteries. Your doctor may do the following:

- Check your blood pressure.
- Calculate your body mass index and measure your waist to see whether you have an unhealthy weight.
- Order blood tests to see whether you have unhealthy blood cholesterol or triglycerides levels or diabetes.

Estimating Your Risk

Talk with your health-care provider about risk factors:

- lifestyle habits, such as smoking or vaping, physical activity, and eating habits
- your personal health history of medical conditions that may affect your risk, including diabetes and inflammatory conditions, such as RA and psoriasis
- your family history if you have blood relatives who had heart attacks or died suddenly before they were 55 years old

A risk estimator app can help assess the risk that you will have a major complication, such as a heart attack, from atherosclerosis. The app estimates your risk over the next 10 years or throughout your lifetime based on your data. If you have all the information, you can use the app yourself. The app shows risk levels as low, borderline, intermediate, or high.

Diagnostic Tests

To diagnose atherosclerosis, your doctor may order tests. Your doctor may recommend tests even if you do not have symptoms. The type of test depends on which arteries are affected by plaque buildup.

BLOOD TESTS

Blood tests check the levels of cholesterol, triglyceride, blood sugar, lipoproteins, or proteins that are signs of inflammation, such as C-reactive protein.

ELECTROCARDIOGRAM

An electrocardiogram ("ECG" or "EKG") is a simple, painless test that detects and records your heart's electrical activity. An EKG can show how fast your heart is beating, whether the rhythm of your heartbeats is steady or irregular, and the strength and timing of the electrical impulses passing through each part of your heart. You may have an EKG as part of a routine exam to screen for heart disease.

An EKG may be recorded in a doctor's office, in an outpatient facility, in a hospital before major surgery, or as part of stress testing. For the test, you will lie still on a table. A nurse or technician will attach up to 12 electrodes to the skin on your chest, arms, and legs. Your skin may need to be shaved to help the electrodes stick. The electrodes are connected by wires to a machine that records your heart's electrical activity on graph paper or on a computer. After the test, the electrodes will be removed.

An EKG has no serious risks. EKGs do not give off electrical charges such as shocks. You may develop a slight rash where the electrodes are attached to your skin. This rash usually goes away on its own without treatment.

HEART IMAGING TESTS

Your doctor may order a heart imaging test to take pictures of your heart and find problems in blood flow in the heart or coronary arteries.

Examples of heart imaging tests used to diagnose atherosclerosis are as follows:

- **Angiography**. This is a special type of x-ray using a dye. This procedure can be used to check the arteries in the heart, neck, brain, or other areas of the body.
- **Cardiac magnetic resonance imaging (MRI)**. This MRI detects tissue damage or problems with blood flow in the heart or coronary arteries. Cardiac MRI can help explain results from other imaging tests such as chest x-rays and computed tomography (CT) scans.
- **Cardiac positron emission tomography (PET) scanning**. PET scan assesses blood flow through the small blood vessels of the heart. This is a type

of nuclear heart scan that can diagnose coronary microvascular disease.

- **Coronary CT angiography**. This shows the insides of your coronary arteries rather than an invasive cardiac catheterization. It is a noninvasive imaging test using CT scanning.

CORONARY CALCIUM SCAN

A coronary calcium scan is a CT scan of your heart that measures the amount of calcium in the walls of your coronary arteries. The buildup of calcium, or calcifications, is a sign of atherosclerosis or coronary heart disease.

A coronary calcium scan may be done in a medical imaging facility or hospital. The test does not use contrast dye and will take about 10–15 minutes to complete. A coronary calcium scan uses a special scanner such as an electron beam CT or a multidetector CT (MDCT) machine. An MDCT machine is a much faster CT scanner that makes high-quality pictures of the beating heart. A coronary calcium scan will determine an Agatston score that reflects the amount of calcium found in your coronary arteries. A score of zero is normal. In general, the higher your score, the more likely you are to have heart disease. If your score is high, your doctor may recommend more tests.

A coronary calcium scan has few risks. There is a slight risk of cancer, particularly in people younger than 40 years old. However, the amount of radiation from one test is similar to the amount of radiation you are naturally exposed to over one year. Talk to your doctor and the technicians performing the test about whether you are or could be pregnant.

STRESS TESTS

A stress test measures how healthy your heart is and how well it works during physical stress. Some heart problems are easier to identify when your heart is working hard to pump blood throughout your body, such as when you exercise.

You may do a stress test in your doctor's office or a hospital. The test usually involves physical exercise such as walking on a treadmill or riding a stationary bicycle. If you are not able to exercise, your doctor will give you medicine that will make your heart work hard and beat faster, as if you were exercising. Your doctor may ask you not to take some of your prescription medicines or to avoid coffee, tea, or any drinks with caffeine on the day of your test because these may affect your results. Your doctor will ask you to wear comfortable clothes and shoes for the test.

ANKLE-BRACHIAL INDEX TEST
Ankle-brachial index (ABI) tests are used to diagnose PAD. This painless test compares the blood pressures in your ankle and your arm using a blood pressure cuff and ultrasound device.

TREATMENT FOR ATHEROSCLEROSIS
If you have a diagnosis of atherosclerosis, work with your healthcare team to set up a treatment plan that works for you based on your lifestyle, your home and neighborhood environment, and your culture. Your 10-year or lifetime risk assessment is a good way to start the conversation.

Heart-Healthy Lifestyle Changes
Heart-healthy living is very important for preventing and treating atherosclerotic plaque buildup throughout your lifetime.
Steps for a healthy lifestyle include the following:
- **Choose heart-healthy foods**. An eating plan such as the Dietary Approaches to Stop Hypertension (DASH) can be chosen for healthy living. A heart-healthy eating plan includes fruits, vegetables, and whole grains and limits saturated fats, sodium (salt), and added sugars.
- **Be physically active**. Routine physical activity can help manage risk factors such as high blood cholesterol, HBP, overweight, and obesity. Adults should engage in a total of 150 minutes or more per week of moderate

physical activity or 75 minutes per week of vigorous physical activity. Before starting any exercise program, ask your doctor what level of physical activity is right for you.

- **Aim for a healthy weight**. Losing just 3–5 percent of your current weight can help you manage some coronary heart disease risk factors, such as high blood cholesterol and diabetes. Greater amounts of weight loss can also improve blood pressure readings.

- **Limit how much alcohol you drink**. Drinking less is better for health than drinking more. Men should limit their intake to two drinks or less in a day. Women should drink one drink or less per day.

- **Manage stress**. Learning how to manage stress, relax, and cope with problems can improve your emotional and physical health.

- **Quit smoking and avoid secondhand smoke**. Visit the Smoking and Your Heart web page (www.nhlbi. nih.gov/health/heart/smoking/effects) and the Your Guide to a Healthy Heart web page (www.nhlbi.nih. gov/health-topics/all-publications-and-resources/your-guide-healthy-heart). Although these resources focus on heart health, they include basic information about how to quit smoking. For free help and support to quit smoking, you can call the National Cancer Institute's Smoking Quitline at 877-44U-QUIT (877-448-7848). Talk to your doctor if you vape. There is scientific evidence that nicotine and flavorings found in vaping products may damage your heart and lungs.

- **Get enough good-quality sleep**. The recommended amount for adults is 7–9 hours of sleep a day.

Medicines

Medicines can help manage risk factors and treat atherosclerosis or its complications. Your doctor may also prescribe medicines to treat other medical conditions, such as HBP, that can worsen plaque buildup.

Atherosclerosis

Medicines often used to treat atherosclerosis or related conditions are as follows:

- Angiotensin-converting enzyme (ACE) inhibitors and beta-blockers help lower blood pressure and lower the heart's workload.
- Antiplatelet or anticlotting medicines may help reduce the risk of complications for some people who have atherosclerosis. Aspirin is not recommended for most people.
- Calcium channel blockers lower blood pressure by relaxing blood vessels.
- Medicines to control blood sugar, such as empagliflozin, canagliflozin, and liraglutide, help lower your risk for complications if you have atherosclerosis and diabetes.
- Metformin helps control plaque buildup if you have diabetes.
- Nitrates, such as nitroglycerin, dilate your coronary arteries and relieve or prevent chest pain from angina.
- Ranolazine treats coronary microvascular disease and the chest pain it may cause.
- Statins treat unhealthy blood cholesterol levels. Your doctor may recommend a statin if you have a higher risk for coronary heart disease or stroke or if you have diabetes and are between the ages of 40 and 75.
- Other cholesterol-lowering medicines, such as ezetimibe, PCSK9 inhibitor, bempedoic acid, and omega-3 fatty acids, may be used if you are unable to take statins or when statins have not worked to treat unhealthy blood cholesterol and triglyceride levels.
- Thrombolytic medicines, sometimes called "clot busters," may be used to treat blood clots resulting from atherosclerosis. These medicines can dissolve blood clots that block arteries, causing a stroke, heart attack, mesenteric ischemia or other problems. Ideally, the medicine should be given as soon as possible.

Complementary and Alternative Treatments

Some dietary supplements and foods have shown signs in studies that they may help manage atherosclerosis risk factors. Talk with your doctor about the possible benefits of nutritional supplements and particular foods. Be sure to discuss any nutritional supplements you are already taking. Some may interfere with other treatments or cause side effects.

Procedures or Surgeries

You may need a procedure, heart surgery, or other types of surgery to treat disease resulting from plaque buildup. The type of procedure or surgery depends on the arteries affected.

- **Percutaneous coronary intervention (PCI)**. PCI opens coronary arteries that are narrowed or blocked by the buildup of plaque. A small mesh tube called a "stent" is usually implanted after PCI to prevent the artery from narrowing again.

- **Coronary artery bypass grafting (CABG)**. CABG improves blood flow to the heart by using normal arteries from the chest wall or veins from the legs to bypass the blocked arteries. Surgeons typically use CABG to treat people who have severe plaque buildup in arteries in the heart. Bypass grafting can also treat arteries in other parts of the body, such as the arteries leading to the intestines.

- **Transmyocardial laser revascularization or coronary endarterectomy**. This treats severe angina associated with coronary heart disease when other treatments are too risky or do not work.

- **Carotid endarterectomy**. This treats carotid artery disease. Other treatment options for this disease may include angioplasty and carotid artery stenting.

- **Weight loss surgery**. This may help reduce inflammation leading to plaque buildup in people who have severe obesity.

- **Angioplasty**. This opens narrowed or blocked arteries. Doctors may use angioplasty to treat PAD affecting the legs, in the arteries of the heart to treat coronary heart disease, or in the neck to treat carotid artery disease. Your doctor may inflate a small balloon in the artery to help flatten the plaque. Sometimes, the balloon is coated with medicine to help the artery heal. Your doctor may also insert a small mesh tube called a "stent" to reduce the chances of the artery narrowing again.

What Other Therapies Might Help?

- To help relieve symptoms of PAD, your doctor will recommend a supervised exercise program in a clinic or a home-based exercise program. Most home programs include health coaching, activity monitors, or regular check-ins with a coach by telephone. Talk with your doctor regularly about your progress.
- If you have had a complication from atherosclerosis, your doctor may recommend a cardiac rehabilitation program.
- Behavioral therapy or coaching support helps many people stick with heart-healthy lifestyle changes. Counseling may also improve people's QOL after they have had a complication.

PREVENTION OF ATHEROSCLEROSIS

Taking action to control your risk factors can help prevent or slow down plaque buildup. If lifestyle changes are not enough, your doctor may prescribe medicine to control your atherosclerosis risk factors. Take all of your medicines as your doctor advises.[1]

---

[1] "What Is Atherosclerosis?" National Heart, Lung, and Blood Institute (NHLBI), March 24, 2022. Available online. URL: www.nhlbi.nih.gov/health/atherosclerosis. Accessed May 25, 2023.

Chapter 33 | Coronary Artery and Heart Disease

Chapter Contents

Section 33.1 | **Coronary Artery Disease**

WHAT IS CORONARY ARTERY DISEASE?

Coronary artery disease (CAD) is the most common type of heart disease. It is the leading cause of death in the United States in both men and women.

CAD happens when the arteries that supply blood to the heart muscle become hardened and narrowed. This is due to the buildup of cholesterol and other material, called "plaque," on their inner walls. This buildup is called "atherosclerosis." As it grows, less blood can flow through the arteries. As a result, the heart muscle cannot get the blood or oxygen it needs. This can lead to chest pain (angina) or a heart attack. Most heart attacks happen when a blood clot suddenly cuts off the heart's blood supply, causing permanent heart damage.

Over time, CAD can also weaken the heart muscle and contribute to heart failure and arrhythmias. Heart failure means that the heart cannot pump blood well to the rest of the body. Arrhythmias are changes in the normal beating rhythm of the heart.[1]

WHAT CAUSES CORONARY ARTERY DISEASE?

Coronary artery disease is caused by plaque buildup in the walls of the arteries that supply blood to the heart (called "coronary arteries") and other parts of the body.

Plaque is made up of deposits of cholesterol and other substances in the artery. Plaque buildup causes the inside of the arteries to narrow over time, which can partially or totally block the blood flow. This process is called "atherosclerosis."

WHAT ARE THE RISK FACTORS FOR CORONARY ARTERY DISEASE?

Being overweight, physical inactivity, unhealthy eating, and smoking tobacco are risk factors for CAD. A family history of heart disease also increases your risk for CAD, especially a family history of having heart disease at an early age (50 or younger).

---

[1] MedlinePlus, "Coronary Artery Disease," National Institutes of Health (NIH), November 1, 2016. Available online. URL: https://medlineplus.gov/coronaryarterydisease.html#top. Accessed June 7, 2023.

To find out your risk for CAD, your health-care team may measure your blood pressure, blood cholesterol, and blood sugar levels.

WHAT ARE THE SYMPTOMS OF CORONARY ARTERY DISEASE?

Angina, or chest pain and discomfort, is the most common symptom of CAD. Angina can happen when too much plaque builds up inside arteries, causing them to narrow. Narrowed arteries can cause chest pain because they can block blood flow to your heart muscle and the rest of your body.

For many people, the first clue that they have CAD is a heart attack. Symptoms of a heart attack include:

- chest pain or discomfort (angina)
- weakness, light-headedness, nausea (feeling sick to your stomach), or a cold sweat
- pain or discomfort in the arms or shoulder
- shortness of breath

Over time, CAD can weaken the heart muscle. This may lead to heart failure, a serious condition where the heart cannot pump blood the way it should.

HOW IS CORONARY ARTERY DISEASE DIAGNOSED?

If you are at high risk for heart disease or already have symptoms, your doctor can use several tests to diagnose CAD, including the following:

- **Electrocardiogram (ECG or EKG)**. ECG measures the electrical activity, rate, and regularity of your heartbeat.
- **Echocardiogram**. It uses ultrasound (a special sound wave) to create a picture of the heart.
- **Exercise stress test**. This test measures your heart rate while you walk on a treadmill. This helps determine how well your heart is working when it has to pump more blood.
- **Chest x-ray**. It uses x-rays to create a picture of the heart, lungs, and other organs in the chest.
- **Cardiac catheterization**. This checks the inside of your arteries for blockage by inserting a thin, flexible tube through an artery in the groin, arm, or neck to

reach the heart. (Health-care professionals can measure blood pressure within the heart and the strength of blood flow through the heart's chambers as well as collect blood samples from the heart or inject dye into the arteries of the heart (coronary arteries).)

- **Coronary angiogram**. This monitors blockage and flow of blood through the coronary arteries and uses x-rays to detect dye injected via cardiac catheterization.
- **Coronary artery calcium scan**. A computed tomography (CT) scan looks into the coronary arteries for calcium buildup and plaque.

WHAT IS CARDIAC REHABILITATION AND RECOVERY?

Cardiac rehabilitation (rehab) is an important program for anyone recovering from a heart attack, heart failure, or other heart problems that require surgery or medical care. In these people, cardiac rehab can help improve their quality of life and can help prevent another cardiac event. Cardiac rehab is a supervised program that includes:

- physical activity
- education about healthy living, including healthy eating; taking medications as prescribed; and ways to quit smoking
- counseling to find ways to relieve stress and improve mental health

A team of people may help you through cardiac rehab, including your health-care team, exercise and nutrition specialists, physical therapists, and counselors or mental health professionals.

HOW CAN YOU BE HEALTHIER IF YOU HAVE CORONARY ARTERY DISEASE?

If you have CAD, your health-care team may suggest the following steps to help lower your risk for heart attack or worsening heart disease:

- lifestyle changes, such as eating a healthier (lower sodium or lower fat) diet, increasing physical activity, reaching a healthy weight, and quitting smoking

- medicines to treat risk factors for CAD, such as high cholesterol, high blood pressure, or an irregular heartbeat
- surgical procedures to help restore blood flow to the heart[2]

Section 33.2 | Angina

WHAT IS ANGINA?

Angina can be a warning sign that you are at increased risk of a heart attack. If you have chest pain that does not go away, call 911 immediately.

Angina is chest pain or discomfort that occurs if an area of your heart muscle does not get enough oxygen-rich blood. It is a common symptom of coronary heart disease (CHD), which limits or cuts off blood flow to the heart.

There are several types of angina, and the symptoms depend on which type you have. Angina chest pain, called an "angina event," can happen when your heart is working hard. It can go away when you stop to rest again, or it can happen at rest. This pain can feel like pressure or squeezing in your chest. It can also spread to your shoulders, arms, neck, jaw, or back, just like a heart attack. Angina pain can even feel like an upset stomach. Symptoms can be different for women and men.

To diagnose angina, your doctor will ask you about your signs and symptoms and may run blood tests, take an x-ray, or order tests, such as an electrocardiogram (EKG), an exercise stress test, or cardiac catheterization, to determine how well your heart is working. With some types of angina, you may need emergency medical treatment to try to prevent a heart attack. To control your condition, your doctor may recommend heart-healthy lifestyle changes, medicines, medical procedures, and cardiac rehabilitation.

---

[2] "Coronary Artery Disease," Centers for Disease Control and Prevention (CDC), July 19, 2021. Available online. URL: www.cdc.gov/heartdisease/coronary_ad.htm. Accessed May 19, 2023.

TYPES OF ANGINA

The types of angina are stable, unstable, microvascular, and variant. The types vary based on their severity or cause.

Stable Angina

Stable angina follows a pattern that has been consistent for at least two months. That means the following factors have not changed:

- how long your angina events last
- how often your angina events occur
- how well angina responds to rest or medicines
- the causes or triggers of your angina

If you have stable angina, you can learn its pattern and predict when an event will occur, such as during physical exertion or mental stress. The pain usually goes away a few minutes after you rest or take your angina medicine. If the condition causing your angina gets worse, stable angina can become unstable angina.

Unstable Angina

Unstable angina does not follow a pattern. It may be new or occur more often and be more severe than stable angina. Unstable angina can also occur with or without physical exertion. Rest or medicine may not relieve the pain.

Unstable angina is a medical emergency since it can progress to a heart attack. Medical attention may be needed right away to restore blood flow to the heart muscle.

Microvascular Angina

Microvascular angina is a sign of CHD affecting the tiny arteries of the heart. Microvascular angina events can be stable or unstable. They can be more painful and last longer than other types of angina, and symptoms can occur during exercise or at rest. Medicine may not relieve symptoms of this type of angina.

Variant Angina

Variant angina, also known as "Prinzmetal's angina," is rare. It occurs when a spasm—a sudden tightening of the muscles within the arteries of your heart—causes angina rather than a blockage. This type of angina usually occurs while you are at rest, and the pain can be severe. It usually happens between midnight and early morning and in a pattern. Medicine can ease symptoms of variant angina.

CAUSES OF ANGINA

Angina happens when your heart muscle does not get enough oxygen-rich blood. Medical conditions, particularly heart disease, or lifestyle habits can cause angina. Understanding the causes of angina helps understand how the heart works.

Coronary Heart Disease

The following are the two types of coronary heart disease that can cause angina:

- **Coronary artery disease (CAD)**. It happens when plaque builds up inside the large arteries that supply blood to the heart. This is called "atherosclerosis." Plaque narrows or blocks the arteries, reducing blood flow to the heart muscle. Sometimes, plaque breaks open and causes blood clots to form. Blood clots can partially or totally block the coronary arteries.
- **Coronary microvascular disease (CMVD)**. It affects the tiny arteries that branch off the larger coronary arteries. Reduced blood flow in these arteries causes microvascular angina. The arteries may be damaged and unable to expand as usual when the heart needs more oxygen-rich blood.

RISKS OF ANGINA

You may have an increased risk for angina because of your age, environment or occupation, family history and genetics, lifestyle, other medical conditions, race, or sex. When speaking with your doctor about potential symptoms, be sure to talk about risk factors. This will help your health-care provider diagnose the condition and prepare a treatment plan specific to your needs.

Age

Genetic or lifestyle factors can cause plaque to build up in your arteries as you age. This means that your risk for coronary heart disease and angina increases as you get older.

Variant angina is rare, but people who have variant angina often are younger than those who have other types of angina.

Environment or Occupation

Angina may be linked to a type of air pollution called "particle pollution." Particle pollution can include dust from roads, farms, dry riverbeds, construction sites, and mines.

Your work life can increase your risk of angina. Examples include work that limits your time available for sleep, involves high stress, requires long periods of sitting or standing, is noisy, or exposes you to potential hazards such as radiation.

Family History and Genetics

CHD often runs in families. Also, people who have no lifestyle-related risk factors can develop heart disease. These factors suggest that genes are involved in CHD and can influence a person's risk of developing angina.

Variant angina has also been linked to specific DNA changes.

Lifestyle Habits

The more heart disease risk factors you have, the greater your risk of developing angina. The main lifestyle risk factors for angina include:

- alcohol use, for variant angina
- illegal drug use, which can cause your heart to race or damage your blood vessels
- lack of physical activity
- smoking tobacco or long-term exposure to secondhand smoke
- stress
- unhealthy eating patterns

Other Medical Conditions

Medical conditions in which your heart needs more oxygen-rich blood than your body can supply increase your risk for angina. They include:

- anemia
- cardiomyopathy, or disease of the heart muscle
- heart problems, such as heart failure, heart valve diseases, or high blood pressure
- inflammation
- metabolic syndrome

Medical Procedures

Heart procedures such as stent placement, percutaneous coronary intervention (PCI), or coronary artery bypass grafting (CABG) can trigger coronary spasms and angina. Although rare, noncardiac surgery can also trigger unstable angina or variant angina.

Race or Ethnicity

Some groups of people are at higher risk for developing coronary heart disease and one of its main symptoms, angina. African Americans who have already had a heart attack are more likely than Whites to develop angina.

Variant angina is more common among people living in Japan, especially men, than among people living in Western countries.

Sex

Angina affects both men and women but at different ages based on men's and women's risk of developing coronary heart disease. In men, heart disease risk starts to increase at age 45. Before age 55, women have a lower risk for heart disease than men. After age 55, the risk rises in both women and men. Women who have already had a heart attack are more likely to develop angina compared with men.

Microvascular angina most often begins in women around the time of menopause.

DIAGNOSIS OF ANGINA

Your doctor may diagnose angina based on your medical history, a physical exam, and diagnostic tests and procedures. These tests can help assess whether you need immediate treatment for a heart attack.

Diagnostic Tests and Procedures

Your doctor may have you undergo some of the following tests and procedures:

- **Blood tests**. These tests check the level of cardiac troponins. Troponin levels can help doctors tell unstable angina from heart attacks. Your doctor may also check levels of certain fats, cholesterol, sugar, and proteins in your blood.
- **Chest x-ray**. It looks for lung disorders and other causes of chest pain not related to heart disease. A chest x-ray alone is not enough to diagnose angina or heart disease, but it can help rule out other causes.
- **Computed tomography angiography**. This test looks at blood flow through the coronary arteries. This test can rapidly diagnose heart disease as the source of your chest pain and help your doctor decide whether a procedure to improve blood flow will benefit your future health.
- **Coronary angiography with cardiac catheterization**. This angiography can help determine whether coronary heart disease is the cause of your chest pain. This test lets your doctor study the flow of blood through your heart and blood vessels to confirm whether plaque buildup is the problem. The results of the scan can also help your doctor assess whether unstable angina might be relieved by surgery or other procedures.
- **Echocardiogram**. This test assesses the strength of your heart beating. It helps the doctor determine your risk of future heart problems.
- **Electrocardiogram (EKG)**. EKG checks for the possibility of a heart attack. Certain EKG patterns are

associated with variant angina and unstable angina. These patterns may indicate serious heart disease or prior heart damage as a cause of angina. However, some people who have angina have normal EKGs.

- **Hyperventilation test**. This test can help diagnose variant angina. Rapid breathing under controlled conditions with careful medical monitoring may bring on EKG changes that help your doctor diagnose variant angina.

- **Magnetic resonance imaging or other noninvasive tests**. These tests check for problems with the heart's movement or with blood flow in the heart's small blood vessels.

- **Provocation tests**. These tests can help diagnose variant angina. Your doctor may give you a medicine such as acetylcholine during coronary angiography to see if the coronary arteries start to spasm.

- **Stress test**. This assesses how well your heart works during exercise. A stress test can show possible symptoms of CHD causing your angina. Stress testing in the early morning can help diagnose variant angina. Stress echocardiography tests can help your doctor diagnose the cause of your angina.

Typically, doctors screen for angina only when you have symptoms. However, your doctor may assess your risk factors for heart disease every few years as part of your regular office visits. If you have two or more risk factors, then your doctor may estimate the chance that you will develop CHD, which may include angina, over the next 10 years.

TREATMENT FOR ANGINA

Your doctor will decide on a treatment approach based on the type of angina you have, your symptoms, test results, and risk of complications. Unstable angina is a medical emergency that requires immediate treatment in a hospital. If your angina is stable and your symptoms are not getting worse, you may be able to control your angina with heart-healthy lifestyle changes and medicines. If lifestyle changes and medicines cannot control your angina, you may need a medical procedure to improve blood flow and relieve your angina.

HOW CAN YOU PREVENT ANGINA?

To prevent angina, your doctor may recommend that you adopt heart-healthy lifestyle changes to lower your risk of heart disease, the most common cause of angina. Heart-healthy lifestyle changes include choosing a heart-healthy eating pattern such as the DASH eating plan, being physically active, aiming for a healthy weight, quitting smoking, and managing stress. You should also avoid using illegal drugs.[3]

Section 33.3 | Heart Attack

WHAT IS A HEART ATTACK?

A heart attack is a life-threatening medical emergency that requires immediate treatment.

A heart attack, also known as a "myocardial infarction," happens when the flow of blood that brings oxygen to a part of your heart muscle suddenly becomes blocked. Your heart cannot get enough oxygen. If blood flow is not restored quickly, the heart muscle will begin to die.

Heart attacks are very common. According to the Centers for Disease Control and Prevention (CDC), more than 800,000 people in the United States have a heart attack each year.

A heart attack is not the same as cardiac arrest, which happens when your heart suddenly and unexpectedly stops beating. A heart attack can cause sudden cardiac arrest (SCA).

---

[3] "Angina (Chest Pain)," National Heart, Lung, and Blood Institute (NHLBI), March 24, 2022. Available online. URL: www.nhlbi.nih.gov/health/angina. Accessed May 18, 2023.

Many people survive and live active, full lives after a heart attack. Getting help and treatment quickly can limit the damage to your heart.

CAUSES OF HEART ATTACK

The most common cause of a heart attack is coronary artery disease (CAD), which is the most common type of heart disease. This is when your coronary arteries cannot carry enough oxygen-rich blood to your heart muscle. Most of the time, CAD happens when a waxy substance called "plaque" builds up inside your arteries, causing the arteries to narrow. The buildup of this plaque is called "atherosclerosis." This can happen over many years, and it can block blood flow to parts of your heart muscle. Plaques that narrow arteries slowly over time cause angina.

Eventually, an area of plaque can break open inside your artery. This causes blood clots to form on the plaque's surface. If the clot becomes large enough, it can block blood flow to your heart. If the blockage is not treated quickly, a part of your heart muscle begins to die.

Other Causes of a Heart Attack

Not all heart attacks are caused by blockages from atherosclerosis. When other heart and blood vessel conditions cause a heart attack, it is called "myocardial infarction in the absence of obstructive coronary artery disease" (MINOCA). MINOCA is more common in women, younger people, and racial and ethnic minorities, including Black, Hispanic/Latino, and Asian people.

Conditions that can cause MINOCA have different effects on the heart.

- Small plaques in your arteries may not block your blood vessels, but they can break open or their outer layer can wear away. This can cause blood clots to form on these plaques. The blood clots can then block blood flow through your coronary arteries. The formation of small plaques is more common in women, people who smoke, and people who have other blood vessel conditions.

- A sudden and serious spasm (tightening) of your coronary artery can block blood flow through your artery, even if there is not a buildup of plaque. Smoking is a risk factor for coronary spasms. If you smoke, you may be more likely to have a spasm triggered by extreme cold or very stressful situations. Drugs like cocaine may also cause coronary spasm.
- A coronary artery embolism occurs when a blood clot travels through your bloodstream and gets stuck in your coronary artery. This can block blood flow through your artery. This is more common in people who have atrial fibrillation or conditions that raise the risk of blood clots, such as thrombocytopenia or pregnancy.
- Spontaneous coronary artery dissection (SCAD) occurs when a tear forms inside your coronary artery. A blood clot can then form at the tear, or the torn tissue itself can block your artery. SCAD can be caused by stress, extreme physical activity, and pregnancy. This condition is more common in women who are under 50 years old or pregnant and in people who have Marfan syndrome (MFS).

Other conditions may cause symptoms similar to a heart attack. Your doctor will look at all of your test results to rule them out.

Heart Attacks in Women
The causes, risk factors, and symptoms of a heart attack can be different in women compared with men.

CAUSES AND RISK FACTORS
Risk factors such as age, lifestyle habits, and other health conditions affect men and women differently.
- Women may get heart attacks at older ages than men.
- Smoking, high blood pressure (HBP), high blood cholesterol, high blood sugar, obesity, and stress raise the risk of a heart attack more in women than in men.

- Women are more likely than men to have heart attacks that are not caused by CAD. This can make it more difficult for health-care providers to diagnose heart attacks in women.
- Women have more health problems after having a heart attack than men.

SYMPTOMS OF A HEART ATTACK IN WOMEN

Both women and men who have a heart attack often have chest pain. However, in addition to chest pain, women are more likely to have these symptoms:

- pain in the shoulder, back, or arm
- shortness of breath
- unusual tiredness and weakness
- upset stomach
- anxiety

These symptoms can happen together with chest pain or without any chest pain.

Many women may not recognize that these are symptoms of a heart attack. Women may not get emergency treatment right away if they downplay their symptoms and delay going to the hospital or if the usual initial screening tests performed at the hospital may not detect an early or atypical heart attack. Because of this, women have a higher risk of serious health problems after a heart attack.

It is important to call 911 if you have these symptoms. Early treatment can limit damage to your heart and can save your life.

PREGNANCY AND HEART ATTACKS

Heart attacks are not common among pregnant women, but they are possible both during and soon after delivery. Normal changes to your body during pregnancy can raise your risk of a heart attack. Your age, lifestyle habits, and other health conditions, such as bleeding disorders, obesity, preeclampsia (HBP during pregnancy), and diabetes, can also raise your risk.

If you already have CAD, being pregnant can raise your risk of a heart attack. CAD is a major cause of heart attacks during pregnancy. Ask your doctor whether it is safe for you to get pregnant and what steps you need to take to keep your heart healthy during your pregnancy.

Heart attacks caused by SCAD, a coronary artery embolus, or a coronary artery spasm are more common in pregnant women than in people who are not pregnant.

If you have symptoms of a heart attack during your pregnancy or at any time, call 911 right away. Your health-care team will take steps to protect your baby during these tests. Your health-care team will also make sure that any treatment you take for a heart attack is safe to use during pregnancy.

RISK FACTORS OF HEART ATTACK

Certain risk factors make it more likely that you will develop CAD and have a heart attack.

Risk Factors You Can Control

- lifestyle habits, such as:
  - an unhealthy diet, including eating too many foods high in saturated fat or sodium
  - lack of regular physical activity
  - smoking
- other medical conditions, such as:
  - high blood cholesterol
  - HBP or preeclampsia (HBP during pregnancy)
  - high blood sugar or diabetes
  - high blood triglycerides
  - overweight and obesity

If you have three or more of these conditions that raise your risk for heart disease, it is called "metabolic syndrome." This greatly increases your risk of a heart attack.

Risk Factors You Cannot Control

- **Age**. The risk of heart disease increases for men after age 45 and for women after age 55 (or after menopause).
- **Family history of early heart disease**. You have a higher risk if your father or brother was diagnosed with coronary artery disease before 55 years of age or if your mother or sister was diagnosed with coronary artery disease before 65 years of age.
- **Infections**. People infected by bacteria and viruses are at risk of developing heart disease.

SYMPTOMS OF HEART ATTACK

Not all heart attacks begin with the sudden and crushing chest pain that comes when the blood flow to the heart gets blocked. Heart attack symptoms can start slowly and can be mild or more serious and sudden. Symptoms may also come and go over several hours. The symptoms of a heart attack can be different from person to person and different between men and women. If you have already had a heart attack, your symptoms may not be the same for another one.

If you are having a heart attack, you may experience one or more of the symptoms below.

- chest pain, heaviness, or discomfort in the center or left side of the chest (which is the most common symptom)
- pain or discomfort in one or both arms, your back, shoulders, neck, jaw, or above your belly button
- shortness of breath when resting or doing a little bit of physical activity (which is more common in older adults)
- sweating a lot for no reason
- feeling unusually tired for no reason, sometimes for days (which is more common in women)
- nausea (feeling sick to the stomach) and vomiting
- light-headedness or sudden dizziness
- rapid or irregular heartbeat

It is also possible to have mild symptoms or even no symptoms at all and still have a heart attack.

When to Call 911

Any time you think you might be having a heart attack, do not ignore it. Call 911 for emergency medical care, even if you are not sure that you are having a heart attack.

- Acting fast can limit damage to your heart and save your life. The 911 operator or emergency medical services (EMS) personnel can give you advice that can help prevent damage to your heart.
- An ambulance is the best and safest way to get to the hospital. Do not drive to the hospital or let someone else drive you. EMS personnel can check how you are doing and start tests and lifesaving medicines right away. People who arrive by ambulance often get faster treatment at the hospital.

Every minute matters. Never delay calling 911, taking aspirin, or doing anything else you think might help.

Knowing the difference between stable angina (chest pain in people who have coronary artery disease) and a heart attack is important.

- The pain from angina usually happens after physical activity and goes away in a few minutes when you rest or take medicine to treat it.
- The pain from a heart attack is more serious than the pain from angina. Heart attack pain does not go away when you rest or take medicine.

DIAGNOSIS OF HEART ATTACK

Once at the hospital, you will likely get tests to see whether you are having a heart attack or whether you have already had one.

An electrocardiogram (EKG) is the most common initial test and may be given within minutes of your arrival at the hospital. An EKG will check whether you may be having a heart attack.

Based on the results of the EKG, your doctor may then order more tests, ask you about your medical history, and do a physical exam.

Blood Tests

During a heart attack, heart muscle cells die and release proteins into your bloodstream. Blood tests can measure the amount of these proteins in your blood. For example, you may get a troponin test to measure the amount of a protein called "troponin" in your blood. Troponin leaks when heart muscle cells die during a heart attack.

Blood tests often are repeated to check for changes over time.

Heart Imaging Tests

Imaging tests, such as a chest x-ray or computed tomography (CT), help your doctor check whether your heart is working properly. You may also need a stress test, which can help your doctor determine the amount of damage to your heart or if the cause of the heart attack is CAD.

TREATMENT FOR HEART ATTACK

Your doctor or emergency medical personnel may start treatment even before they confirm that you are having a heart attack. Early treatment to remove the blood clot or plaque can prevent or limit damage to your heart, help your heart work better, and save your life.

STEPS TO PREVENT ANOTHER HEART ATTACK

Once you have had a heart attack, you have a higher risk of another one. Your doctor may prescribe medicines or talk to you about steps you can take, including heart-healthy lifestyle changes.

Medicines

- **Angiotensin-converting enzyme (ACE) inhibitors**. These medicines lower your blood pressure and make it easier for your heart to pump blood. Side effects may include pain in your stomach area and swelling in your face and neck.
- **Anticlotting medicines**. Medicines such as aspirin and clopidogrel stop platelets from clumping together to form blood clots.

- **Anticoagulants, or blood thinners**. These medicines help prevent blood clots from forming in your blood vessels. These medicines also keep existing clots from getting larger. Both anticlotting medicines and anticoagulants can cause bleeding problems.
- **Beta-blockers**. They make it easier for your heart to pump blood. These medicines are also used to treat irregular heartbeats and chest pain and discomfort. Side effects include an irregular heartbeat and worsening heart failure.
- **Statins**. These medicines control or lower your blood cholesterol. Serious side effects include muscle pain and muscle damage.

Take all your medicines as instructed by your doctor. Do not change the amount of your medicine or skip a dose unless your doctor tells you to. If you find it hard to get your medicines or complete your cardiac rehabilitation program, talk to your doctor.

The symptoms of a second heart attack may not be the same as those of your first heart attack. Do not take a chance if you are not sure. Always call 911 right away if you or someone else has heart attack symptoms.[4]

---

[4] "Heart Attack," National Heart, Lung, and Blood Institute (NHLBI), March 24, 2022. Available online. URL: www. nhlbi.nih.gov/health/heart-attack. Accessed May 18, 2023.

Chapter 34 | **Stroke**

WHAT IS A STROKE?

A stroke, also known as a "transient ischemic attack" (TIA) or "cerebrovascular accident," happens when blood flow to the brain is blocked. This prevents the brain from getting oxygen and nutrients from the blood. Without oxygen and nutrients, brain cells begin to die within minutes. Sudden bleeding in the brain can also cause a stroke if it damages brain cells.

A stroke is a medical emergency. A stroke can cause lasting brain damage, long-term disability, or even death. If you think you or someone else is having a stroke, call 911 right away. Do not drive to the hospital or let someone else drive you. Call an ambulance so that medical personnel can begin lifesaving treatment on the way to the emergency room. During a stroke, every minute counts.

CAUSES AND RISK FACTORS OF STROKE

Strokes are caused by blocked blood flow to the brain (ischemic stroke) or sudden bleeding in the brain (hemorrhagic stroke). Many things raise your risk of stroke, and many of these can be changed to help prevent a stroke or prevent another stroke.

Causes
ISCHEMIC STROKE

Ischemic strokes are usually caused by a piece of plaque or a blood clot that blocks blood flow to the brain.

When plaque builds up on the inner walls of the arteries, it can lead to a disease called "atherosclerosis." Plaque hardens and narrows the arteries, which limits blood flow to tissues and organs. Plaque can build up in any artery in the body, including arteries in the brain and neck. Carotid artery disease (CAD) is when plaque builds up in the carotid arteries in the neck that supply blood to the brain. It is a common cause of ischemic stroke.

Plaque in an artery can also break open. Blood platelets stick to the site of the plaque injury and clump together to form blood clots. These clots can partly or fully block an artery.

A blood clot that forms in one part of the body can also break loose and travel to the brain. This type of ischemic stroke is called an "embolic stroke." Certain heart and blood conditions, such as atrial fibrillation and sickle cell disease (SCD), can cause blood clots that lead to stroke.

INFLAMMATION

Chronic (long-term) inflammation contributes to ischemic stroke. Researchers are still trying to understand this fully. It is known that inflammation can damage the blood vessels and contribute to atherosclerosis, however. In addition, ischemic stroke can lead to inflammation that further damages brain cells.

TRANSIENT ISCHEMIC ATTACK

A TIA is caused by a blockage in the brain, just like an ischemic stroke. But the blockage breaks up before there is any damage to your brain. It typically lasts less than an hour but can come and go. Eventually, it can progress to a full stroke. A TIA is also called a "ministroke."

Hemorrhagic Stroke

Sudden bleeding can cause a hemorrhagic stroke. This can happen when an artery in or on top of the brain breaks open. The leaked blood causes the brain to swell, putting pressure on it that can damage brain cells.

Some conditions make blood vessels in the brain more likely to bleed.

- Aneurysm is a balloon-like bulge in an artery that can stretch and burst.

- Arteriovenous malformations (AVMs) are tangles of poorly formed arteries and veins that can break open in the brain.
- High blood pressure (HBP) puts pressure on the inside walls of the arteries. This pressure makes them more likely to break open, especially when they are weakened because of an aneurysm or AVM.

WHAT ARE THE RISK FACTORS OF STROKE?

There are many risk factors for stroke. You can treat or control some of your risk factors, such as HBP and smoking. But you cannot control others, such as your age or sudden changes in your health—for example, if you have an aneurysm.

The major risk factors for stroke include:

- HBP
- diabetes
- heart and blood vessel diseases (Conditions that can cause blood clots or other blockages include coronary heart disease, atrial fibrillation, heart valve disease, and CAD.)
- high low-density lipoprotein (LDL) cholesterol levels
- smoking
- brain aneurysms or AVMs (which are tangles of poorly formed arteries and veins that can break open in the brain)
- viral infections or conditions that cause inflammation, such as lupus or rheumatoid arthritis (RA)
- age (A stroke can happen at any age, but the risk is higher for babies under the age of one and for adults. In adults, the risk increases with age.)
- sex (At younger ages, men are more likely than women to have a stroke. But women tend to live longer, so their lifetime risk of having a stroke is higher. Women who take birth control pills or use hormone replacement therapy are at higher risk. Women are also at higher risk during pregnancy and in the weeks after giving birth. HBP during pregnancy—such as from preeclampsia—raises the risk of stroke later in life.)

- race and ethnicity (In the United States, stroke occurs more often in African American, Alaska Native, American Indian, and Hispanic adults than in White adults.)
- family history and genetics (Your risk of having a stroke is higher if a parent or other family member has had a stroke, particularly at a younger age. Certain genes affect your stroke risk, including those that determine your blood type. People with blood type AB (which is not common) have a higher risk.)

Other risk factors for stroke—some of which you can control—include:
- anxiety, depression, and high stress levels, as well as working long hours and not having much contact with friends, family, or others outside the home
- living or working in areas with air pollution
- other medical conditions, such as certain bleeding disorders, sleep apnea, kidney disease, migraine headaches, and SCD
- blood thinners or other medicines that can lead to bleeding
- other unhealthy lifestyle habits, including eating unhealthy foods, not getting regular physical activity, drinking alcohol, getting too much sleep (more than nine hours), and using illegal drugs such as cocaine
- overweight and being obese or carrying extra weight around your waist and stomach

SYMPTOMS OF STROKE
The signs and symptoms of a stroke often develop quickly. However, they can develop over hours or even days, such as when a TIA turns into a stroke.

The type of symptoms depends on the type of stroke and the area of the brain that is affected.

Signs of a TIA or stroke may include:
- sudden numbness or weakness, especially on one side of the body

- sudden confusion or trouble speaking or understanding speech
- sudden trouble seeing in one or both eyes
- sudden trouble walking, dizziness, or loss of balance or coordination
- sudden severe headache with no known cause

The FAST test can help you remember what to do if you think someone may be having a stroke:

- **F—Face**. Ask the person to smile. Does one side of the face droop?
- **A—Arms**. Ask the person to raise both arms. Does one arm drift downward?
- **S—Speech**. Ask the person to repeat a simple phrase. Is their speech slurred or strange?
- **T—Time**. If you observe any of these signs, call 911 right away. Early treatment is essential.

COMPLICATIONS OF STROKE

A stroke can cause lasting brain damage, long-term disability, or even death. When you have a stroke, your doctor may rate how severe it is. A more severe stroke means more brain tissue was damaged. When there has been significant damage, your doctor may call it a massive stroke. This can mean more severe complications.

After having a stroke, you may develop the following complications:

- **Dangerous blood clots**. Being unable to move around for a long time can raise your risk of developing blood clots in the deep veins of the legs. In some cases, blood clots can break loose and travel to the lungs. Your stroke care team may try to prevent these complications with medicine or a device that puts pressure on your calves to keep your blood flowing.
- **Difficulty speaking**. If a stroke affects the muscles you use to speak, you may have trouble communicating as easily as before.

- **Loss of bladder or bowel control**. Some strokes affect the muscles used to urinate and have bowel movements. You may need a urinary catheter (a tube placed into the bladder) until you can urinate on your own. The use of these catheters can lead to urinary tract infections (UTIs). You may also lose control of your bowels or be constipated.
- **Loss of bone density or strength**. This usually happens on one side of the body. Physical activity as part of rehabilitation can help prevent this loss. Your care team may also evaluate you for osteoporosis.
- **Loss of vision, hearing, or touch**. Your ability to feel pain or temperature may be affected after a stroke, or you may have trouble seeing or hearing as well as before. Some of these changes could affect your ability to cook, read, change your clothes, or do other tasks.
- **Muscle weakness or inability to move**. A stroke can make your muscles become weak and stiff or cause them to spasm. This can be painful or make it hard to stand or walk around on your own. You may also have problems with balance or controlling your muscles. This puts you at risk of falling.
- **Problems swallowing and pneumonia**. If a stroke affects the muscles used for swallowing, you may have a hard time eating or drinking. You may also be at risk of inhaling food or drink into your lungs. If this happens, you may develop pneumonia.
- **Problems with language, thinking, or memory**. A stroke may affect your ability to focus on a task or make decisions quickly. It also raises the risk of dementia.
- **Seizures**. This is more common in the weeks after a stroke and is less likely as time goes on. If you have seizures, your stroke team may give you medicine.
- **Swelling in the brain**. After a stroke, fluid may build up between the brain and the skull or in the cavities of the brain, causing swelling. Doctors may drain fluid from the brain or cut away part of the skull to relieve the pressure on your brain.

DIAGNOSIS OF STROKE

Your doctor will diagnose a stroke based on your symptoms, your medical history, a physical exam, and test results. Your doctor will want to find out the type of stroke you have had, its cause, the part of the brain that is affected, and whether you have bleeding in the brain. If your doctor thinks you have had a TIA, he or she will look for its cause to help prevent a future stroke.

TREATMENT FOR STROKE

A stroke requires emergency care. You will probably receive treatment in a specialized stroke unit of the hospital. A team of specialists will oversee your care. Treatment will depend on whether the stroke was ischemic or hemorrhagic, how much time has passed since symptoms began, and whether you have other medical conditions.

Treating an Ischemic Stroke

Treatment for an ischemic stroke or transient ischemic stroke (TIA) may include medicines and medical procedures.

MEDICINES

The main treatment for an ischemic stroke is a medicine called "tissue plasminogen activator" (tPA). It breaks up the blood clots that block blood flow to your brain. A doctor will inject tPA into a vein in your arm. This type of medicine must be given within three hours after your symptoms start. In some cases, it is given up to 4.5 hours. The sooner treatment begins, the better your chances of recovery.

If you cannot have tPA, your doctor may give you an anticoagulant or blood-thinning medicine, such as aspirin or clopidogrel. This helps stop blood clots from forming or getting larger. The main side effect of these medicines is bleeding.

MEDICAL PROCEDURES

You may need a procedure to open up blocked arteries and restore blood flow to the brain. This can be done in several ways.

A thrombectomy removes the clot from the blood vessel. A surgeon will put a long, flexible tube called a "catheter" into your groin (upper thigh) and thread it to the blocked artery in your neck or brain. They will then use angioplasty and stenting or a device called a "stent retriever" to open up the blocked artery.

- Angioplasty and stenting procedures use a thin tube to deliver a balloon or small mesh tube into the artery. Inflating the balloon or expanding the mesh tube clears space for blood to flow more easily to the brain.
- The stent retriever is a wire mesh inside the catheter that traps the clot. The stent retriever and the blood clot are then pulled out through the tube.

If CAD causes your stroke, your doctor may suggest carotid endarterectomy, a surgery to remove plaque from the carotid artery in your neck.

Treating a Hemorrhagic Stroke

Hemorrhagic stroke can happen suddenly and grow worse quickly. Just as with an ischemic stroke, getting treatment as quickly as possible is essential for a full recovery. The type of treatment you receive depends on what part of your brain is bleeding and how severe it is.

MEDICINES

You may be given blood pressure medicine to lower the pressure and strain on blood vessels in the brain. You will also be taken off any anticoagulant or blood-thinning medicines that may have led to bleeding. Depending on the type of medicine you are taking, you may be given vitamin K to help stop bleeding.

MEDICAL PROCEDURES

Procedures may include:

- **Aneurysm clipping to block off the aneurysm from the blood vessels in the brain**. This surgery helps stop bleeding from an aneurysm. It can also help prevent the aneurysm from bursting again. During the procedure, a surgeon places a tiny clamp at the base of the aneurysm.

- **Coil embolization to block blood flow to or seal an aneurysm**. The surgeon will insert a tube called a "catheter" into an artery in the groin. He or she will thread the tube to the aneurysm in your brain. A tiny coil will be pushed through the tube and into the aneurysm. The coil will cause a blood clot to form, which will block blood flow through the aneurysm and prevent it from bursting again.
- **Blood transfusion to replace the blood that is lost through surgery or injury**. A blood transfusion is a common, safe medical procedure in which healthy donor blood is given to you through an intravenous (IV) line inserted in one of your blood vessels.
- **Draining excess fluid that collects in the brain**. Fluid can build up after a stroke, pushing the brain against the skull and causing damage. Draining the fluid can relieve that pressure.
- **Surgery or radiation to remove or shrink an AVM**. An AVM is a tangle of arteries and veins that can break open in the brain.
- **Surgery to remove pooled blood**. Typically, the stroke team will use surgery only if you show signs of getting worse.
- **Surgery to temporarily remove part of the skull**. This is done if you have a lot of swelling. This allows room for the brain to swell without putting pressure on the brain.

OTHER CARE YOU MAY RECEIVE IN THE HOSPITAL

In addition to treating the blockage or bleeding causing the stroke, your health-care team may suggest additional treatments or tests.

- **Breathing support**. If your stroke makes it difficult to breathe or your oxygen levels are low, you may receive ventilator support.

- **Compression therapy**. A sleeve can be placed on your leg and filled with air to reduce the risk of venous thromboembolism.
- **Feeding tube**. If it is difficult for you to swallow on your own, your team may set up a feeding tube to provide you with nutrients.
- **Fluids**. If you have low blood pressure or low blood volume, you may get fluids to restore proper levels.
- **Medicine to reduce fever**. Your team will monitor your body temperature and may give you acetaminophen or another medicine to reduce fever and prevent additional brain damage.
- **Rehabilitation plan**. Before you leave the hospital, your medical team will test how well you can speak, swallow, and walk. You and your medical team can work together to set up a rehabilitation plan.
- **Skin care**. To prevent skin irritation or sores from forming, your team will help make sure that you have enough cushioning, your skin stays dry, and that you change positions often if you cannot move well on your own.

A stroke is a life-threatening condition that can cause severe disability. Palliative care or hospice care may help some patients have a better quality of life with fewer symptoms.[1]

[1] "Stroke," National Heart, Lung, and Blood Institute (NHLBI), March 24, 2022. Available online. URL: www.nhlbi.nih.gov/health/stroke. Accessed May 22, 2023.

Chapter 35 | Peripheral Vascular Disease

Chapter Contents

Section 35.1 | Peripheral Artery Disease

WHAT IS PERIPHERAL ARTERY DISEASE?

In the United States, more than 8 million people aged 40 and older have peripheral artery disease (PAD). Also called "peripheral arterial disease," PAD is caused by atherosclerosis, or plaque buildup, that reduces the flow of blood in peripheral arteries—the blood vessels that carry blood away from the heart to other parts of the body. This section focuses on the most common type of PAD, called "lower extremity PAD," which reduces blood flow to the legs and feet.

You may have lower extremity PAD if you have muscle pain or weakness that begins with physical activity, such as walking, and stops within minutes after resting. About one in four people who have PAD experiences these symptoms. But you may experience other symptoms or no symptoms at all. If you smoke or have high blood pressure (HBP) or other risk factors for PAD, even without symptoms, ask your health-care provider about getting tested. It is important to be aware that if you have lower extremity PAD, you may also have plaque buildup in other arteries leading to and from your heart and brain, putting you at higher risk of stroke or heart attack.

Early diagnosis and management of PAD can help treat your symptoms and reduce your risk for serious complications.

CAUSES AND RISK FACTORS OF PERIPHERAL ARTERY DISEASE
What Causes Peripheral Artery Disease?

Atherosclerosis is the main cause of PAD.

Atherosclerosis is a disease in which a waxy substance called "plaque" builds up on the inner lining of arteries. Plaque is made up of fat, cholesterol, fibrous tissue, and calcium. In PAD, plaque may reduce or fully block the flow of oxygen-rich blood through arteries to the body's vital organs and limbs. A person may have atherosclerosis in just a single artery or in many.

What Raises the Risk of Peripheral Artery Disease?

You may have a higher risk of lower extremity PAD because of your age, family history and genetics, lifestyle habits, other

483

medical conditions, race, ethnicity, and sex. The risk factors for PAD are mostly the same as those for coronary heart disease (CHD) and carotid artery disease (CAD), which are also caused by atherosclerosis.

AGE

You can develop PAD at any age, but your risk goes up as you get older. Most people in the United States who have PAD are aged 65 or older.

Worldwide, the age group for PAD is younger (aged 45–49) in countries with lower incomes when compared with high-income countries.

FAMILY HISTORY AND GENETICS

A family history of PAD, heart disease, stroke, or blood vessel disease, such as some types of vasculitis, raises your risk of PAD. Researchers are studying gene variations that seem to increase the risk of PAD or could make the disease worse.

Genetic studies have found that certain gene variations are found in different types of atherosclerotic diseases, such as PAD, CAD, and CHD. An example is the gene variation that is found in factor V Leiden disorder, a specific gene mutation that leads to an increased risk of blood clots.

LIFESTYLE HABITS

Over time, unhealthy lifestyle habits can lead to plaque buildup in the leg and foot arteries, causing PAD. These habits may include the following:

- Smoking or regularly breathing in secondhand smoke damages your blood vessels, raises your blood pressure, and causes unhealthy cholesterol levels. The nicotine in tobacco also makes your blood vessels tighten and reduces blood flow in your legs. Quitting smoking is a very important step in lowering your risk of PAD.
- Not getting enough physical activity can make other PAD risk factors worse.

- Stress can make your arteries tighten and narrow.
- Eating foods high in saturated fats and following other unhealthy eating patterns can also increase your risk of PAD. Butter, palm and coconut oils, cheese, and red meat have high amounts of saturated fat.

OTHER MEDICAL CONDITIONS

Medical conditions that raise your risk of developing PAD include the following:

- diabetes
- chronic kidney disease (CKD)
- disorders that cause blood clots, such as thrombocytosis or antiphospholipid syndrome (APS)
- fibromuscular dysplasia (FMD), a condition that occurs when cells in the artery walls grow too much, making the artery narrow
- HBP
- metabolic syndrome
- obesity
- unhealthy blood cholesterol levels or high blood triglycerides

Also, if you had preeclampsia or gestational diabetes during pregnancy, you have a higher risk of developing PAD later in life.

RACE OR ETHNICITY

African Americans have a higher risk of PAD than people of other races or ethnicities. African Americans are also more likely to have complications of PAD, such as problems walking or loss of a limb.

Additionally, American Indian women have a higher risk of PAD than White or Asian American women. Hispanic or Latino people and White people have similar risk levels. However, the National Heart, Lung, and Blood Institute (NHLBI) research found that rates of lower extremity PAD are higher among Hispanic and Latino adults who have highly sedentary lifestyles, even when they do not have any other risk factors.

SEX

Men and women have a similar risk of developing PAD, but PAD affects men and women differently.

Women are more likely than men to have PAD without symptoms. However, women also frequently have more PAD complications, such as problems walking.

SYMPTOMS OF PERIPHERAL ARTERY DISEASE

About one in four people with PAD experiences common symptoms of the condition. More than half have nontypical symptoms, and about one in five people who have PAD does not report any symptoms. No matter the symptoms, everyone with PAD shares the same high risk of cardiovascular disease (CVD). Without treatment, PAD may cause sores, infections, and even the loss of a limb.

Symptoms of PAD can vary, but the following are a few common ones:

- Pain, aching, heaviness, or cramping in your legs that comes when walking or climbing stairs and goes away after rest is called "intermittent claudication." It is the most common PAD symptom. The pain is often in the calf, but you may also feel it in your buttocks, thigh, or foot.
- Your toenails and leg hair may stop growing.
- One foot may feel colder than the other.
- Your foot or leg may become pale, discolored, or blue.
- Leg weakness or numbness may make you feel off-balance or make it harder to walk.
- You may have pain or a feeling of pins and needles in your leg or foot.
- In severe PAD, pain in your leg and foot when at rest is called "critical limb ischemia."
- Sores or wounds on your toes, feet, or legs may appear, may heal slowly, or may not heal at all. The sores may become infected.

DIAGNOSIS OF PERIPHERAL ARTERY DISEASE

Your health-care provider will diagnose PAD based on your medical and family history, a physical exam, and the results from tests and procedures.

Medical History and Physical Exam

To help diagnose PAD, your provider will want to learn about your symptoms, risk factors, personal health history, and family health history. This discussion may include questions about the following:

- other medical conditions, including diabetes, heart disease, and CKD
- pain or cramps in your legs while walking or exercising
- problems with your legs and feet, including swelling, redness, trouble with walking, and wounds that are slow to heal
- smoking, either current or past
- your family history of PAD, heart disease, and other blood vessel diseases

During an exam to look for signs of PAD, your provider will:
- check for weak pulses in your legs
- listen for poor blood flow in your legs (Your provider will use a stethoscope to listen for an abnormal whooshing sound, called a "bruit.")
- look for problems on your legs and feet, including swelling, sores, or pale skin

Conditions That Can Seem Like Peripheral Artery Disease

Some conditions, such as arthritis or vein problems, can cause leg pain, but the symptoms are different from those of PAD. A physical exam and your medical history can help your provider rule out these conditions.

However, problems with nerves can cause pain that may be confused with PAD. Sometimes, a nerve is squeezed where it exits the spinal column. The result is pain that radiates, or spreads, from the hips or buttocks and down the leg.

487

To confirm that your pain is the result of PAD, your provider may ask you to stand up or change your position. Those movements often trigger nerve-related pain. In contrast, PAD pain is often brought on by leg exercise and is quickly relieved by rest with no need to change position.

Diagnostic Tests and Procedures

The ankle-brachial index (ABI) test is usually the first test used to diagnose PAD. The test compares the blood pressure in your ankle with the blood pressure in your arm. Your provider uses a blood pressure cuff and ultrasound device for this painless test.

A healthy ABI result is 1.00 or greater. If you have an ABI of less than 0.90 while resting, you may have PAD. An ABI of less than 0.40 is a sign of severe PAD. If there are problems with the arteries in your ankle, your provider may do a toe-brachial index (TBI) test instead, which measures the blood pressure in your big toe. A TBI less than 0.7 is abnormal. Be aware of your ABI, just as you know, keep track of your blood pressure numbers.

TREATMENT FOR PERIPHERAL ARTERY DISEASE

Treatment depends on how severe your PAD is and what complications you may develop or already have. Your treatment plan will be designed to help you reach the following key goals:
- reducing your risk of a major health problem such as a heart attack or stroke
- reducing symptoms of PAD
- improving your ability to walk, climb stairs, and perform other daily activities
- lowering your risk of losing a limb
- improving your quality of life

To treat PAD, your provider may recommend heart-healthy lifestyle changes, an exercise program, medicine, or a procedure to open or bypass blockages in your arteries.

HOW CAN YOU PREVENT PERIPHERAL ARTERY DISEASE?

To help you prevent PAD, your provider may talk to you about heart-healthy lifestyle changes and managing conditions that may lead to PAD.

Heart-healthy lifestyle changes include quitting smoking, choosing a heart-healthy eating pattern (such as the Dietary Approaches to Stop Hypertension (DASH) eating plan), being physically active, aiming for a healthy weight, and managing stress.

Follow your provider's advice about preventing and treating conditions that raise your risk of PAD, such as diabetes, HBP, and high blood cholesterol.[1]

Section 35.2 | Raynaud Phenomenon

Raynaud phenomenon is a condition that causes the blood vessels in the extremities to narrow, restricting blood flow. The episodes or "attacks" usually affect the fingers and toes. In rare cases, attacks occur in other areas, such as the ears or nose. An attack usually happens from exposure to cold or emotional stress.

There are two types of Raynaud phenomenon—primary and secondary. The primary form has no known cause, but the secondary form is related to another health issue, especially autoimmune diseases such as lupus or scleroderma. The secondary form tends to be more serious and needs more aggressive treatment.

In most people, lifestyle changes such as staying warm keep symptoms under control, but in severe cases, repeated attacks lead to skin sores or gangrene (death and decay of tissue). The treatment depends on how serious the condition is and whether it is in the primary or secondary form.

---

[1] "Peripheral Artery Disease," National Heart, Lung, and Blood Institute (NHLBI), March 24, 2022. Available online. URL: www.nhlbi.nih.gov/health/peripheral-artery-disease. Accessed May 22, 2023.

WHO GETS RAYNAUD PHENOMENON?

Anyone can get Raynaud phenomenon, but some people are more likely to have it than others. There are two types, and the risk factors for each are different.

The primary form of Raynaud phenomenon, which is of unknown cause, has been linked to the following:

- **Sex**. Women get it more often than men.
- **Age**. It usually occurs in people younger than age 30 and often starts in the teenage years.
- **Family history of Raynaud phenomenon**. People with a family member who has Raynaud phenomenon have a higher risk of getting it themselves, suggesting a genetic link.

The secondary form of Raynaud phenomenon occurs in combination with another disease or environmental exposure. Factors that have been linked to the secondary Raynaud phenomenon include the following:

- **Diseases**. Among the most common ones are lupus, scleroderma, inflammatory myositis, rheumatoid arthritis (RA), and Sjögren syndrome. Conditions such as certain thyroid disorders, clotting disorders, and carpal tunnel syndrome (CTS) have also been linked to the secondary form.
- **Medications**. Medicines used to treat high blood pressure (HBP), migraines, or attention deficit hyperactivity disorder (ADHD) may cause symptoms similar to Raynaud phenomenon or make the underlying Raynaud phenomenon worse.
- **Work-related exposures**. Repeated use of vibrating machinery (such as a jackhammer) or exposure to cold or certain chemicals can cause Raynaud phenomenon.

CAUSES OF RAYNAUD PHENOMENON

Scientists do not know exactly why Raynaud phenomenon develops in some people, but they do understand how attacks happen. When a person is exposed to cold, the body tries to slow the loss of heat and maintain its temperature. To do so, blood vessels in the surface layer of the skin constrict (narrow), moving blood from vessels near the surface to those deeper in the body.

In people with Raynaud phenomenon, blood vessels in the hands and feet react to cold or stress, narrowing quickly and staying constricted for a long period. This causes the skin to turn pale or white, then bluish as the blood left in the vessels becomes depleted of oxygen. Eventually, when you warm up and the vessels expand again, the skin flushes and may tingle or burn.

Many factors, including nerve and hormonal signals, control blood flow in the skin, and Raynaud phenomenon happens when this complex system gets disrupted. Emotional stress releases signaling molecules that cause blood vessels to narrow, which is why anxiety can trigger an attack.

More women than men are affected by primary Raynaud phenomenon, suggesting that estrogen may play a role in this form. Genes may also be involved: The risk of the condition is higher in people with a relative who has it, but the specific genetic factors have not yet been definitively identified.

In secondary Raynaud phenomenon, damage to the blood vessels from certain diseases, such as lupus or scleroderma, or work-related exposures likely underlies the condition.

SYMPTOMS OF RAYNAUD PHENOMENON

Raynaud phenomenon happens when episodes or "attacks" affect certain parts of the body, especially the fingers and toes, causing them to become cold and numb, and change colors. Exposure to cold is the most common trigger, such as grabbing hold of a glass of ice water or taking something out of the freezer. Sudden changes in ambient temperature, such as entering an air-conditioned supermarket on a warm day, can lead to an attack.

Emotional stress, cigarette smoking, and vaping can also trigger symptoms. Parts of the body besides the fingers and toes, such as the ears or nose, may be affected as well.

- **Raynaud attacks**. A typical attack progresses as follows:
  - The skin of the affected part of the body turns pale or white due to a lack of blood flow.

- The area then turns blue and feels cold and numb as the blood that is left in the tissue loses its oxygen.
- Finally, as you warm up and circulation returns, the area turns red and may swell, tingle, burn, or throb.
- Only one finger or toe may be affected at first; then, it may move to other fingers and toes. The thumbs are less likely to be affected than the other fingers. An attack may last a few minutes or a few hours, and the pain associated with each episode can vary.
- **Skin ulcers and gangrene**. People with severe Raynaud phenomenon can develop small, painful sores, especially at the tips of the fingers or toes. In rare cases, an extended episode (days) of a lack of oxygen to tissues can lead to gangrene (cellular death and decay of body tissues).

For many people, especially those with the primary form of Raynaud phenomenon, the symptoms are mild and not highly troublesome. People with the secondary form tend to have more severe symptoms.

DIAGNOSIS OF RAYNAUD PHENOMENON

There is no single test to diagnose Raynaud phenomenon. Doctors usually diagnose it based on symptoms, in particular, on a description of a typical attack upon exposure to cold. Your doctor will also likely take a medical history and perform a physical exam.

Your doctor may perform additional tests to distinguish between the two forms of the condition. These include the following:

- **Nailfold capillary microscopy**. During this test, your doctor uses a magnifier to look at the base of your fingernails for signs of changes in capillaries (extremely small blood vessels), a sign of secondary Raynaud phenomenon.
- **Blood tests**. If your doctor suspects that you have the secondary form, they may order blood tests that may indicate you have a disease that has been linked to

Raynaud phenomenon, such as lupus or scleroderma. One of the more common of these tests is the antinuclear antibody (ANA) test.

TREATMENT FOR RAYNAUD PHENOMENON

The goals of treatment for Raynaud phenomenon are to:
- reduce how many attacks you have
- make attacks less severe
- prevent tissue damage

For most people with Raynaud phenomenon, avoiding getting cold prevents attacks and keeps symptoms under control. But, if this is not enough, medications and, in some cases, surgical procedures can help.

Secondary Raynaud phenomenon is more likely to be serious and to need more aggressive therapy. If you have the secondary form, you may need to seek treatment for an underlying condition if you have not already done so.

Preventing Attacks

- **Medications**. While there are no medications approved by the U.S. Food and Drug Administration (FDA) for Raynaud phenomenon, medications that have been approved for other conditions are routinely used to treat it.
- **Surgery**. If you have severe Raynaud phenomenon, your doctor may recommend a procedure called a "sympathectomy" to destroy the nerves that trigger blood vessel narrowing in the affected areas. This is usually done by incision or injections. The procedure often relieves symptoms, but it may need to be repeated after a few years.

Treating Tissue Damage

In serious cases, repeated attacks can lead to skin sores or gangrene (death and decay of tissue). If this happens, you may need to be admitted to the hospital for a few days and receive intravenous medications to rapidly improve blood flow and treat the infection. In rare cases, you may need surgery to remove dead tissue.[2]

Section 35.3 | Buerger Disease

WHAT IS BUERGER DISEASE?

Buerger disease (also known as "thromboangiitis obliterans") affects blood vessels in the body, most commonly in the arms and legs. Blood vessels swell, which can prevent blood flow, causing clots to form. This can lead to pain, tissue damage, and even gangrene (the death or decay of body tissues). In some cases, amputation may be required.

CAUSES OF BUERGER DISEASE

The exact cause of Buerger disease is unknown; however, tobacco use is strongly linked to its development. Researchers believe that chemicals in tobacco may irritate the lining of the blood vessels, causing them to swell. Almost everyone diagnosed with Buerger disease smokes cigarettes or uses other forms of tobacco, such as cigars and chewing tobacco.

SYMPTOMS OF BUERGER DISEASE

The most common symptoms of Buerger disease are:
- pale, red, or bluish fingers or toes
- cold hands or feet
- pain in the hands and feet that may feel like burning or tingling
- pain in the legs, ankles, or feet when walking—often located in the arch of the foot
- skin changes or small painful sores on the fingers or toes

[2] "Raynaud's Phenomenon," National Institute of Arthritis and Musculoskeletal and Skin Diseases (NIAMS), May 2021. Available online. URL: www.niams.nih.gov/health-topics/raynauds-phenomenon. Accessed May 22, 2023.

HOW IS BUERGER DISEASE TREATED?

There is no cure for Buerger disease. The only way to keep Buerger disease from getting worse is to stop using all tobacco products. Medicines do not usually work well to treat the disease but can help control the symptoms.

Surgery may help restore blood flow to some areas. It may be necessary to amputate the hand or foot if infection or widespread tissue death occurs.

HOW CAN BUERGER DISEASE BE PREVENTED?

If you want to prevent getting Buerger disease, do not smoke cigarettes or use any other tobacco products.[3]

Section 35.4 | Erythromelalgia

WHAT IS ERYTHROMELALGIA?

Erythromelalgia (EM) is a condition characterized by episodes of pain, redness, and swelling in various parts of the body, particularly in the hands and feet. These episodes are usually triggered by increased body temperature, which may be caused by exercise or entering a warm room. Ingesting alcohol or spicy foods may also trigger an episode. Wearing warm socks, tight shoes, or gloves can cause a pain episode so debilitating that it can impede everyday activities, such as wearing shoes and walking. Pain episodes can prevent an affected person from going to school or work regularly.

CAUSES OF ERYTHROMELALGIA

Mutations in the *SCN9A* gene can cause EM. The *SCN9A* gene provides instructions for making one part (the alpha subunit) of a sodium channel called "NaV1.7." Sodium channels transport positively charged sodium atoms (sodium ions) into cells and play a

---

[3] "Smoking and Buerger's Disease," Centers for Disease Control and Prevention (CDC), May 5, 2022. Available online. URL: www.cdc.gov/tobacco/campaign/tips/diseases/buergers-disease.html. Accessed May 22, 2023.

key role in a cell's ability to generate and transmit electrical signals. NaV1.7 sodium channels are found in nerve cells called "nociceptors" that transmit pain signals to the spinal cord and brain.

The *SCN9A* gene mutations that cause EM result in NaV1.7 sodium channels that open more easily than usual and stay open longer than normal, increasing the flow of sodium ions into nociceptors. This increase in sodium ions enhances the transmission of pain signals, leading to the signs and symptoms of EM. It is unknown why the pain episodes associated with EM mainly occur in the hands and feet.

An estimated 15 percent of cases of EM are caused by mutations in the *SCN9A* gene. Other cases are thought to have a nongenetic cause or may be caused by mutations in one or more as-yet-unidentified genes.

SIGNS AND SYMPTOMS OF ERYTHROMELALGIA

The signs and symptoms of EM typically begin in childhood; however, mildly affected individuals may have their first pain episode later in life. As individuals with EM get older and the disease progresses, the hands and feet may be constantly red, and the affected areas can extend from the hands to the arms, shoulders, and face and from the feet to the entire legs.

EM is often considered a form of peripheral neuropathy because it affects the peripheral nervous system, which connects the brain and spinal cord to muscles and to cells that detect sensations, such as touch, smell, and pain.

INHERITANCE OF ERYTHROMELALGIA

Some cases of EM occur in an autosomal dominant pattern, which means one copy of the altered gene in each cell is sufficient to cause the disorder. In some of these instances, an affected person inherits the mutation from one affected parent. Other cases result from new mutations in the gene and occur in people with no history of the disorder in their family.[4]

---

[4] MedlinePlus, "Erythromelalgia," National Institutes of Health (NIH), February 1, 2016. Available online. URL: https://medlineplus.gov/genetics/condition/erythromelalgia/#inheritance. Accessed June 14, 2023.

Chapter 36 | **Renal Artery Stenosis**

WHAT ARE RENAL ARTERY STENOSIS AND RENOVASCULAR HYPERTENSION?

Renal artery stenosis (RAS) is the narrowing of one or both renal arteries. "Renal" means "kidney," and "stenosis" means "narrowing." The renal arteries are blood vessels that carry blood to the kidneys from the aorta—the main blood vessel that carries blood from the heart to arteries throughout the body.

Renovascular hypertension (RVH) is high blood pressure (HBP) caused by RAS. Blood pressure is written with two numbers separated by a slash, 120/80, and is said as "120 over 80." The top number is called the "systolic pressure" and represents the pressure as the heart beats and pushes blood through the blood vessels. The bottom number is called the "diastolic pressure" and represents the pressure as blood vessels relax between heartbeats. A person's blood pressure is considered normal if it stays at or below 120/80. HBP is a systolic pressure of 140 or above or a diastolic pressure of 90 or above.

WHAT ARE THE KIDNEYS, AND WHAT DO THEY DO?

The kidneys are two bean-shaped organs, each about the size of a fist. They are located just below the rib cage, one on each side of the spine. Every day, the two kidneys filter about 120–150 quarts of blood to produce about 1–2 quarts of urine, composed of wastes and extra fluid.

WHAT CAUSES RENAL ARTERY STENOSIS?

About 90 percent of RAS is caused by atherosclerosis—clogging, narrowing, and hardening of the renal arteries. In these cases, RAS develops when plaque—a sticky substance made up of fat, cholesterol, calcium, and other material found in the blood—builds up on the inner wall of one or both renal arteries. Plaque buildup is what makes the artery wall hard and narrow.

Most other cases of RAS are caused by fibromuscular dysplasia (FMD)—the abnormal development or growth of cells on the renal artery walls—which can cause blood vessels to narrow. Rarely, RAS is caused by other conditions.

WHO IS AT RISK OF RENAL ARTERY STENOSIS?

People at risk of atherosclerosis are also at risk of RAS. Risk factors for RAS caused by atherosclerosis include the following:

- high blood cholesterol levels
- HBP
- smoking
- insulin resistance
- diabetes
- being overweight or having obesity
- lack of physical activity
- a diet high in fat, cholesterol, sodium, and sugar
- being a man older than 45 or a woman older than 55
- a family history of early heart disease

The risk factors for RAS caused by FMD are unknown, but FMD is most common in women and people 25–50 years of age. FMD can affect more than one person in a family, indicating that it may be caused by an inherited gene.

WHAT ARE THE SYMPTOMS OF RENAL ARTERY STENOSIS?

In many cases, RAS has no symptoms until it becomes severe.

The signs of RAS are usually either HBP or decreased kidney function, or both, but RAS is often overlooked as a cause of HBP. RAS should be considered as a cause of HBP in people who:

- are older than age 50 when they develop HBP or have a marked increase in blood pressure
- have no family history of HBP

- cannot be successfully treated with at least three or more different types of blood pressure medications

Symptoms of a significant decrease in kidney function include the following:
- increase or decrease in urination
- edema—swelling, usually in the legs, feet, or ankles and less often in the hands or face
- drowsiness or tiredness
- generalized itching or numbness
- dry skin
- headaches
- weight loss
- appetite loss
- nausea
- vomiting
- sleep problems
- trouble concentrating
- darkened skin
- muscle cramps

WHAT ARE THE POSSIBLE COMPLICATIONS OF RENAL ARTERY STENOSIS?

People with RAS are at increased risk for the following complications resulting from loss of kidney function or atherosclerosis occurring in other blood vessels:
- **Chronic kidney disease (CKD)**. Reduced kidney function over a period of time.
- **Coronary artery disease**. Narrowing and hardening of arteries that supply blood to the heart.
- **Stroke**. Brain damage caused by a lack of blood flow to the brain.
- **Peripheral vascular disease**. Blockage of blood vessels that restricts the flow of blood from the heart to other parts of the body, particularly the legs.

RAS can lead to kidney failure, described as end-stage renal disease, when treated with blood-filtering treatments called "dialysis" or a "kidney transplant," though this is uncommon in people who receive ongoing treatment for RAS.

HOW IS RENAL ARTERY STENOSIS DIAGNOSED?

A health-care provider can diagnose RAS by listening to the abdomen with a stethoscope and performing imaging tests. When blood flows through a narrow artery, it sometimes makes a whooshing sound called a "bruit." The health-care provider may place a stethoscope on the front or the side of the abdomen to listen for this sound. The absence of this sound, however, does not exclude the possibility of RAS.

In some cases, RAS is found when a person has a test for another reason. For example, a health-care provider may find RAS during a coronary angiogram for diagnosis of heart problems. A coronary angiogram is a procedure that uses a special dye called "contrast medium" and x-rays to see how blood flows through the heart.

The following imaging tests are used to diagnose RAS:

- **Duplex ultrasound**. It combines traditional ultrasound with Doppler ultrasonography. Traditional ultrasound uses a device called a "transducer" that bounces safe, painless sound waves off organs to create an image of their structure. Doppler ultrasonography records sound waves reflected off of moving objects, such as blood, to measure their speed and other aspects of how they flow. The procedure is performed in a health-care provider's office, outpatient center, or hospital by a specially trained technician, and the images are interpreted by a radiologist—a doctor who specializes in medical imaging. Anesthesia is not needed. The images can show blockage in the renal artery or blood moving through nearby arteries at a lower-than-normal speed. Ultrasound is noninvasive and cost-effective.

- **Catheter angiogram**. A catheter angiogram, also called a "traditional angiogram," is a special kind of x-ray in which a thin, flexible tube called a "catheter" is threaded through the large arteries, often from the groin, to the artery of interest—in this case, the renal artery. The procedure is performed in a hospital or outpatient center by a radiologist. Anesthesia is not needed though a sedative may be given to lessen anxiety during the procedure. A contrast medium is injected through the catheter, so the renal artery shows up more clearly on the x-ray. A catheter angiogram is the "gold standard" for diagnosing RAS due to the high quality of the image produced. In addition, severe RAS can be treated during the same visit. However, a catheter angiogram is an invasive procedure, and a person may have side effects from the sedative or contrast medium or may have bleeding or injury to the artery from the catheter. The procedure is also more expensive than other imaging tests.

- **Computerized tomographic angiography (CTA) scan**. CTA scans use a combination of x-rays and computer technology to create images. The procedure is performed in an outpatient center or hospital by an x-ray technician, and the images are interpreted by a radiologist. Anesthesia is not needed. A contrast medium is injected into a vein in the person's arm to better see the structure of the arteries. CTA scans require the person to lie on a table that slides into a tunnel-shaped device where the x-rays are taken. CTA scans are less invasive than catheter angiograms and take less time. However, the risks from the x-ray radiation still exist, and the test often requires more contrast medium than a catheter angiogram, so it may not be recommended for a person with poor kidney function.

- **Magnetic resonance angiogram (MRA)**. MRA uses radio waves and magnets to produce detailed pictures of the body's internal organs and soft tissues without using x-rays. The procedure is performed in an outpatient center or hospital by an x-ray technician, and the images are interpreted by a radiologist. Anesthesia is not needed though light sedation may be used for people with a fear of confined spaces. A contrast medium may be injected into a vein in the person's arm to better see the structure of the arteries. With most MRA scans, the person lies on a table that slides into a tunnel-shaped device that may be open-ended or closed at one end; some newer machines are designed to allow the person to lie in a more open space. In addition to providing high-quality images noninvasively, MRA can provide a functional assessment of blood flow and organ function. However, the use of a contrast medium for an MRA is not advised for people with poor kidney function because of the risk of complications to the skin and other organs if the kidneys do not remove the contrast medium well enough.

HOW IS RENAL ARTERY STENOSIS TREATED?

Treatment for RAS includes lifestyle changes, medications, and surgery and aims to:

- prevent RAS from getting worse
- treat RVH
- relieve the blockage of the renal arteries

RAS that has not led to RVH or caused a significant block-age of the artery may not need treatment. RAS that needs to be treated, also called "critical RAS," is defined by the American Heart Association (AHA) as a reduction by more than 60 percent in the diameter of the renal artery. However, health-care providers are not exactly sure what degree of blockage will cause significant problems.

Lifestyle Changes

The first step in treating RAS is making lifestyle changes that promote healthy blood vessels throughout the body, including the renal arteries. The best ways to keep plaque from building up in the arteries are to exercise, maintain healthy body weight, and choose healthy foods. People who smoke should quit to help protect their kidneys and other internal organs.

Medications

People with RVH may need to take medications that—when taken as prescribed by their health-care provider—lower blood pressure and can also significantly slow the progression of kidney disease. Two types of blood pressure-lowering medications, angiotensin-converting enzyme (ACE) inhibitors and angiotensin receptor blockers (ARBs), have proven effective in slowing the progression of kidney disease. Many people require two or more medications to control their blood pressure. In addition to an ACE inhibitor or an ARB, a diuretic—a medication that helps the kidneys remove fluid from the blood—may be prescribed. Beta-blockers, calcium channel blockers, and other blood pressure medications may also be needed. Some people with RAS cannot take an ACE inhibitor or ARB due to the effects on the kidneys. People with RAS who are prescribed an ACE inhibitor or ARB should have their kidney function checked within a few weeks of starting the medication.

A cholesterol-lowering medication to prevent plaque from building up in the arteries and a blood thinner, such as aspirin, to help the blood flow more easily through the arteries may also be prescribed.

Surgery

Although surgery has been used in the past for the treatment of RAS due to atherosclerosis, recent studies have not shown improved outcomes with surgery compared with medication. However, surgery may be recommended for people with RAS caused by FMD or RAS that does not improve with medication. Different types of surgery for RAS include the following. The procedures are performed in a hospital by a vascular surgeon—a doctor who specializes in repairing blood vessels. Anesthesia is needed.

- **Angioplasty and stenting**. Angioplasty is a procedure in which a catheter is put into the renal artery, usually through the groin, just as in a catheter angiogram. In addition, for angioplasty, a tiny balloon at the end of the catheter can be inflated to flatten the plaque against the artery wall. A small mesh tube, called a "stent," may then be positioned inside the artery to keep plaque flattened and the artery open. People with RAS caused by FMD may be successfully treated with angioplasty alone, while angioplasty with stenting has a better outcome for people with RAS caused by atherosclerosis.

- **Endarterectomy or bypass surgery**. In an endarterectomy, the plaque is cleaned out of the artery, leaving the inside lining smooth and clear. To create a bypass, a vein or synthetic tube is used to connect the kidney to the aorta. This new path serves as an alternate route for blood to flow around the blocked artery into the kidney. These procedures are not performed as often as in the past due to a high risk of complications during and after the procedure.

EATING, DIET, AND NUTRITION

Limiting the intake of fats, cholesterol, sodium, and sugar can help prevent atherosclerosis, which can lead to RAS. Most sodium in the diet comes from salt. A healthy diet that prevents people from becoming overweight or developing obesity can also help prevent atherosclerosis. People with RAS that has caused decreased kidney function should limit their intake of protein, cholesterol, sodium, and potassium to slow the progression of kidney failure.[1]

[1] "Renal Artery Stenosis," National Institute of Diabetes and Digestive and Kidney Diseases (NIDDK), July 2014. Available online. URL: www.niddk.nih.gov/health-information/kidney-disease/renal-artery-stenosis. Accessed May 24, 2023.

Chapter 37 | Vasculitis

Chapter Contents

Vasculitis, also known as "angiitis" or "arteritis," includes a group of rare conditions that can occur when swelling affects the walls of your blood vessels. Swelling is your body's response to tissue injury. Autoimmune disorders or diseases that make your body attack itself, infections, and trauma are some examples of potential causes of swelling in the blood vessels. Swelling in the blood vessels can lead to serious problems, including organ damage and aneurysms, a bulge in the wall of a blood vessel.

TYPES OF VASCULITIS

The following are a few types of vasculitis:

- **Antiglomerular basement membrane disease**. This disease affects blood vessels in the lungs and kidneys.
- **Behçet disease**. This disease can cause damage to many areas of your body.
- **Buerger disease**. Also known as "thromboangiitis obliterans," Buerger disease usually affects blood flow to the arms and legs.
- **Central nervous system (CNS) vasculitis**. Also called "primary angiitis," this vasculitis affects the blood vessels in the CNS, or the brain and spinal cord. This type of vasculitis may also occur as the result of another type of vasculitis.
- **Cogan syndrome**. This syndrome is an autoimmune disorder associated with a particular type of vasculitis that affects the whole body.
- **Cryoglobulinemic vasculitis**. This vasculitis affects the small blood vessels. It prevents proper blood flow and causes pain and damage to the skin, joints, peripheral nerves, kidneys, and liver.
- **Eosinophilic granulomatosis with polyangiitis**. Also known as "Churg-Strauss syndrome," this disease often affects the respiratory tract.

- **Giant cell arteritis (GCA)**. GCA mostly affects the aorta or its major branches. The condition often affects the temporal artery in the head.
- **Granulomatosis with polyangiitis**. This type usually affects the nose and throat area, lungs, and kidneys.
- **Hypersensitivity vasculitis**. It affects the skin. This condition is also known as "allergic vasculitis," "cutaneous vasculitis," or "leukocytoclastic vasculitis."
- **Hypocomplementemic urticarial vasculitis**. This type of vasculitis is associated with swelling in the small blood vessels and low levels of complement proteins, which affect the body's ability to develop defenses against infection.
- **Immunoglobulin A (IgA) vasculitis**. Also known as "Henoch-Schönlein purpura," this is one of the most common types of vasculitis in children but can also affect adults. It develops when IgA, which is a type of antibody that usually helps defend the body against infections, builds up in blood vessels in the skin, joints, intestines, and kidneys.
- **Kawasaki disease**. This disease is a rare childhood disease that develops when the walls of the blood vessels throughout the body swell. Kawasaki disease is also known as "mucocutaneous lymph node syndrome."
- **Microscopic polyangiitis**. This vasculitis affects small blood vessels, often including those in the kidneys and lungs.
- **Polyarteritis nodosa**. This type causes swelling and damage, most often to medium-sized arteries. This type of vasculitis may cause muscle pain or symptoms related to the stomach or intestines, such as heartburn.
- **Takayasu arteritis**. This arteritis most often affects the aorta and its branches. The condition can also affect medium-sized arteries.

CAUSES OF VASCULITIS

Vasculitis occurs when your immune system hurts your blood vessels by mistake. What causes this to happen is not fully known, but when it occurs, your blood vessels swell and can narrow or close off. Rarely, the blood vessel wall may weaken, causing it to expand or bulge. This bulge is known as an "aneurysm."

WHAT ARE THE RISK FACTORS FOR VASCULITIS?
Age
Vasculitis can happen at any age. However, some types of vasculitis are more common among people of certain ages:
- Buerger disease usually affects men younger than 45 who smoke or have smoked.
- IgA vasculitis is diagnosed more often in children than adults.
- GCA affects adults 50 years and older and is most common in people who are in their 70s and 80s.
- Kawasaki disease affects only children and is most common under the age of five.

Family History
The following types of vasculitis may run in families:
- Behçet disease
- granulomatosis with polyangiitis
- Kawasaki disease

Lifestyle Habits
- Smoking raises your risk of vasculitis.
- Using illegal drugs, such as cocaine, also raises your risk.

Medicines
The risk of vasculitis is higher if you take certain medicines, including:
- hydralazine, used to treat high blood pressure
- levamisole, used for infections but also added to most cocaine
- propylthiouracil, used to treat some thyroid disorders

- tumor necrosis factor inhibitors, a treatment for some immune diseases

Other Medical Conditions
- autoimmune disorders, such as lupus, rheumatoid arthritis, and scleroderma
- hepatitis B or C, infections that sometimes trigger vasculitis inflammation
- lymphoma, a cancer of the blood

Race or Ethnicity
- Behçet disease is most common in Turkey and is relatively common in other countries in the Mediterranean, the Middle East, Central Asia, China, and Japan. It is relatively uncommon in Northern and Western Europe and the United States.
- GCA is most common in Scandinavia and Minnesota.
- Kawasaki disease is more common among children of Japanese descent.

Sex
- Behçet disease is more common in men in some countries and more common in women in other countries.
- Buerger disease is more common in men.
- GCA affects women two to four times more often than men.
- Microscopic polyangiitis affects men slightly more often than women.

SYMPTOMS OF VASCULITIS
The symptoms of vasculitis are different depending on the type of vasculitis you have, the blood vessels and organs involved, and whether your condition is serious. Some people may have few symptoms. Other people may become very sick.

Sometimes, the symptoms develop slowly over months. The symptoms may also develop very quickly over days or weeks. Not

everyone will experience the common symptoms below. Some people will experience some, but not all of them. General symptoms of vasculitis include:
- tiredness
- fever
- general aches and pains
- loss of appetite
- weight loss

Others may experience common, more specific problems that are caused by vasculitis.

What Problems Can Vasculitis Cause?
- Ear and nose problems, including sinus infections, inner ear infections, open sores in the nose, a runny nose, dizziness, ringing in the ears, hearing loss, and deafness, may occur.
- Eye problems, including redness, itching, burning, and changes in vision, may also occur. Blindness in one eye may be the first sign of GCA. The risk of blindness with GCA is higher for people who have had a stroke or have peripheral artery disease (PAD).
- Gastrointestinal tract problems, such as open sores in the mouth or stomach area, diarrhea, vomiting blood, and pain in the stomach area, are also sometimes caused by vasculitis.
- Genital ulcers, which are open sores in the genital area, may also occur.
- Headache, scalp tenderness, and pain may develop after chewing.
- Heart palpitations, or the feeling that your heart is racing, can occur with vasculitis.
- Joint pain is another common condition caused by vasculitis.
- Lung problems, including shortness of breath, bleeding within the lung, and coughing up blood, may also occur when you have vasculitis.

- Nerve problems, including numbness, tingling, pain, and weakness in various parts of the body, can occur. Loss of strength in the hands and feet and shooting pains in the arms and legs can also occur with vasculitis.
- Skin rashes, purple or red spots or bumps, clusters of small dots, splotches, bruises, hives, and itching also sometimes develop.
- Problems with the hands and feet, including swelling or hardening of the palms and soles or pain, ulcers, and gangrene, can show up in some people.
- Swollen, dry lips or tongue or swelling in the mouth and throat may occur.
- Problems during pregnancy can develop if a person has vasculitis.

Blood vessels damaged by vasculitis can narrow and block normal blood flow, which may cause problems in other parts of the body. Some problems can be life-threatening. They include:

- aneurysm or a tear inside the aorta called an "aortic dissection"
- arrhythmia
- coronary heart disease (CHD)
- deep vein thrombosis (DVT), a type of venous thromboembolism
- heart attack
- high blood pressure
- low blood pressure
- kidney disease
- myocarditis, a type of heart inflammation
- stroke and transient ischemic attack (TIA, which, also known as a "ministroke," occurs if blood flow to a part of the brain is blocked only for a short time. A TIA may happen and may develop into a stroke later.)

DIAGNOSIS OF VASCULITIS

Your health-care provider may be able to diagnose the type of vasculitis that you have and how serious it is. Depending on your symptoms, your provider may recommend you see a specialist for more tests or procedures.

TREATMENT FOR VASCULITIS

The goal of treatment is usually to reduce inflammation. People who have mild vasculitis may find relief with over-the-counter (OTC) pain medicines. For severe vasculitis, you may receive prescription medicines. With treatment, vasculitis can go into remission, which is a period of time when you do not have symptoms.

PREVENTION OF VASCULITIS

Some types of vasculitis cannot be prevented, as they are caused by autoimmune disorders. However, depending on what caused the vasculitis, some types can be prevented from flaring up.

Medicines may be used to reduce the symptoms of vasculitis.

- Anticlotting medicines treat blood clots or prevent blood clots from forming. You may need them if you have an aneurysm.
- Beta-blockers lower blood pressure. You may need them if you have an aneurysm.
- Statins control or lower high blood cholesterol levels.

Healthy lifestyle changes may also be recommended.

- Adopt a heart-healthy lifestyle.
- Avoid illegal drugs, including cocaine. If you use illegal or street drugs, ask your provider how to get help to stop. You can also call the National Helpline of the Substance Abuse and Mental Health Services Administration (SAMHSA) at 1-800-662-HELP.
- Quit smoking and tobacco. Visit the Smoking and Your Heart web page (https://www.nhlbi.nih.gov/health/heart/smoking) and the National Heart, Lung, and Blood Institute's Your Guide to a Healthy Heart web page (https://www.nhlbi.nih.gov/resources/your-guide-healthy-heart). Although these resources focus on heart health, they include basic information about how to quit

smoking. For free help and support to quit smoking, you may call the National Cancer Institute's Smoking Quitline at 1-877-44U-QUIT (1-877-448-7848).[1]

Section 37.2 | Kawasaki Disease

WHAT IS KAWASAKI DISEASE?

Kawasaki disease (KD) is a rare illness that usually affects small children. It is also called "Kawasaki syndrome" or "mucocutaneous lymph node syndrome." It is a type of vasculitis, which is inflammation of the blood vessels. KD is serious, but most children can fully recover if they are treated right away.

WHAT CAUSES KAWASAKI DISEASE?

Kawasaki disease happens when the immune system injures the blood vessels by mistake. Researchers do not fully know why this happens. But, when it does, the blood vessels become inflamed and can narrow or close off.

Genetics may play a role in KD. There may also be environmental factors, such as infections. It does not seem to be contagious. This means that it cannot be passed from one child to another.

WHO IS AT RISK OF KAWASAKI DISEASE?

Kawasaki disease usually affects children under the age of five. But older children and adults can sometimes get it. It is more common in boys than girls. It can affect children of any race, but those of Asian or Pacific Islander descent are more likely to get it.

---

[1] "Vasculitis," National Heart, Lung, and Blood Institute (NHLBI), March 24, 2022. Available online. URL: www.nhlbi.nih.gov/health/vasculitis. Accessed June 16, 2023.

WHAT ARE THE SYMPTOMS OF KAWASAKI DISEASE?

The symptoms of KD may include:
- high fever lasting at least five days
- a rash, often on the back, chest, and groin
- swollen hands and feet
- redness of the lips, lining of the mouth, tongue, palms of the hand, and soles of the feet
- pink eye
- swollen lymph nodes

WHAT OTHER PROBLEMS CAN KAWASAKI DISEASE CAUSE?

Sometimes, KD can affect the walls of the coronary arteries. These arteries supply blood and oxygen to your heart. This can lead to:
- an aneurysm (bulging and thinning of the walls of the arteries; this can raise the risk of blood clots in the arteries. If the blood clots are not treated, they could lead to a heart attack or internal bleeding.)
- inflammation in the heart
- heart valve problems

KD can also affect other parts of the body, including the brain and nervous system, the immune system, and the digestive system.

HOW IS KAWASAKI DISEASE DIAGNOSED?

There is no specific test for KD. To make a diagnosis, your child's health-care provider may use many tools:
- a physical exam, which includes looking at the signs and symptoms
- blood and urine tests to rule out other diseases and check for signs of inflammation
- tests to check for damage to the heart, such as an echocardiogram and electrocardiogram (EKG)

WHAT ARE THE TREATMENTS FOR KAWASAKI DISEASE?

Kawasaki disease is usually treated in the hospital with an intravenous (IV) dose of immunoglobulin (IVIG). Aspirin may also be part of the treatment. But do not give your child aspirin unless the health-care provider tells you to. Aspirin can cause Reye syndrome in children. This is a rare, serious illness that can affect the brain and liver.

Usually, treatment works. But, if it is not working well enough, the provider may also give your child other medicines to fight the inflammation. If the disease affects your child's heart, he or she might need additional medicines, surgery, or other medical procedures.[2]

Section 37.3 | **Behçet Disease**

Behçet disease is an inflammatory condition that affects many parts of the body. The health problems associated with Behçet disease result from widespread inflammation of blood vessels (vasculitis). This inflammation most commonly affects small blood vessels in the mouth, genitals, skin, and eyes.

CAUSES OF BEHÇET DISEASE

The cause of Behçet disease is unknown. The condition probably results from a combination of genetic and environmental factors, most of which have not been identified. However, a particular variation in the *HLA-B* gene has been associated with the risk of developing Behçet disease.

The *HLA-B* gene provides instructions for making a protein that plays an important role in the immune system. The *HLA-B* gene is part of a family of genes called the "human leukocyte antigen" (HLA) complex. The HLA complex helps the immune system distinguish the body's own proteins from proteins made by foreign invaders (such as viruses and bacteria). The *HLA-B* gene has many different normal variations, allowing each person's immune system to react to a wide range of foreign proteins. A variation of the

---

[2] MedlinePlus, "Kawasaki Disease," National Institutes of Health (NIH), June 20, 2021. Available online. URL: https://medlineplus.gov/kawasakidisease.html. Accessed May 23, 2023.

HLA-B gene called "*HLA-B51*" increases the risk of developing Behçet disease by about a factor of six although the mechanism is not well understood. One-third to two-thirds of people with Behçet disease have the *HLA-B51* variation, but most people with this version of the *HLA-B* gene never develop the disorder.

Other genetic and environmental factors likely contribute to the risk of Behçet disease. Researchers are studying several genes related to immune system function. It also appears likely that environmental factors, such as certain bacterial or viral infections, play a role in triggering the disease in people who are at risk. However, the influence of genetic and environmental factors on the development of this complex disorder remains unclear.

SIGNS AND SYMPTOMS OF BEHÇET DISEASE

Painful mouth sores called "aphthous ulcers" are usually the first sign of Behçet disease. These sores can occur on the lips, tongue, roof of the mouth, throat, and tonsils and inside the cheeks. The ulcers look like common canker sores, and they typically heal within one to two weeks. About 75 percent of all people with Behçet disease develop similar ulcers on the genitals. These ulcers occur most frequently on the scrotum in men and on the labia in women.

Behçet disease can also cause painful bumps and sores on the skin. Most affected individuals develop pus-filled bumps that resemble acne. These bumps can occur anywhere on the body. Some affected people also have red, tender nodules called "erythema nodosum." These nodules usually develop on the legs but can also occur on the arms, face, and neck.

An inflammation of the eye called "uveitis" is found in more than half of people with Behçet disease. Eye problems are more common in younger people with the disease and affect men more often than women. Uveitis can result in blurry vision and an extreme sensitivity to light (photophobia). Rarely, inflammation can also cause eye pain and redness. If untreated, the eye problems associated with Behçet disease can lead to blindness.

Joint involvement is also common in Behçet disease. Often, this affects one joint at a time, with each affected joint becoming swollen and painful and then getting better.

Less commonly, Behçet disease can affect the brain and spinal cord (central nervous system (CNS)), gastrointestinal (GI) tract, large blood vessels, heart, lungs, and kidneys. CNS abnormalities can lead to headaches, confusion, personality changes, memory loss, impaired speech, and problems with balance and movement. Involvement of the GI tract can lead to a hole in the wall of the intestine (intestinal perforation), which can cause serious infection and may be life-threatening.

The signs and symptoms of Behçet disease usually begin in a person's 20s or 30s although they can appear at any age. Some affected people have relatively mild symptoms that are limited to sores in the mouth and on the genitals. Others have more severe symptoms affecting various parts of the body, including the eyes and the vital organs. The features of Behçet disease typically come and go over a period of months or years. In most affected individuals, the health problems associated with this disorder improve with age.

FREQUENCY OF BEHÇET DISEASE

Behçet disease is most common in Mediterranean countries, the Middle East, Japan, and other parts of Asia. However, it has been found in populations worldwide.

The highest prevalence of Behçet disease has been reported in northern Turkey, where the disorder affects up to 420 in 100,000 people. The disorder is rare in northern European countries and the United States, where it generally affects fewer than 1 in 100,000 people.

INHERITANCE OF BEHÇET DISEASE

Most cases of Behçet disease are sporadic, which means they occur in people with no history of the disorder in their family. A small percentage of all cases have been reported to run in families; however, the condition does not have a clear pattern of inheritance.[3]

[3] MedlinePlus, "Behçet Disease," National Institutes of Health (NIH), June 1, 2017. Available online. URL: https://medlineplus.gov/genetics/condition/behcet-disease. Accessed May 23, 2023.

Section 37.4 | **Other Types of Vasculitis**

Polyarteritis nodosa (PAN) and Takayasu arteritis are types of vasculitis that affect the medium-sized arteries in the body.

POLYARTERITIS NODOSA

Polyarteritis nodosa is a blood vessel disease characterized by inflammation of small and medium-sized arteries (vasculitis), preventing them from bringing oxygen and food to organs.

When Does Polyarteritis Nodosa Occur?

Most cases occur in the fourth or fifth decade of life although it can occur at any age. PAN most commonly affects vessels related to the skin, joints, peripheral nerves, gastrointestinal tract, heart, eyes, and kidneys.

Symptoms of Polyarteritis Nodosa

Symptoms are caused by damage to affected organs and may include fever, fatigue, weakness, loss of appetite, weight loss, muscle and joint aches, rashes, numbness, and abdominal pain.

Cause of Polyarteritis Nodosa

The underlying cause of PAN is unknown.[4]

TAKAYASU ARTERITIS

Takayasu arteritis is a condition that causes inflammation of the main blood vessel that carries blood from the heart to the rest of the body (aorta) and its associated branched blood vessels. As a result of the inflammation, the blood vessel walls become thick and make it difficult for blood to flow. Over time, impaired blood flow causes damage to the heart and various other organs of the body.

---

[4] Genetic and Rare Diseases Information Center (GARD), "Polyarteritis Nodosa," National Center for Advancing Translational Sciences (NCATS), February 2023. Available online. URL: https://rarediseases.info.nih.gov/diseases/7360/polyarteritis-nodosa. Accessed May 23, 2023.

When Do Symptoms of Takayasu Arteritis Begin?

Symptoms of this disease may start to appear as a teenager and as an adult.

Symptoms of Takayasu Arteritis

The following symptoms have been linked to Takayasu arteritis:
- abnormal heart valve morphology (any structural abnormality of a cardiac valve)
- arterial stenosis (narrowing or constriction of the inner surface (lumen) of an artery)
- fatigue
- hyperhidrosis (abnormal excessive perspiration (sweating) despite the lack of appropriate stimuli, such as hot and humid weather)
- subcutaneous nodule (slightly elevated lesions on or in the skin with a diameter of over 5 mm)
- vascular dilatation (abnormal outpouching or sac-like dilatation in the wall of an artery, vein, or heart)
- vasculitis
- weight loss
- abnormal aortic valve morphology
- abnormal pattern of respiration
- anemia
- anorexia (a lack or loss of appetite for food (as a medical condition))
- arthritis (inflammation of a joint)
- ascending tubular aorta aneurysm (an abnormal localized widening (dilatation) of the tubular part of the ascending aorta)
- chest pain
- gangrene (a serious and potentially life-threatening condition that arises when a considerable mass of body tissue dies (necrosis))
- hypertension
- hypertrophic cardiomyopathy (HCM, which is defined by the presence of increased ventricular wall

thickness or mass in the absence of loading conditions (hypertension, valve disease) sufficient to cause the observed abnormality.)
- increased inflammatory response (an abnormal increase in the inflammatory response to injury or infection)
- inflammatory abnormality of the eye (inflammation of the eye, parts of the eye, or the periorbital region)
- migraine
- muscle weakness
- myalgia (pain in muscle)
- myocardial infarction (necrosis of the myocardium caused by an obstruction of the blood supply to the heart and often associated with chest pain, shortness of breath, palpitations, and anxiety, as well as characteristic electrocardiogram (EKG) findings and elevation of serum markers, including creatine kinase–myocardial band fraction and troponin)
- pulmonary arterial hypertension (Pulmonary hypertension is defined as a mean pulmonary artery pressure of 25 mm Hg or more and pulmonary capillary wedge pressure of 15 mm Hg or less when measured by right heart catheterization at rest and in a supine position.)
- seizure
- skin ulcer
- abnormal endocardium morphology (an abnormality of the endocardium)
- amaurosis fugax (a transient visual disturbance that is typically caused by a circulatory, ocular, or neurological underlying condition)
- arthralgia (joint pain)
- hemoptysis (coughing up (expectoration) of blood or blood-streaked sputum from the larynx, trachea, bronchi, or lungs)
- retinopathy (any noninflammatory disease of the retina)

- hypertensive crisis
- cerebral ischemia
- gastrointestinal infractions
- neurological speech impairment
- reduced consciousness/confusion

Cause of Takayasu Arteritis

Although the cause remains unknown, Takayasu arteritis appears to be an autoimmune condition in which cells that fight infection and disease are wrongly targeted against the body's own tissues.[5]

---

[5] Genetic and Rare Diseases Information Center (GARD), "Takayasu Arteritis," National Center for Advancing Translational Sciences (NCATS), February 2023. Available online. URL: https://rarediseases.info.nih.gov/diseases/7730/takayasu-arteritis. Accessed May 23, 2023.

Chapter 38 | Giant Cell Arteritis

Giant cell arteritis (GCA) is a form of vasculitis, a group of disorders that cause inflammation of blood vessels. GCA most commonly affects the arteries of the head (especially the temporal arteries, located on each side of the head), but arteries in other areas of the body can also become inflamed. The inflammation causes the arteries to narrow, resulting in poor blood flow. The cause of GCA is still being studied, but it is thought to involve the immune system mistakenly attacking the artery walls. Several genetic and environmental factors may increase a person's risk of developing GCA. GCA may develop with or after another inflammatory disorder known as "polymyalgia rheumatica."[1]

WHO GETS GIANT CELL ARTERITIS?

You are more likely to get GCA if you have certain risk factors that include the following:

- **Age**. GCA occurs almost exclusively in people older than age 50, typically in people in their late 60s and in their 70s.
- **Sex**. Women get this disorder more frequently than men.
- **Ethnic and racial background**. GCA is more common in Caucasians, especially people of Northern European ancestry but is also observed in patients of other ethnic and racial backgrounds.

[1] Genetic and Rare Diseases Information Center (GARD), "Giant Cell Arteritis," National Center for Advancing Translational Sciences (NCATS), February 16, 2023. Available online. URL: https://rarediseases.info.nih.gov/diseases/9615/giant-cell-arteritis. Accessed May 23, 2023.

CAUSES OF GIANT CELL ARTERITIS
Inflammation causes GCA, but scientists do not know what triggers it. Some studies have linked certain gene variants with the disorders, but these genetic links have not been consistent across different populations. Because the disorder occurs in older people, the aging process may contribute to the disease onset.

SYMPTOMS OF GIANT CELL ARTERITIS
Symptoms of GCA include the following:
- **Headaches and scalp tenderness**. These are the most common symptoms. The headache pain may be severe and is usually located in the temple areas. Some people notice tenderness of the scalp, often prior to the onset of headaches.
- **Jaw pain**. People sometimes experience jaw pain, especially when chewing.
- **Visual disturbances**. Many people have episodes of double vision or vision loss in one or both eyes. At first, the visual disturbances may last only a few minutes and resolve on their own. It is important to see a health-care provider right away if you develop visual symptoms because, if left untreated, they can lead to permanent vision loss within hours or days.
- **Flu-like symptoms**. These include low-grade fever, weakness, loss of appetite, and weight loss.
- **Arteric aneurysms**. Large artery involvement, including inflammation of the aorta and its major branches, can lead to bulging of the artery (aneurysms) or, due to blockages in the arteries, cause cramping or aching pain in the arms or legs with activity. At times, inflammation of the aorta does not cause any symptoms but is detected by chance in imaging studies (such as computed tomography (CT) or magnetic resonance imaging (MRI)).

In most people, symptoms of GCA develop over the course of weeks or months, but in some cases, the onset is more abrupt. It is important to seek treatment right away if you have visual symptoms because, if left untreated, they may potentially lead to permanent blindness. Some people may have only large artery involvement (such as the aorta) and not have any symptoms in the head or scalp; these people may experience flu-like symptoms or no symptoms at all. GCA is also known as "temporal arteritis" and "Horton disease."

GCA generally responds well to treatment although it is common for symptoms to recur after decreasing or stopping therapy.

DIAGNOSIS OF GIANT CELL ARTERITIS

There is no single test to tell if you have GCA. The doctors usually do the following:

- **Take your medical history and perform a physical exam**. He or she will likely examine the temporal arteries for evidence of swelling or tenderness and signs of GCA.
- **Order blood tests**. They include the erythrocyte sedimentation rate (ESR) or "sed" rate and the C-reactive protein (CRP) test. These tests are to measure inflammation, but they are not specific to GCA. They can indicate any inflammatory disorder.

The doctors may also do the following:

- **Obtain a biopsy of the temporal artery if GCA is suspected**. The procedure is performed using local anesthetic. A pathologist will examine the sample under a microscope and look for signs of inflammation.
- **Order imaging tests**. An ultrasound, positron emission tomography (PET), CT, or MRI scan can reveal changes consistent with the disorders, such as swelling and inflammation in large vessels, or may help rule out other diseases and conditions.
- **Request consultation from specialists**. If visual symptoms are occurring, consult an ophthalmologist.

TREATMENT FOR GIANT CELL ARTERITIS

The primary goal of treatment for GCA is to alleviate symptoms and prevent vision loss and other potential complications.

GCA is primarily treated with the following:

- **Corticosteroids**. These anti-inflammatory medications are a mainstay of treatment for both disorders. Doctors usually prescribe high doses for GCA. Most people respond to these medications within days to weeks, and once symptoms resolve, the dosage is usually gradually decreased. You may remain on a maintenance dose for a year or possibly longer. Because these are potent drugs, your doctor will prescribe the lowest dose possible to achieve the desired benefit.

Other medications your doctor may prescribe include the following:

- **Disease-modifying antirheumatic drugs (DMARDs)**. These medications, approved for other conditions, are small molecules that act on inflammation at the cellular level. Doctors may prescribe them in combination with corticosteroids, especially in people who experience side effects from these medications, to quell a flare of symptoms.
- **Biologic response modifiers**. These medications, which are also DMARDs, target specific immune messages and interrupt the signal, helping to decrease or stop inflammation. They are sometimes prescribed in combination with corticosteroids in people with GCA.

Osteoporosis, a condition characterized by weak and brittle bones, can be a complication of taking corticosteroids, so your doctor may also prescribe medications to strengthen the bones.[2]

---

[2] "Polymyalgia Rheumatica and Giant Cell Arteritis," National Institute of Arthritis and Musculoskeletal and Skin Diseases (NIAMS), February 1, 2022. Available online. URL: www.niams.nih.gov/health-topics/polymyalgia-rheumatica-giant-cell-arteritis. Accessed May 23, 2023.

Chapter 39 | **Venous Disorders**

Chapter Contents

Section 39.1 | **Arteriovenous Malformations**

WHAT ARE ARTERIOVENOUS MALFORMATIONS?

Arteriovenous malformations (AVMs) are abnormal, snarled tangles of blood vessels that cause multiple irregular connections between your arteries and veins. These malformations most often occur in the spinal cord and in any part of your brain or on its surface but can develop elsewhere in the body.

Normally, arteries carry oxygen-rich blood away from your heart to the body's cells, organs, and tissues; veins return blood with less oxygen to the lungs and heart. But in AVMs, the absence of capillaries—a network of small blood vessels that connect arteries to veins and deliver oxygen to cells—creates a shortcut for blood to pass directly from arteries to veins and bypass tissue, which can lead to tissue damage and the death of nerve cells and other cells. Over time, some AVMs get progressively larger as the amount of blood flow increases.

In most cases, people with neurological AVMs experience few, if any, significant symptoms. In some cases, a weakened blood vessel may burst, spilling blood into the brain (hemorrhage) that can cause stroke and brain damage. Most malformations tend to be discovered only incidentally, usually during treatment for an unrelated disorder or at autopsy.

Treatment options depend on your type of AVM, its location, noticeable symptoms, and your general health.

Symptoms, which vary greatly in severity, may include the following:

- **Seizures**. They can be focal (meaning they involve a small part of the brain) or generalized (widespread), involving convulsions, a loss of control over movement, or a change in your level of consciousness. No particular type of seizure has been identified.
- **Headache**. They can vary greatly in frequency, duration, and intensity, sometimes becoming as severe as migraines. No specific pattern of headache has been identified.

529

- **Pain**. You may have pain on either one side of the head or on both sides. Sometimes, a headache consistently affecting one side of the head may be closely linked to the site of an AVM. Most often, the location of the pain is not specific to the malformation and may encompass most of the head. Back pain in the lower extremities may be caused by a spinal AVM.
- **Visual problems**. An AVM can cause problems such as a loss of part of the visual field, inability to control eye movement, or swelling of a part of the optic nerve.
- **Muscle weakness**. You may have muscle weakness or paralysis in one part of your body.
- **Problems with speech**. A neurological AVM can cause difficulty speaking or understanding language (aphasia).
- **Problems with movement**. You may notice a loss of coordination (ataxia) that can lead to problems such as gait disturbances (your manner of walking).
- **Abnormal sensations**. You may feel sensations such as numbness, tingling, or spontaneous pain.

AVMs can also cause a wide range of more specific neurological symptoms that vary from person to person, depending primarily upon the location of the AVM. Such symptoms may include the following:
- difficulties carrying out tasks that require planning (apraxia)
- dizziness
- loss of consciousness
- memory deficits
- subtle learning or behavioral disorders during childhood or adolescence
- confusion, hallucinations, or dementia

Symptoms caused by AVMs can appear at any age. Because the abnormalities tend to result from a slow buildup of neurological damage over time, they are most often noticed when people are in their 20s or older. If AVMs do not become symptomatic by the time people reach their late 40s or early 50s, they tend to remain stable and are less likely to produce symptoms. Some pregnant women may experience a sudden onset or worsening of symptoms due to accompanying cardiovascular changes, especially increases in blood volume and blood pressure.

Although most neurological AVMs have very few, if any, significant symptoms, one particularly severe type of AVM causes symptoms to appear at, or very soon after, birth. Called a "vein of Galen defect" (named after the major blood vessel involved), this lesion is located deep inside the brain. It is frequently associated with hydrocephalus (an accumulation of fluid within certain spaces in the brain, often with visible enlargement of the head), swollen veins visible on the scalp, seizures, failure to thrive, and congestive heart failure. Children born with this condition who survive past infancy often remain developmentally impaired.

How Do Arteriovenous Malformations Damage the Brain and Spinal Cord?

AVMs damage the brain or spinal cord through three basic mechanisms: by reducing the amount of oxygen reaching neurological tissues, by causing bleeding (hemorrhage) into surrounding tissues, and by compressing or displacing parts of the brain or spinal cord.

- AVMs affect oxygen delivery to the brain or spinal cord by altering normal patterns of blood flow using the arteries, veins, and capillaries. In AVMs, arteries pump blood directly into veins through a passageway called a "fistula," rather than using the network of tiny vessels called "capillaries," which help the blood flow to slow down. The uncontrolled blood flow into the veins is too rapid to allow oxygen and nutrients to be distributed to surrounding tissues, causing the cells that make up these tissues to become oxygen-depleted and begin to deteriorate, sometimes dying off completely.
- This abnormally rapid rate of blood flow frequently causes blood pressure inside the vessels to rise to dangerously high levels. The arteries feeding blood into the AVM often become swollen and distorted;

the veins that drain blood away from it often become abnormally constricted (a condition called "stenosis"). Also, the walls of the involved arteries and veins are often abnormally thin and weak. This can cause aneurysms—balloon-like bulges in blood vessel walls that are susceptible to bursting—to develop.

- Bleeding into the brain, called "intracranial hemorrhage," can result from the combination of high internal pressure and vessel wall weakness. Such hemorrhages are often microscopic in size (called "microbleeds") and cause limited damage and few significant symptoms. Generally, microbleeds do not have short-term consequences on brain function, but microbleeds, over time, can lead to an increased risk of dementia and cognitive disruption. But massive hemorrhages can occur if the physical stresses caused by extremely high blood pressure, rapid blood flow rates, and vessel wall weakness are great enough. A burst aneurysm can release a large volume of blood into the surrounding brain and cause a catastrophic stroke. AVMs account for approximately 2 percent of all hemorrhagic strokes that occur each year.

- Large AVMs can press on the surrounding brain or spinal cord structures and cause damage. They can range in size from a fraction of an inch to more than 2.5 inches in diameter, depending on the number and size of the blood vessels making up the lesion. The largest lesions may compress several inches of the spinal cord or distort the shape of an entire hemisphere (one-half) of the brain. Massive AVMs can also constrict the flow of cerebrospinal fluid (CSF)—a clear liquid that normally nourishes and protects the brain and spinal cord—by distorting or closing the passageways and open chambers (ventricles) inside the brain that allow this fluid to circulate freely. The buildup of CSF can cause hydrocephalus and further increase the amount of pressure on fragile neurological structures, adding to the damage caused by the AVM itself.

AVMs can form virtually anywhere in the brain or spinal cord—wherever arteries and veins exist. Some are formed from blood vessels located in the dura mater or in the pia mater, the outermost and innermost membrane, respectively, of the three membranes surrounding the brain and spinal cord. (The third membrane, called the "arachnoid," lacks blood vessels.)

Arteriovenous Malformations in the Spinal Cord

AVMs can affect how the spinal cord functions by causing hemorrhage, reducing blood flow to the spinal cord, or causing excess pressure in the blood vessels. Spinal AVMs frequently cause attacks of sudden, severe back pain and can also cause sensory disturbances, muscle weakness, or paralysis in the parts of the body served by the spinal cord or the damaged nerve fibers. A spinal cord AVM can lead to degeneration of the nerve fibers within the spinal cord below the level of the lesion, causing widespread paralysis in parts of the body controlled by those nerve fibers.

Arteriovenous Malformations in the Brain

AVMs on the surface of the cerebral hemispheres—the uppermost portions of the brain—exert pressure on the cerebral cortex, the brain's "gray matter" that is made up mostly of nerve cells. AVMs may damage portions of the cerebral cortex involved with thinking, speaking, understanding language, hearing, taste, touch, or initiating and controlling voluntary movements. AVMs located on the frontal lobe close to the optic nerve or on the occipital lobe (the rear portion of the cerebrum where images are processed) may cause a variety of visual disturbances.

AVMs can also form from blood vessels located deep inside the interior of the cerebrum (the main portion of the brain). These AVMs may compromise the functions of three vital structures: the thalamus, which transmits nerve signals between the spinal cord and upper regions of the brain; the basal ganglia surrounding the thalamus, which coordinate complex movements and play a role in learning and memory; and the hippocampus, which plays a major role in memory.

AVMs can affect other parts of the brain besides the cerebrum. The hindbrain is formed from two major structures: the cerebellum, which is nestled under the rear portion of the cerebrum, and the brain stem, which serves as the bridge linking the upper portions of the brain with the spinal cord. These structures control finely coordinated movements, maintain balance, and regulate some functions of internal organs, including those of the heart and lungs. AVM damage to these parts of the hindbrain can result in dizziness, giddiness, vomiting, a loss of the ability to coordinate complex movements, such as walking, or uncontrollable muscle tremors.

Health Consequences of Arteriovenous Malformations

The greatest potential danger posed by AVMs is hemorrhage. Most episodes of bleeding remain undetected at the time they occur because they are not severe enough to cause significant neurological damage. But massive, even fatal, bleeding episodes do occur.

A few physical characteristics appear to indicate a greater-than-usual likelihood of clinically significant hemorrhage:

- Smaller AVMs have a greater likelihood of bleeding than larger ones.
- Impaired drainage by unusually narrow or deeply situated veins increases the chances of hemorrhage.
- Pregnancy appears to increase the likelihood of clinically significant hemorrhage, mainly because of increases in blood pressure and blood volume.
- AVMs that have hemorrhaged once are about nine times more likely to bleed again during the first year after the initial hemorrhage than are lesions that have never bled.

Bleeding from AVMs located deep inside the interior tissues of the brain typically causes more severe neurological damage than hemorrhage by lesions that have formed in the membranes or on the surface of the brain or spinal cord. (Deeply located bleeding is usually referred to as an intracerebral or parenchymal hemorrhage; bleeding within the membranes or on the surface of the brain is known as "subdural" or "subarachnoid hemorrhage.")

Other Vascular Lesions That Affect the Central Nervous System

Besides AVMs, the following three are the other main types of vascular lesions that can arise anywhere in the brain or spinal cord. Unlike AVMs, these lesions involve only one type of blood vessel and do not pose the same relatively high risk of significant hemorrhage. In general, low blood flow lesions tend to cause fewer troubling neurological symptoms and require less aggressive treatment than AVMs.

- **Cavernous malformations**. These are formed from groups of tightly packed, abnormally thin-walled, small blood vessels that displace normal neurological tissue in the brain or spinal cord. The vessels are filled with slow-moving or stagnant blood that is usually clotted or in a state of decomposition. Like AVMs, cavernous malformations can range in size from a few fractions of an inch to several inches in diameter, depending on the number of blood vessels involved. Some people develop multiple lesions. Cavernous malformations sometimes leak blood into surrounding tissues because the walls of the involved blood vessels are extremely fragile. They can cause seizures in some people. After AVMs, cavernous malformations are the type of vascular lesion most likely to require treatment.

- **Capillary telangiectases**. These are groups of abnormally swollen capillaries and usually measure less than an inch in diameter. They are usually benign and rarely cause extensive damage to surrounding brain or spinal cord tissues. Any isolated hemorrhages that occur are microscopic in size. However, in some inherited disorders in which people develop large numbers of these lesions, telangiectases can contribute to the development of headaches or seizures.

535

- **Venous malformations**. These consist of abnormally enlarged veins. They usually do not interfere with the function of the blood vessels and rarely hemorrhage. Most venous malformations do not produce symptoms and remain undetected.

WHO IS MORE LIKELY TO GET ARTERIOVENOUS MALFORMATIONS?

It is unclear why AVMs form. Most often, AVMs are congenital (you are born with them), but they can appear shortly after birth or later in life. In some cases, the AVM may be inherited, but it is more likely that other inherited conditions increase the risk of having an AVM. It is estimated that brain AVMs occur in less than 1 percent of the general population; each year, about 1 percent of those with AVMs will die as a direct result of the AVM.

Causes of Vascular Lesions

The cause of vascular anomalies of the central nervous system (CNS) is not yet well understood. Scientists believe the anomalies most often result from mistakes that occur during embryonic or fetal development. These mistakes may be linked to genetic mutations in some cases. A few types of vascular malformations are known to be hereditary and thus are known to have a genetic basis. Some evidence also suggests that at least some of these lesions are acquired later in life as a result of injury to the CNS.

During fetal development, new blood vessels continuously form and then disappear as the human body changes and grows. These changes in the body's vascular map continue after birth and are controlled by angiogenic factors, chemicals produced by the body that stimulate new blood vessel formation and growth. Researchers have identified changes in the chemical structures of various angiogenic factors in some people who have AVMs or other vascular abnormalities of the CNS. However, it is not yet clear how these chemical changes actually cause changes in blood vessel structure.

By studying patterns of occurrence in families, researchers have established that one type of cavernous malformation involving multiple lesion formation is caused by a genetic mutation in chromosome 7. This genetic mutation appears in many ethnic groups, but it is especially frequent in a large population of Hispanic Americans living in the Southwest; these individuals share a common ancestor in whom the genetic change occurred. Some other types of vascular defects of the CNS are part of larger medical syndromes known to be hereditary. They include hereditary hemorrhagic telangiectasia (HHT), Sturge-Weber syndrome (SWS), and Klippel-Trenaunay syndrome (KTS).

HOW ARE ARTERIOVENOUS MALFORMATIONS DIAGNOSED AND TREATED?
Diagnosing Arteriovenous Malformations

One of the more distinctive signs clinicians use to diagnose an AVM is an auditory phenomenon called a "bruit"—a rhythmic, whooshing sound caused by excessively rapid blood flow through the arteries and veins of an AVM. The sound is similar to that made by a torrent of water rushing through a narrow pipe. A bruit can sometimes become a symptom when it is especially severe. When audible to individuals, the bruit may compromise hearing, disturb sleep, or cause significant psychological distress.

An array of imaging technologies can be used to uncover the presence of AVMs.

- **Cerebral angiography**. Also called "cerebral arteriography," this imaging provides the most accurate pictures of blood vessel structure in brain AVMs. A special water-soluble dye, called a "contrast agent," is injected into an artery and highlights the structure of blood vessels so that it can be seen on x-rays.
- **Computed tomography (CT) scans**. CT scans use x-rays to create an image of the head, brain, or spinal cord and are especially useful in revealing the presence of hemorrhage. Magnetic resonance imaging (MRI) uses magnetic fields and radio waves to create detailed images that can show subtle changes in neurological tissues.
- **Magnetic resonance angiography (MRA)**. MRA can record the pattern and velocity of blood flow through

vascular lesions as well as the flow of CSF throughout the brain and spinal cord.

- **Transcranial Doppler ultrasound**. This can diagnose medium-sized to large AVMs and also detect the presence and extent of hemorrhage. It evaluates blood flow through the brain by directing high-frequency sound waves through the skull at particular arteries. The resulting sound wave signals that bounce back from blood cells are interpreted by a computer to make an image of the velocity of blood flow.

Treating Arteriovenous Malformations

Whenever an AVM is detected, the individual should be carefully and consistently monitored for any signs of instability that may indicate an increased risk of hemorrhage.

There are several options for treating AVMs. Although medication can often lessen general symptoms such as headache, back pain, and seizures caused by AVMs and other vascular lesions, the definitive treatment for AVMs is either surgery or focused radiation therapy. Venous malformations and capillary telangiectases rarely require surgery. Cavernous malformations are usually well-defined enough for surgical removal, but surgery on these lesions is less common than for AVMs because they do not pose the same risk of hemorrhage.

Because so many variables are involved in treating AVMs, doctors must assess the danger posed to individuals largely on a case-by-case basis. A hemorrhage from an untreated AVM can cause serious neurological deficits or death, leading many clinicians to recommend surgical intervention whenever the physical characteristics of an AVM appear to indicate a greater-than-usual likelihood of significant bleeding and subsequent neurological damage. However, surgery on any part of the CNS carries some risk of serious complications or death. There is no easy formula that can allow physicians and individuals to reach a decision on the best course of therapy.

Three surgical options are used to treat AVMs: conventional surgery, endovascular embolization, and radiosurgery. The choice of treatment depends largely on the size and location of an AVM. Endovascular embolization and radiosurgery are less invasive than conventional surgery and offer safer treatment options for some AVMs located deep inside the brain.

- **Conventional surgery**. This involves entering the brain or spinal cord and removing the central portion of the AVM, including the fistula, while causing as little damage as possible to surrounding neurological structures. This surgery is most appropriate when an AVM is located in a superficial portion of the brain or spinal cord and is relatively small in size. AVMs located deep inside the brain generally cannot be approached through conventional surgical techniques because there is too great a possibility that functionally important brain tissue will be damaged or destroyed.

- **Endovascular embolization**. In endovascular embolization, the surgeon guides a catheter through the arterial network until the tip reaches the site of the AVM. The surgeon then injects a substance (such as fast-drying glue-like substances, fibered titanium coils, and tiny balloons) that will travel through blood vessels and create an artificial blood clot in the center of an AVM. Since embolization usually does not permanently obliterate the AVM, it is usually used as an adjunct to surgery or to radiosurgery to reduce the blood flow through the AVM and make the surgery safer.

- **Radiosurgery**. This is an even less invasive therapeutic approach often used to treat small AVMs that have not ruptured. A beam of highly focused radiation is aimed directly at the AVM and damages the walls of the blood vessels making up the lesion. Over the course of the next several months, the irradiated vessels gradually degenerate and eventually close, leading to the resolution of the AVM.

Embolization frequently proves incomplete or temporary, although new embolization materials have led to improved results. Radiosurgery often has incomplete results as well, particularly when an AVM is large, and it poses the additional risk of radiation damage to surrounding normal tissues. Even when successful, complete closure of an AVM takes place over the course of many months following radiosurgery. During that period, the risk of hemorrhage is still present. However, both techniques can treat deeply situated AVMs that had previously been inaccessible. And in many individuals, staged embolization followed by conventional surgical removal or by radiosurgery is now performed, resulting in further reductions in death and complication rates.[1]

Section 39.2 | Chronic Venous Insufficiency

The veins in the legs carry blood toward the heart. When these veins do not function properly, the blood flows backward, thus causing accumulation in the legs. This is known as "chronic venous insufficiency" (CVI). Although this condition is not a serious health threat, it may be painful and disabling.

CAUSES AND RISK FACTORS OF CHRONIC VENOUS INSUFFICIENCY

The following are a few risk factors that contribute to CVI:
- a history of leg injury, surgery, or blood clots
- inflammation of veins
- standing or sitting for long durations
- smoking or use of tobacco
- lack of exercise
- overweight
- pregnancy
- being above 50 years of age

---

[1] "Arteriovenous Malformations (AVMs)," Centers for Disease Control and Prevention (CDC), February 7, 2023. Available online. URL: www.ninds.nih.gov/health-information/disorders/arteriovenous-malformations-avms. Accessed May 23, 2023.

SYMPTOMS OF CHRONIC VENOUS INSUFFICIENCY

Some of the symptoms of CVI are as follows:

- swelling of ankles and legs
- itchy and painful legs
- tight or heavy feeling in the calves
- pain experienced while walking
- tingling, burning, or pins and needles sensation in the legs
- reddish-brown or tan pigmentation of skin near the ankles
- flaky skin on legs and feet
- leg ulcers
- leg cramps or muscle spasms
- varicose veins

The symptoms of this condition may be similar to other health conditions. It is best to visit a doctor and get a diagnosis if any of the symptoms mentioned above are experienced.

STAGES OF CHRONIC VENOUS INSUFFICIENCY

The following are the six stages of CVI based on clinical signs and physical examination. Individuals are diagnosed with CVI if they reach the third stage or above.

- **Stage 0**. No signs are visible at this stage. A healthy diet and lifestyle changes could slow down the progression of CVI.
- **Stage 1**. Blood vessels are visible, including "spider veins," which are blue, purple, or red. They are also known as "thread veins." At this stage, compression stockings or bandages may help.
- **Stage 2**. Varicose veins are now at least 3 mm wide. In this stage, an injection containing a sclerosant or laser therapy may help, but the condition may return even after treatment. Compression stockings must be continued.
- **Stage 3**. Edema or swelling, caused by water retention, is visible without changes in the skin. Compression garments must be continued.

- **Stage 4**. The skin becomes itchy, thick with gray or brown marks. Skin care is also necessary along with the treatment for varicose veins.
- **Stage 5**. Ulcers or open wounds begin to form. Treatment is required to prevent further ulcers.
- **Stage 6**. Acute or active ulcers are evident. The open wounds are treated with creams and ointments.

DIAGNOSIS OF CHRONIC VENOUS INSUFFICIENCY

To form a diagnosis, a doctor takes the patient's history and checks for blood clots, ulcers, or discoloration. This is followed by a duplex or vascular ultrasound that uses high-frequency sound waves to check the following:

- structure of veins
- damaged areas of the veins
- speed and direction of the blood flow in the legs

TREATMENT FOR CHRONIC VENOUS INSUFFICIENCY

Doctors provide a treatment plan based on the age, overall health, and medical history of the patient; the severity of the case, based on the signs and symptoms; and the patient's overall health to determine if certain medicines, therapies, and treatments are suitable. Based on these parameters, surgical or nonsurgical methods of treatment may be used as follows:

- **Exercise**. Regular exercises and keeping legs elevated while sitting or sleeping are recommended to reduce swelling and help increase blood flow.
- **Medication**. Medicines (such as antibiotics, anticoagulants, or blood thinners), an Unna boot (medicated wrap), and zinc oxide gel-based multilayer compression can increase blood flow and help heal leg ulcers.
- **Radio frequency ablation**. This treatment uses sound waves to create heat and destroy tissues. A tube or catheter sends heat into the affected vein to close the vein. After the vein is closed, less blood pools in the leg, improving the overall blood flow.

- **Endovenous laser ablation**. This uses laser heat passed through a thin catheter to damage the vein and form a scar. The scar closes the vein, stopping it from functioning by cutting its source of blood and preventing pooling.
- **Sclerotherapy**. This treatment is used for severe cases where a chemical (sclerosant) is injected into the affected veins, causing scarring, so these veins can no longer carry blood. Blood then returns to the heart through the other veins.
- **Surgery**. Different surgeries are available based on the severity of the condition. Ligation and vein stripping are done in very severe cases. Ligation is a surgery in which the affected vein is tied, so blood does not flow through it. If the vein or valves are heavily damaged, the vein is removed through vein stripping.
  - **Subfascial endoscopic perforator surgery (SEPS)**. SEPS uses clips to block the affected veins that lie above the ankles.
  - **Microincision phlebectomy**. This is carried out when the varicose veins are near the skin's surface. Small incisions are made to remove the affected veins.
  - **Vein bypass surgery**. This is done when no other treatment has been effective. A healthy vein from another part of the body is used to reroute the blood around the blocked veins.

PREVENTION OF CHRONIC VENOUS INSUFFICIENCY

Chronic venous insufficiency cannot be prevented, but lifestyle changes can help lower the risk. They include the following:

- Avoid wearing high heels and tight clothing, as they hinder blood flow.
- Wear compression garments to help blood flow toward the heart.
- Eat a heart-healthy diet that includes reducing sodium or salt intake since salt contributes to water retention, resulting in swelling of veins and weakening of vein walls.

- Develop a healthy exercise routine to maintain body weight, as obesity causes blocked leg veins.
- Do not sit or stand for too long.
- Avoid sitting cross-legged; keep your legs elevated to increase blood flow.
- Avoid smoking and tobacco use.

References

Abby Sikorcin and John Bassham, "Venous Insufficiency," Healthline, September 17, 2018. Available online. URL: www.healthline.com/health/venous-insufficiency. Accessed July 4, 2023.

"Chronic Venous Insufficiency," The Johns Hopkins University, July 21, 2012. Available online. URL: www. hopkinsmedicine.org/health/conditions-and-diseases/ chronic-venous-insufficiency. Accessed July 4, 2023.

"Chronic Venous Insufficiency (CVI)," Cleveland Clinic, July 17, 2022. Available online. URL: https:// my.clevelandclinic.org/health/diseases/16872-chronic-venous-insufficiency-cvi. Accessed July 4, 2023.

Deepak Sudheendra and David Zieve, MedlinePlus, "Venous Insufficiency," National Institutes of Health (NIH), May 10, 2022. Available online. URL: https://medlineplus. gov/ency/article/000203.htm. Accessed July 4, 2023.

Teresa Dumain and Nayana Ambardekar, "What Is Chronic Venous Insufficiency?" WebMD, November 19, 2022. Available online. URL: www.webmd.com/dvt/dvt-venous-insufficiency. Accessed July 4, 2023.

Section 39.3 | **Varicose Veins and Spider Veins**

WHAT ARE VARICOSE VEINS?

Varicose veins are twisted veins that can be blue, red, or skin-colored. The larger veins may appear rope-like and make the skin bulge out.

Varicose veins are often on the thighs, the backs and fronts of the calves, or the inside of the legs, near the ankles and feet. During pregnancy, varicose veins can happen around the inner thigh, lower pelvic area, and buttocks.

WHAT ARE SPIDER VEINS?

Spider veins, or thread veins, are smaller than varicose veins. They are usually red. They may look like tree branches or spider webs. Spider veins can usually be seen under the skin, but they do not make the skin bulge out as varicose veins do.

Spider veins are usually found on the legs or the face.

WHO GETS VARICOSE VEINS AND SPIDER VEINS?

Varicose veins affect almost twice as many women as men and are more common in older women. Spider veins may affect more than half of women.

WHAT CAUSES VARICOSE VEINS AND SPIDER VEINS?

Problems in the valves in your veins can prevent blood from flowing normally and cause varicose veins or spider veins.

Your heart pumps blood filled with oxygen and nutrients through your arteries to your whole body. Veins then carry the blood from different parts of your body back to your heart. Normally, your veins have valves that act as one-way flaps. But, if the valves do not close correctly, blood can leak back into the lower part of the vein rather than going toward the heart. Over time, more blood gets stuck in the vein, building pressure that weakens the walls of the vein. This causes the vein to grow larger.

ARE SOME WOMEN MORE LIKELY AT RISK OF VARICOSE VEINS AND SPIDER VEINS?

Yes. Varicose veins and spider veins are caused by damaged valves in the veins that prevent blood from flowing normally. Many things can damage your valves, but your risk of varicose veins and spider veins may be higher in case of the following instances:

- **Having a family or personal history of varicose veins or spider veins**. In one small study, more than half of women with varicose veins had a parent with varicose veins, too.

- **Sitting or standing for long periods**. Sitting or standing for a long time, especially for more than four hours at a time, may make your veins work harder against gravity to pump blood to your heart.

- **Being overweight or obese**. Being overweight or obese can put extra pressure on your veins. Women who are obese are more likely to get varicose veins than women at a healthy weight.

- **Being pregnant**. During pregnancy, the amount of blood pumping through your body increases to support the fetus. The extra blood causes your veins to swell. Your growing uterus (womb) also puts pressure on your veins. Varicose veins may go away within a few months after childbirth, or they may remain and continue to cause symptoms. More varicose veins and spider veins may appear with each additional pregnancy.

- **Being older**. As you get older, the valves in your veins may weaken and not work as well. Your calf muscles also weaken as you age. Your calf muscles normally help squeeze veins and send blood back toward the heart as you walk.

- **Using hormonal birth control or menopausal hormone therapy (MHT)**. The hormone estrogen may weaken vein valves and lead to varicose veins. Using hormonal birth control, including the pill or a patch, shot, vaginal ring, or intrauterine device (IUD), with estrogen and progesterone, or taking MHT may raise your risk of varicose or spider veins.

- **Having a condition that damaged the valves**. Blood clots in the legs or scarring of the veins can damage the valves.

WHAT ARE THE SYMPTOMS OF VARICOSE VEINS AND SPIDER VEINS?

Some women do not have any symptoms of varicose veins and spider veins. If you do have symptoms, your legs may feel extremely tired, heavy, or achy. Your symptoms may get worse after sitting or standing for long periods of time. Your symptoms may get better after resting and putting your legs up.

Other symptoms that may be more common with varicose veins include the following:

- throbbing or cramping
- swelling
- itching

Changing hormone levels may affect your symptoms. Because of this, you may notice more symptoms during certain times in your menstrual cycle or during pregnancy or menopause.

WHY DO VARICOSE VEINS AND SPIDER VEINS USUALLY APPEAR IN THE LEGS?

Varicose veins and spider veins appear most often in the legs. This is because the veins in your legs carry blood to your heart against gravity and for the longest distance from anywhere in the body.

SHOULD YOU CALL YOUR DOCTOR OR NURSE IF YOU HAVE VARICOSE VEINS OR SPIDER VEINS?

Maybe. If you think you have varicose veins or spider veins and they cause you pain or discomfort, talk to your doctor or nurse. Varicose veins and spider veins usually do not cause symptoms. But you may want to remove or close varicose veins or spider veins if you have symptoms or if you do not like the way they look.

Talk to your doctor or nurse if varicose veins or spider veins cause you pain or if:

- the vein has become swollen, red, or very tender or warm to the touch, which can be a sign of a blood clot
- you have sores or a rash on your leg or near your ankle
- the skin on your ankle or calf changes color
- one of the varicose veins begins to bleed
- your symptoms keep you from doing daily activities

WILL YOU GET VARICOSE VEINS DURING PREGNANCY?

Maybe. During pregnancy, you have more blood pumping through your body to support the fetus. The extra blood can cause your veins to get larger. Your growing uterus also puts pressure on the veins. Varicose veins may appear around the vagina and buttocks.

For some women, varicose veins shrink or disappear after childbirth. For others, varicose veins stay after childbirth, and symptoms continue to get worse. Women may also get more varicose veins or spider veins with each additional pregnancy.[2]

---

[2] Office on Women's Health (OWH), "Varicose Veins and Spider Veins," U.S. Department of Health and Human Services (HHS), February 15, 2021. Available online. URL: www.womenshealth.gov/a-z-topics/varicose-veins-and-spider-veins. Accessed June 7, 2023.

Chapter 40 | **Aneurysm**

Chapter Contents

WHAT IS AN AORTIC ANEURYSM?

An aortic aneurysm is a balloon-like bulge in the aorta, the large artery that carries blood from the heart through the chest and torso.

Aortic aneurysms can dissect or rupture:

- The force of blood pumping can split the layers of the artery wall, allowing blood to leak in between them. This process is called a "dissection."
- The aneurysm can burst completely, causing bleeding inside the body. This is called a "rupture."
- Dissections and ruptures are the cause of most deaths from aortic aneurysms.

FACTS ABOUT AORTIC ANEURYSMS IN THE UNITED STATES

- A history of smoking accounts for about 75 percent of all abdominal aortic aneurysms.
- The U.S. Preventive Services Task Force (USPSTF) recommends that men 65–75 years old who have ever smoked should get an ultrasound screening for abdominal aortic aneurysms, even if they have no symptoms.

WHAT ARE THE TYPES OF AORTIC ANEURYSMS?

Thoracic Aortic Aneurysm

A thoracic aortic aneurysm happens in the chest. Men and women are equally likely to get thoracic aortic aneurysms, which become more common with increasing age.

Thoracic aortic aneurysms are usually caused by high blood pressure (HBP) or sudden injury. Sometimes, people with inherited connective tissue disorders, such as Marfan syndrome (MFS) and Ehlers-Danlos syndrome (EDS), get thoracic aortic aneurysms.

Signs and symptoms of thoracic aortic aneurysms can include the following:

- sharp, sudden pain in the chest or upper back
- shortness of breath
- trouble breathing or swallowing

Abdominal Aortic Aneurysm

An abdominal aortic aneurysm happens below the chest. Abdominal aortic aneurysms happen more often than thoracic aortic aneurysms.

Abdominal aortic aneurysms are more common in men and among people aged 65 and older. Abdominal aortic aneurysms are more common among White people than among Black people.

Abdominal aortic aneurysms are usually caused by atherosclerosis (hardened arteries), but infection or injury can also cause them.

Abdominal aortic aneurysms do not often have any symptoms. If an individual does have symptoms, they can include the following:

- throbbing or deep pain in the back or side
- pain in the buttocks, groin, or legs

Other Types of Aneurysms

Aneurysms can happen in other parts of your body. A ruptured aneurysm in the brain can cause a stroke. Peripheral aneurysms—those found in arteries other than the aorta—can happen in the neck, in the groin, or behind the knees. These aneurysms are less likely to rupture or dissect than aortic aneurysms, but they can form blood clots. These clots can break away and block blood flow through the artery.

WHAT ARE THE RISK FACTORS FOR AORTIC ANEURYSMS?

Diseases and unhealthy behaviors that damage your heart and blood vessels also increase your risk of aortic aneurysms. Smoking is the most important behavior related to aortic aneurysms.

Other factors include the following:

- HBP
- high blood cholesterol
- atherosclerosis (hardened arteries)

Some inherited connective tissue disorders, such as MFS and EDS, can also increase your risk of aortic aneurysms. Your family may also have a history of aortic aneurysms that can increase your risk.

HOW ARE AORTIC ANEURYSMS TREATED?

The two main treatments for aortic aneurysms are medicines and surgery. Medicines can lower blood pressure and reduce the risk of an aortic aneurysm. Surgery can repair or replace the affected section of the aorta.[1]

Section 40.2 | Cerebral Aneurysm

WHAT IS A CEREBRAL ANEURYSM?

A cerebral aneurysm (also known as a "brain aneurysm") is a weak or thin spot on an artery in the brain that balloons or bulges out and fills with blood. The bulging aneurysm can put pressure on the nerves or brain tissue. It may also burst or rupture, spilling blood into the surrounding tissue (called a "hemorrhage"). A ruptured aneurysm can cause serious health problems such as hemorrhagic stroke, brain damage, coma, and even death.

Some cerebral aneurysms, particularly those that are very small, do not bleed or cause other problems. These types of aneurysms are usually detected during imaging tests for other medical conditions. Cerebral aneurysms can occur anywhere in the brain, but most form in the major arteries along the base of the skull. All cerebral aneurysms have the potential to rupture and cause bleeding within the brain or surrounding area.

CLASSIFICATION OF CEREBRAL ANEURYSMS
Types of Cerebral Aneurysms

The following are the three types of cerebral aneurysms:
- **Saccular aneurysm**. A saccular aneurysm is a rounded sac containing blood that is attached to a main artery or one of its branches. Also known as a "berry aneurysm" (because it resembles a berry hanging from a vine),

---

[1] "Aortic Aneurysm," Centers for Disease Control and Prevention (CDC), September 27, 2021. Available online. URL: www.cdc.gov/heartdisease/aortic_aneurysm.htm. Accessed May 23, 2023.

this is the most common form of cerebral aneurysm. It is typically found on arteries at the base of the brain. Saccular aneurysms occur most often in adults.
- **Fusiform aneurysm**. A fusiform aneurysm balloons or bulges out on all sides of the artery.
- **Mycotic aneurysm**. A mycotic aneurysm occurs as the result of an infection that can sometimes affect the arteries in the brain. The infection weakens the artery wall, causing a bulging aneurysm to form.

Size of Cerebral Aneurysms
Aneurysms are also classified by size as follows:
- **Small aneurysms**. These aneurysms are less than 11 millimeters in diameter (about the size of a large pencil eraser).
- **Large aneurysms**. These aneurysms are 11–25 millimeters (about the width of a dime).
- **Giant aneurysms**. These aneurysms are greater than 25 millimeters in diameter (more than the width of a quarter).

WHO IS MORE LIKELY TO GET A CEREBRAL ANEURYSM?
Cerebral aneurysms form when the walls of the arteries in the brain become thin and weaken. Aneurysms typically form at branch points in arteries because these sections are the weakest. Occasionally, cerebral aneurysms may be present from birth, usually resulting from an abnormality in an artery wall.

Brain aneurysms can occur in anyone and at any age. They are most common in adults between the ages of 30 and 60 and are more common in women than in men. People with certain inherited disorders are also at higher risk.

RISK FACTORS FOR DEVELOPING AN ANEURYSM
Sometimes, cerebral aneurysms are the result of inherited risk factors, including the following:
- genetic connective tissue disorders that weaken artery walls

- polycystic kidney disease (in which numerous cysts form in the kidneys)
- arteriovenous malformations (AVMs; these are snarled tangles of arteries and veins in the brain that disrupt blood flow. Some AVMs develop sporadically or on their own.)
- history of aneurysm in a first-degree family member (child, sibling, or parent)

Other risk factors develop over time and include the following:
- untreated high blood pressure (HBP)
- cigarette smoking
- drug abuse, especially cocaine or amphetamines, which raise blood pressure to dangerous levels (Intravenous drug abuse is a cause of infectious mycotic aneurysms.)
- age over 40

Less common risk factors include the following:
- head trauma
- brain tumor
- infection in the arterial wall (mycotic aneurysm)

Additionally, HBP, cigarette smoking, diabetes, and high cholesterol put one at risk of atherosclerosis (a blood vessel disease in which fats build up on the inside of artery walls), which can increase the risk of developing a fusiform aneurysm.

Risk Factors for an Aneurysm to Rupture

Not all aneurysms will rupture. Aneurysm characteristics such as size, location, and growth during follow-up evaluation may affect the risk that an aneurysm will rupture. In addition, medical conditions may influence aneurysm rupture.

Risk factors include the following:
- **Smoking**. It is linked to both the development and rupture of cerebral aneurysms. Smoking may even cause multiple aneurysms to form in the brain.
- **HBP**. HBP damages and weakens arteries, making them more likely to form and rupture.

- **Size**. The largest aneurysms are the ones most likely to rupture in a person who previously did not show symptoms.
- **Location**. Aneurysms located on the posterior communicating arteries (a pair of arteries in the back part of the brain) and possibly those on the anterior communicating artery (a single artery in the front of the brain) have a higher risk of rupturing than those at other locations in the brain.
- **Growth**. Aneurysms that grow, even if they are small, are at increased risk of rupture.
- **Family history**. A family history of aneurysm rupture suggests a higher risk of rupture for aneurysms detected in family members.

The greatest risk occurs in individuals with multiple aneurysms who have already suffered a previous rupture or sentinel bleed.

SYMPTOMS OF CEREBRAL ANEURYSM
Unruptured Aneurysm
Most cerebral aneurysms do not show symptoms until they either become very large or rupture. Small unchanging aneurysms generally will not produce symptoms.

A larger aneurysm that is steadily growing may press on tissues and nerves, causing:
- pain above and behind the eye
- numbness
- weakness
- paralysis on one side of the face
- a dilated pupil in the eye
- vision changes or double vision

Ruptured Aneurysm
When an aneurysm ruptures (bursts), one always experiences a sudden and extremely severe headache (e.g., the worst headache of one's life) and may also develop the following:
- double vision
- nausea

- vomiting
- stiff neck
- sensitivity to light
- seizures
- loss of consciousness (which may happen briefly or may be prolonged)
- cardiac arrest

Leaking Aneurysm

Sometimes, an aneurysm may leak a small amount of blood into the brain (called a "sentinel bleed"). Sentinel or warning headaches may result from an aneurysm that suffers a tiny leak days or weeks prior to a significant rupture. However, only a minority of individuals have a sentinel headache prior to rupture.

If you experience a sudden, severe headache, especially when it is combined with any other symptoms, you should seek immediate medical attention.

COMPLICATIONS OF A RUPTURED CEREBRAL ANEURYSM

Aneurysms may rupture and bleed into the space between the skull and the brain (subarachnoid hemorrhage) and sometimes into the brain tissue (intracerebral hemorrhage). These are forms of stroke called "hemorrhagic stroke." The bleeding into the brain can cause a wide spectrum of symptoms, from a mild headache to permanent damage to the brain or even death.

After an aneurysm has ruptured, it may cause the following serious complications:

- **Rebleeding**. Once it has ruptured, an aneurysm may rupture again before it is treated, leading to further bleeding into the brain and causing more damage or death.
- **Change in the sodium level**. Bleeding in the brain can disrupt the balance of sodium in the blood supply and cause swelling in brain cells. This can result in permanent brain damage.
- **Hydrocephalus**. Subarachnoid hemorrhage can cause hydrocephalus. Hydrocephalus is a buildup of too

much cerebrospinal fluid (CSF) in the brain, which causes pressure that can lead to permanent brain damage or death. Hydrocephalus occurs frequently after subarachnoid hemorrhage because the blood blocks the normal flow of CSF. If left untreated, increased pressure inside the head can cause coma or death.

- **Vasospasm**. This frequently occurs after subarachnoid hemorrhage when the bleeding causes the arteries in the brain to contract and limit blood flow to vital areas of the brain. This can cause strokes from lack of adequate blood flow to parts of the brain.

- **Seizures**. Aneurysm bleeding can cause seizures (convulsions), either at the time of bleed or in the immediate aftermath. While most seizures are evident, on occasion, they may only be seen by sophisticated brain testing. Untreated seizures or those that do not respond to treatment can cause brain damage.

HOW ARE CEREBRAL ANEURYSMS DIAGNOSED AND TREATED?
Diagnosing Cerebral Aneurysms

Most cerebral aneurysms go unnoticed until they rupture or are detected during medical imaging tests for another condition.

If you have experienced a severe headache or have any other symptoms related to a ruptured aneurysm, your doctor will order tests to determine if blood has leaked into the space between the skull bone and brain.

Several tests are available to diagnose brain aneurysms and determine the best treatment. These include the following:

- **Computed tomography (CT)**. This is often the first test a physician will order to determine if blood has leaked into the brain. CT uses x-rays to create two-dimensional images, or "slices," of the brain and skull. Occasionally a contrast dye is injected into the bloodstream prior to scanning to assess the arteries and look for a possible aneurysm. This process, called "CT angiography" (CTA), produces sharper, more detailed images of blood flow in the brain arteries. CTA can show the size, location, and shape of an unruptured or ruptured aneurysm.

- **Magnetic resonance imaging (MRI)**. An MRI uses computer-generated radio waves and a magnetic field to create two- and three-dimensional detailed images of the brain and can determine if there has been bleeding into the brain. Magnetic resonance angiography (MRA) produces detailed images of the brain arteries and can show the size, location, and shape of an aneurysm.
- **Cerebral angiography**. This imaging technique can find blockages in arteries in the brain or neck. It can also identify weak spots in an artery, such as an aneurysm. The test is used to determine the cause of the bleeding in the brain and the exact location, size, and shape of an aneurysm. Your doctor will pass a catheter (long, flexible tube), typically from the groin arteries, to inject a small amount of contrast dye into your neck and brain arteries. The contrast dye helps the x-ray create a detailed picture of the appearance of an aneurysm and a clear picture of any blockage in the arteries.
- **Cerebrospinal fluid (CSF) analysis**. This test measures the chemicals in the fluid that cushions and protects the brain and spinal cord (CSF). Most often, a doctor will collect the CSF by performing a spinal tap (lumbar puncture), in which a thin needle is inserted into the lower back (lumbar spine) and a small amount of fluid is removed and tested. The results will help detect any bleeding around the brain. If bleeding is detected, additional tests would be needed to identify the exact cause of the bleeding.

Treating Cerebral Aneurysms

Not all cerebral aneurysms require treatment. Some very small unruptured aneurysms that are not associated with any factors suggesting a higher risk of rupture may be safely left alone and monitored with MRA or CTA to detect any growth. It is important to aggressively treat any coexisting medical problems and risk factors.

Treatments for unruptured cerebral aneurysms that have not shown symptoms have some potentially serious complications and should be carefully weighed against the predicted rupture risk.

A doctor will consider a variety of factors when determining the best option for treating an unruptured aneurysm, including the following:
- type, size, and location of the aneurysm
- risk of rupture
- the person's age and health
- personal and family medical history
- risk of treatment

Individuals should also take the following steps to reduce the risk of aneurysm rupture:
- Carefully control blood pressure.
- Stop smoking.
- Avoid cocaine use or other stimulant drugs.

Surgery, endovascular treatments, or other therapies are often recommended to manage symptoms and prevent damage from unruptured and ruptured aneurysms.

SURGERY

There are a few surgical options available for treating cerebral aneurysms. These procedures carry some risks, such as possible damage to other blood vessels, the potential for aneurysm recurrence and rebleeding, and risk of stroke.
- **Microvascular clipping**. This procedure involves cutting off the flow of blood to the aneurysm and requires open brain surgery. A doctor will locate the blood vessels that feed the aneurysm and place a tiny, metal, clothespin-like clip on the aneurysm's neck to stop its blood supply. Clipping has been shown to be

highly effective, depending on the location, size, and shape of the aneurysm. In general, aneurysms that are completely clipped do not recur.

Endovascular treatment includes the following:

- **Platinum coil embolization**. This procedure is a less invasive procedure than microvascular surgical clipping. A doctor will insert a hollow plastic tube (a catheter) into an artery, usually in the groin, and thread it through the body to the brain aneurysm. Using a wire, the doctor will pass detachable coils (tiny spirals of platinum wire) through the catheter and release them into the aneurysm. The coils block the aneurysm and reduce the flow of blood into the aneurysm. The procedure may need to be performed more than once during the person's lifetime because aneurysms treated with coiling can sometimes recur.
- **Flow diversion devices**. Other endovascular treatment options include placing a small stent (flexible mesh tube), similar to those placed for heart blockages, in the artery to reduce blood flow into the aneurysm. A doctor will insert a hollow plastic tube (a catheter) into an artery, usually in the groin, and thread it through the body to the artery on which the aneurysm is located. This procedure is used to treat very large aneurysms and those that cannot be treated with surgery or platinum coil embolization.

Other treatments for a ruptured cerebral aneurysm aim to control symptoms and reduce complications. These treatments include the following:

- **Antiseizure drugs (anticonvulsants)**. These drugs may be used to prevent seizures related to a ruptured aneurysm.
- **Calcium channel-blocking drugs**. These drugs may reduce the risk of stroke by vasospasm.
- **Shunt**. It funnels CSF from the brain to elsewhere in the body and may be surgically inserted into

the brain following rupture if the buildup of CSF (hydrocephalus) is causing harmful pressure on surrounding brain tissue.

- **Rehabilitative therapy**. Individuals who have suffered a subarachnoid hemorrhage often need physical, speech, and occupational therapy to regain lost function and learn to cope with any permanent disability.[2]

[2] "Cerebral Aneurysms," Centers for Disease Control and Prevention (CDC), March 8, 2023. Available online. URL: www.ninds.nih.gov/health-information/disorders/cerebral-aneurysms. Accessed May 24, 2023.

Chapter 41 | **Vascular Birthmarks: Hemangiomas and Vascular Malformations**

Vascular birthmarks or vascular anomalies occur due to the improper formation of the blood vessels. These birthmarks take many forms, differing in size, shape, and location on the body. The color of birthmarks varies from shades of brown or blue to red or pink. The following are the two main types of vascular birthmarks:
- hemangiomas
- vascular malformations

HEMANGIOMAS

Hemangiomas are noncancerous tumors formed due to the extra blood vessels in the skin. They affect female children about three times more often than boys. Due to their distinctive color, these birthmarks are also sometimes known as "strawberry marks" or "salmon patches." They most often appear on the surface of the skin on parts such as the head or neck but can develop anywhere on the body, including internal organs. In general, hemangiomas do not require treatment unless they affect the vision, breathing, or other vital functions.

VASCULAR MALFORMATIONS

Vascular malformations are lesions that are present at birth. These birthmarks grow with the child throughout life without involution. There are four main types of vascular malformations. Lesions that are typically flat and colored pink, purple, or red are called "port-wine stains." They can appear anywhere on the body. Venous birthmarks are most commonly found on the jaw, cheek, tongue, and lips. These birthmarks are soft to the touch, and their color disappears when compressed (such as by pressing on the birthmark with a finger). Lymphatic birthmarks form as a result of excess fluid in the lymphatic vessels. Arteriovenous birthmarks appear when blood pools in capillary veins.

CAUSES OF VASCULAR MALFORMATIONS

A tendency to develop hemangiomas and vascular malformations can be inherited, though most birthmarks of this type seem to form by chance. Hemangiomas and vascular malformations develop as a result of many different genetic syndromes with many variables affecting the chance of a child being born with a birthmark. If one parent has or had a hemangioma or vascular malformation, there is a 50 percent chance that their baby will also have such a birthmark.

TREATMENT FOR VASCULAR MALFORMATIONS

Some birthmarks can result in serious complications if the location of the birthmark impairs the body's critical functions such as breathing or blood flow. Most hemangiomas do not require treatment. Treatment is usually required for hemangiomas that interfere with vision, breathing, hearing, and ability to feed or result in other medical problems. Treatment options include surgery, laser treatment, medication, or a combination of approaches.

Treatment for vascular malformations depends upon the location and type of birthmark. Venous and lymphatic malformations are typically treated by injection therapy, in which a clotting medication is used to remove excessive blood or lymphatic fluid. Capillary malfunctions such as port-wine stains are usually treated with laser surgery. Arterial malformations can be treated with a process known as "embolization," in which blood flow is blocked by injection of medication near the lesion. Treatments can also include oral medications such as steroids, radiology treatment, surgery, or a combination of approaches.

References

"Hemangioma," OrthoInfo, August 2018. Available online. URL: https://orthoinfo.aaos.org/en/diseases--conditions/ hemangioma. Accessed June 29, 2023.

"Vascular Birthmarks," Harvard Health Publishing, March 22, 2019. Available online. URL: www.health. harvard.edu/a_to_z/vascular-birthmarks-a-to-z. Accessed June 29, 2023.

"Vascular Malformations and Hemangiomas," Stanford Children's Health, 2016. Available online. URL: www. stanfordchildrens.org/en/topic/default?id=vascular-malformations-and-hemangiomas-90-P01841. Accessed June 29, 2023.

"What Is a Vascular Birthmark?" University of Rochester Medical Center (URMC), 2016. Available online. URL: www.urmc.rochester.edu/childrens-hospital/craniofacial/ vascular-birthmark.aspx. Accessed June 29, 2023.

Chapter 42 | **Fibromuscular Dysplasia**

WHAT IS FIBROMUSCULAR DYSPLASIA?

Fibromuscular dysplasia (FMD) is the abnormal development or growth of cells in the walls of arteries that can cause the vessels to narrow or bulge. The carotid arteries, which pass through the neck and supply blood to the brain, are commonly affected. Arteries within the brain and kidneys can also be affected. A characteristic "string of beads" pattern caused by the alternating narrowing and enlarging of the artery can block or reduce blood flow to the brain, causing a stroke or ministroke.

CAUSE OF FIBROMUSCULAR DYSPLASIA

The cause of FMD is unknown.

WHO IS AT RISK OF FIBROMUSCULAR DYSPLASIA?

Fibromuscular dysplasia is most often seen in people 25–50 years of age and more often affects women than men. More than one family member may be affected by the disease.

SYMPTOMS OF FIBROMUSCULAR DYSPLASIA

Some people experience no symptoms of the disease, while others may have:
- high blood pressure
- dizziness or vertigo
- chronic headache
- intracranial aneurysm

- ringing in the ears
- weakness or numbness in the face
- neck pain
- vision problems

DIAGNOSIS OF FIBROMUSCULAR DYSPLASIA

An angiogram can detect the degree of narrowing or obstruction of the artery and identify changes such as a tear (dissection) or weak area (aneurysm) in the vessel wall. FMD can also be diagnosed using computed tomography (CT), magnetic resonance imaging (MRI), or ultrasound.

TREATMENT FOR FIBROMUSCULAR DYSPLASIA

There is no standard treatment for FMD. Any treatment to improve blood flow is based on the arteries affected and the progression and severity of the disease. The carotid arteries should be tested if FMD is found elsewhere in the body since carotid involvement is linked to an increased risk of stroke. People with minimal narrowing may take a daily antiplatelet such as an aspirin or an anticoagulant to thin the blood and reduce the chances that a clot might form. Medications such as aspirin can also be taken for headaches and neck pain associated with FMD.

People with arterial disease who smoke should be encouraged to quit as smoking worsens the disease. Further treatment may include angioplasty, in which a small balloon is inserted through a catheter and inflated to open the artery. Small tubes called "stents" may be inserted to keep arteries open. Surgery may be needed to treat aneurysms that have the potential to rupture and cause bleeding within the brain.

CAN FIBROMUSCULAR DYSPLASIA BE PREVENTED?

Currently, there is no cure for FMD. Medicines and angioplasty can reduce the risk of initial or recurrent stroke. In rare cases, FMD-related aneurysms can burst and bleed into the brain, causing stroke, permanent nerve damage, or death.

HOW CAN YOU OR YOUR LOVED ONE HELP IMPROVE CARE FOR PEOPLE WITH FIBROMUSCULAR DYSPLASIA?

Consider participating in a clinical trial, so clinicians and scientists can learn more about FMD and related disorders. All types of volunteers are needed—those who are healthy or may have an illness or disease—of all different ages, sexes, races, and ethnicities to ensure that study results apply to as many people as possible and that treatments will be safe and effective for everyone who will use them.[1]

[1] "Fibromuscular Dysplasia," National Heart, Lung, and Blood Institute (NHLBI), January 20, 2023. Available online. URL: www.ninds.nih.gov/health-information/disorders/fibromuscular-dysplasia. Accessed May 25, 2023.

Chapter 43 | **Klippel-Trenaunay Syndrome**

Klippel-Trenaunay syndrome (KTS) is a condition that affects the development of blood vessels, soft tissues (such as skin and muscles), and bones.

CAUSES OF KLIPPEL-TRENAUNAY SYNDROME

Klippel-Trenaunay syndrome can be caused by mutations in the *PIK3CA* gene. This gene provides instructions for making the p110 alpha (p110α) protein, which is one piece (subunit) of an enzyme called "phosphatidylinositol 3-kinase" (PI3K). PI3K plays a role in chemical signaling that is important for many cell activities, including cell growth and division (proliferation), movement (migration) of cells, and cell survival. These functions make PI3K important for the development of tissues throughout the body.

The *PIK3CA* gene mutations associated with KTS alter the p110α protein. The altered subunit makes PI3K abnormally active, which allows cells to grow and divide continuously. Increased cell proliferation leads to abnormal growth of the bones, soft tissues, and blood vessels.

KTS is one of several overgrowth syndromes, including megalencephaly-capillary malformation syndrome, that are caused by mutations in the *PIK3CA* gene. Together, these conditions are known as the "*PIK3CA*-related overgrowth spectrum" (PROS).

Because not everyone with KTS has a mutation in the *PIK3CA* gene, it is possible that mutations in unidentified genes may also cause this condition.

SYMPTOMS OF KLIPPEL-TRENAUNAY SYNDROME

The disorder has three characteristic features: a red birthmark called a "port-wine stain," "abnormal overgrowth of soft tissues and bones," and "vein malformations."

Most people with KTS are born with a port-wine stain. This type of birthmark is caused by swelling of small blood vessels near the surface of the skin. Port-wine stains are typically flat and can vary from pale pink to deep maroon in color. In people with KTS, the port-wine stain usually covers part of one limb. The affected area may become lighter or darker with age. Occasionally, port-wine stains develop small red blisters that break open and bleed easily.

KTS is also associated with the overgrowth of bones and soft tissues beginning in infancy. Usually, this abnormal growth is limited to one limb, most often one leg. However, the overgrowth can also affect the arms or, rarely, the torso. The abnormal growth can cause pain, a feeling of heaviness, and reduced movement in the affected area. If the overgrowth causes one leg to be longer than the other, it can also lead to problems with walking.

Malformations of veins are the third major feature of KTS. These abnormalities include varicose veins, which are swollen and twisted veins near the surface of the skin that often cause pain. Varicose veins usually occur on the sides of the upper legs and calves. Veins deep in the limbs can also be abnormal in people with KTS. Malformations of deep veins increase the risk of a type of blood clot called "deep vein thrombosis" (DVT). If a DVT travels through the bloodstream and lodges in the lungs, it can cause a life-threatening blood clot known as "pulmonary embolism" (PE).

COMPLICATIONS OF KLIPPEL-TRENAUNAY SYNDROME

Complications of KTS can include a type of skin infection called "cellulitis," swelling caused by a buildup of fluid (lymphedema), and internal bleeding from abnormal blood vessels. Less commonly, this condition is also associated with the fusion of certain fingers or toes (syndactyly) or the presence of extra digits (polydactyly).

FREQUENCY OF KLIPPEL-TRENAUNAY SYNDROME

Klippel-Trenaunay syndrome is estimated to affect at least 1 in 100,000 people worldwide.

INHERITANCE OF KLIPPEL-TRENAUNAY SYNDROME

Klippel-Trenaunay syndrome is almost always sporadic, which means that it occurs in people with no history of the disorder in their family. Studies suggest that the condition results from gene mutations that are not inherited. These genetic changes, which are called "somatic mutations," arise randomly in one cell during the early stages of development before birth. As cells continue to divide during development, cells arising from the first abnormal cell will have the mutation, and other cells will not. This mixture of cells with and without a genetic mutation is known as "mosaicism."[1]

[1] MedlinePlus, "Klippel-Trenaunay Syndrome," National Institutes of Health (NIH), May 17, 2021. Available online. URL: https://medlineplus.gov/genetics/condition/klippel-trenaunay-syndrome/#diagnosis. Accessed May 25, 2023.

Part 6 | Diagnosing and Treating Blood and Circulatory Disorders

Chapter 44 | **Blood Tests**

Chapter Contents

Section 44.1 | Blood Tests: An Overview

Blood tests are very common. They help doctors check for certain diseases and conditions. They also help check the function of your organs and show how well treatments are working.

TYPES OF BLOOD TESTS
Complete Blood Count

The complete blood count (CBC) is one of the most common blood tests. It is often done as part of a routine checkup. This test measures many different parts of your blood, including red blood cells (RBCs), white blood cells (WBCs), and platelets:

- RBC levels that are higher or lower than normal could be a sign of dehydration, anemia, or bleeding. RBCs carry oxygen from your lungs to the rest of your body.
- WBC levels that are higher or lower than normal could be a sign of infection, blood cancer, or an immune system disorder. WBCs are part of your immune system, which fights infections and diseases.
- Platelet levels that are higher or lower than normal may be a sign of a clotting disorder or a bleeding disorder. Platelets are blood cell fragments that help your blood clot. They stick together to seal cuts or breaks on blood vessel walls and stop bleeding.
- Hemoglobin levels that are lower than normal may be a sign of anemia, sickle cell disease (SCD), or thalassemia. Hemoglobin is an iron-rich protein in RBCs that carries oxygen.
- Hematocrit levels that are too high might mean you are dehydrated. Low hematocrit levels may be a sign of anemia. Hematocrit is a measure of how much space RBCs take up in your blood.
- Mean corpuscular volume (MCV) levels that are lower than normal may be a sign of anemia or thalassemia. MCV is a measure of the average size of your RBCs.

Table 44.1 shows some normal adult ranges for different parts of the CBC test. Some of the normal ranges differ between men and women. Other factors, such as age, high altitude, and race, may also affect normal ranges.

Your health-care provider should discuss your results with you. They will advise you further if your results are outside the normal range for your group.

Table 44.1. Complete Blood Count

Test	Normal Range Results*
Red blood cell	• Adult men: 5–6 million cells/mcL • Adult women: 4–5 million cells/mcL
White blood cell	• 4,500–10,000 cells/mcL
Platelets	• 140,000–450,000 cells/mcL
Hemoglobin (varies with altitude)	• Adult men: 14–17 gm/dL • Adult women: 12–15 gm/dL
Hematocrit (varies with altitude)	• Adult men: 41–50% • Adult women: 36–44%
Mean corpuscular volume	• 0–95 femtoliter†

* Cells/mcL = cells per microliter; gm/dL = grams per deciliter.
† A femtoliter is a measure of volume.

Blood Chemistry Tests/Basic Metabolic Panel

The basic metabolic panel (BMP) is a group of tests that measure different naturally occurring chemicals in the blood. These tests are usually done on the fluid (plasma) part of the blood. The tests can give providers information about your organs, such as the heart, kidneys, and liver.

The BMP includes blood glucose, calcium, and electrolyte tests, as well as blood tests that measure kidney function. Some of these tests require you to fast (not eat any food) before the test, and others do not. Your provider will tell you how to prepare for the test(s) you are having.

Blood Enzyme Tests

Blood enzyme tests may be used to check for a heart attack. Enzymes are chemicals that help control chemical reactions in your body. There are many types of blood enzyme tests. The ones for heart attack include troponin and creatine kinase (CK) tests.

Blood levels of troponin go up when a person has muscle damage, including damage to the heart muscle. In addition, an enzyme called "creatine kinase-myocardial band" (CK-MB) is released into the blood when the heart muscle is damaged. High levels of CK-MB in the blood can mean that you have had a heart attack.

Lipoprotein Panel

A lipoprotein panel, also called a "lipid panel" or "lipid profile," measures the levels of low-density lipoprotein (LDL) and high-density lipoprotein (HDL) cholesterol and triglycerides in your blood. Cholesterol and triglyceride levels that are higher or lower than normal may be signs of higher risk of coronary heart disease (CHD).

A lipoprotein panel gives information about your:
- total cholesterol
- LDL ("bad") cholesterol, which is the main source of cholesterol buildup and blockages in the arteries
- HDL ("good") cholesterol, which helps decrease cholesterol blockages in the arteries
- triglycerides, which are a type of fat in your blood

Most people will need to fast for 9–12 hours before a lipoprotein panel.

Blood Clotting Tests

Blood clotting tests are sometimes called a "coagulation panel." These tests check proteins in your blood that affect the blood clotting process. Levels that are higher or lower than normal might suggest that you are at risk of bleeding or developing clots in your blood vessels.

Blood clotting tests are also used to monitor people who are taking medicines to lower the risk of blood clots. Warfarin and heparin are two examples of such medicines.[1]

Section 44.2 | Fibrinogen Test

A fibrinogen test, also known as "factor I," measures the level of fibrinogen in a person's blood. Fibrinogen is a blood plasma protein that is produced by the liver. It is 1 of 13 blood elements that help to form blood clots to stop bleeding after an injury. Low fibrinogen affects the body's ability to form blood clots, which can result in excessive bleeding.

Fibrinogen tests are usually performed on people who experience problems with blood clotting, excessive bleeding, or excessive bruising after an injury. Fibrinogen tests are also performed on people who experience blood in their urine or stool or have had a ruptured spleen or gastrointestinal tract hemorrhage. The test is an important tool in the diagnosis of disseminated intravascular coagulation, a condition in which small blood clots form inside the blood vessels throughout the body.

Testing for elevated levels of fibrinogen is also used to help diagnose or determine the risk of cardiovascular disease (heart disease) or brain aneurysm (stroke). Elevated fibrinogen levels can result from certain health conditions, including acute infections, cancer, coronary heart disease, heart attack, stroke, rheumatoid arthritis, kidney disease, liver disease, peripheral artery disease, and pregnancy. Receiving a blood transfusion, taking certain drugs, and smoking can also cause elevated fibrinogen levels in the body.

METHODS OF CONDUCTING FIBRINOGEN TEST

Fibrinogen tests can be conducted using one of four methods. In the Clauss method, plasma drawn from the person being tested is

---

[1] "Blood Tests," National Heart, Lung, and Blood Institute (NHLBI), March 24, 2022. Available online. URL: www.nhlbi.nih.gov/health/blood-tests. Accessed May 18, 2023.

mixed with concentrated thrombin (an enzyme in blood plasma) and analyzed. The time it takes for the blood clot to form is noted and compared against standard measures. Automated equipment senses when the blood clot has formed based on the optical density of the plasma/thrombin mixture.

In prothrombin-time-derived fibrinogen tests, a baseline measurement for known fibrinogen levels in various diluted plasma samples (the control group) is compared to the fibrinogen levels found in equivalent plasma dilutions created from the blood plasma being tested.

Immunological fibrinogen tests are conducted to measure the fibrinogen protein concentration in the blood rather than fibrinogen function.

Gravimetric fibrinogen tests are used to measure the weight of a clot produced using the Clauss method instead of measuring the optical density of the clot. Another type of gravimetric fibrinogen test measures the amount of fibrinogen protein present in a blood clot created using the Clauss method.

RESULTS OF THE FIBRINOGEN TEST

A normal fibrinogen blood level is typically between 1.5 and 3.0 g/L.
Normal reference ranges are as follows:
- adult: 200–400 mg/dl
- new born: 125–300 mg/dl

Fibrinogen levels are considered abnormal if the level is higher or lower than the normal range. An abnormal result may be due to one of the following inherited or acquired conditions:
- **Afibrinogenemia**. It is the absence of fibrinogen in the body.
- **Disseminated intravascular coagulation**. This condition is characterized by the presence of too much fibrinogen used by the body.
- **Dysfibrinogenemia**. A malfunction in fibrinogen performance results in dysfibrinogenemia.
- **Fibrinolysis**. It is the excessive breakdown of fibrinogen in the body.
- **Hemorrhage**. Excessive bleeding leads to hemorrhage.

- **Hypofibrinogenemia**. This condition is characterized by the presence of too little fibrinogen in the body.
- **Placental abruption**. In this condition, the placenta separates from the uterus wall during pregnancy.
- **Spontaneous bleeding**. It will occur when the fibrinogen level falls below 100 mg/dl.

Fibrinogen deficiency is treatable through the use of blood products that act as a replacement or substitute for the fibrinogen protein in the body. Fibrinogen concentrate may be used to prevent excessive bleeding in people during surgery, during or after childbirth, before dental surgery, or after traumatic injury.

References

"Fibrinogen," Lab Tests Online, April 10, 2014. Available "Fibrinogen," Lab Tests Online, April 10, 2014. Available online. URL: https://labtestsonline.org/understanding/analytes/fibrinogen/tab/test. Accessed June 29, 2023.

"Fibrinogen Assays," Practical Haemostasis, 2017. Available online. URL: https://practical-haemostasis.com/Screening%20Tests/fibrinogen.html. Accessed June 29, 2023.

Chen Yi-Bin, MedlinePlus, "Fibrinogen Blood Test," National Institutes of Health (NIH), January 27, 2015. Available online. URL: www.nlm.nih.gov/medlineplus/ency/article/003650.htm. Accessed June 29, 2023.

Corinna Underwood, "Fibrinogen," HealthLine, January 4, 2016. Available online. URL: www.healthline.com/health/fibrinogen. Accessed June 29, 2023.

Section 44.3 | Hemoglobin Electrophoresis

WHAT IS HEMOGLOBIN ELECTROPHORESIS?

Hemoglobin is a protein in your red blood cells (RBCs) that carries oxygen from your lungs to the rest of your body. There are several different types of hemoglobin. Hemoglobin electrophoresis is a test that measures the different types of hemoglobin in the blood. It also looks for abnormal types of hemoglobin.

Normal types of hemoglobin include the following:
- **Hemoglobin A (HgbA).** This is the most common type of hemoglobin in healthy adults.
- **Hemoglobin F (HgbF; fetal hemoglobin).** This type of hemoglobin is found in unborn babies and newborns. HgbF is replaced by HgbA shortly after birth.

If levels of HgbA or HgbF are too high or too low, it can indicate certain types of anemia.

Abnormal types of hemoglobin include the following:
- **Hemoglobin S (HgbS).** This type of hemoglobin is found in sickle cell disease (SCD). SCD is an inherited disorder that causes the body to make stiff, sickle-shaped RBCs. Healthy RBCs are flexible, so they can move easily through blood vessels. Sickle cells can get stuck in the blood vessels, causing severe and chronic pain, infections, and other complications.
- **Hemoglobin C (HgbC).** This type of hemoglobin does not carry oxygen well. It can cause a mild form of anemia.
- **Hemoglobin E (HgbE).** This type of hemoglobin is mostly found in people of Southeast Asian descent. People with HgbE usually have no symptoms or mild symptoms of anemia.

A hemoglobin electrophoresis test applies an electric current to a blood sample. This separates normal and abnormal types of hemoglobin. Each type of hemoglobin can then be measured individually.

WHAT IS HEMOGLOBIN ELECTROPHORESIS USED FOR?
Hemoglobin electrophoresis measures hemoglobin levels and looks for abnormal types of hemoglobin. It is most often used to help diagnose anemia, SCD, and other hemoglobin disorders.

WHY DO YOU NEED HEMOGLOBIN ELECTROPHORESIS?

You may need testing if you have symptoms of a hemoglobin disorder. These include the following:

- fatigue
- pale skin
- jaundice, a condition that causes your skin and eyes to turn yellow
- severe pain (SCD)
- growth problems (in children)

If you have just had a baby, your newborn will be tested as part of newborn screening. Newborn screening is a group of tests given to most American babies shortly after birth. The screening checks for a variety of conditions. Many of these conditions can be treated if found early.

You may also want testing if you are at risk of having a child with SCD or another inherited hemoglobin disorder. Risk factors include the following:

- family history
- ethnic background
  - In the United States, most people with SCD are of African ancestry.
  - Thalassemia, another inherited hemoglobin disorder, is most common among people of Italian, Greek, Middle Eastern, Southern Asian, and African descent.

ARE THERE ANY RISKS IN HEMOGLOBIN ELECTROPHORESIS?

There is very little risk in having a blood test. You may have slight pain or bruising at the spot where the needle was put in, but most symptoms go away quickly.

Your baby may feel a little pinch when the heel is poked, and a small bruise may form at the site. This should go away quickly.

WHAT HAPPENS DURING HEMOGLOBIN ELECTROPHORESIS?

A health-care professional will take a blood sample from a vein in your arm using a small needle. After the needle is inserted, a small amount of blood will be collected into a test tube or vial. You may feel a little sting when the needle goes in or out. This usually takes less than five minutes.

To test a newborn, a health-care provider will clean your baby's heel with alcohol and poke the heel with a small needle. The provider will collect a few drops of blood and put a bandage on the site.

WILL YOU NEED TO DO ANYTHING TO PREPARE FOR THE TEST?

You do not need any special preparations for a hemoglobin electrophoresis test.

WHAT DO THE RESULTS MEAN?

Your results will show the types of hemoglobin found and their levels.

Hemoglobin levels that are too high or too low may mean:

- **Thalassemia**. A condition that affects the production of hemoglobin.
- **Sickle cell trait**. A condition in which you have one sickle cell gene and one normal gene.
- **SCD**. A group of disorders that affects hemoglobin.
- **HgbC disease**. A condition that causes a mild form of anemia and sometimes an enlarged spleen and joint pain.
- **Hemoglobin S-C disease**. A condition that causes a mild or moderate form of SCD.

Your results may also show whether a specific disorder is mild, moderate, or severe.

There are several options for treating thalassemia and other hemoglobin disorders. Until recently, treatment options for SCD were limited. But now promising new therapies have become available. If you or your child was diagnosed with an SCD or other hemoglobin disorder, talk to your provider about treatment options.

Hemoglobin electrophoresis test results are often compared with other tests, including a complete blood count and a blood smear. If you have questions about your results, talk to your health-care provider.[2]

---

[2] MedlinePlus, "Hemoglobin Electrophoresis," National Institutes of Health (NIH), November 15, 2021. Available online. URL: https://medlineplus.gov/lab-tests/hemoglobin-electrophoresis. Accessed May 17, 2023.

Chapter 45 | **Bone Marrow Tests**

WHAT ARE BONE MARROW TESTS?

Bone marrow is a soft, spongy tissue found in the center of most bones. Bone marrow makes different types of blood cells, including the following:

- **Red blood cells (RBCs; also called "erythrocytes").** RBCs carry oxygen from your lungs to every cell in your body.
- **White blood cells (WBCs; also called "leukocytes").** WBCs help you fight infections.
- **Platelets.** These blood cells help with blood clotting.

Bone marrow tests check to see if your bone marrow is working correctly and making normal amounts of blood cells. The tests can help diagnose and monitor bone marrow disorders, blood disorders, and certain types of cancer.

The following are the two types of procedures used to collect bone marrow samples for testing:

- **Bone marrow aspiration.** This procedure removes a small amount of bone marrow fluid and cells.
- **Bone marrow biopsy.** This procedure removes a small piece of bone and bone marrow.

Bone marrow aspiration and bone marrow biopsy are usually done at the same time.

WHAT ARE BONE MARROW TESTS USED FOR?

Bone marrow tests are used to:
- find out the cause of problems with RBCs, WBCs, or platelets
- diagnose and monitor blood disorders, such as:
  - anemia (when the cause is unknown)
  - polycythemia vera
  - thrombocytopenia
- diagnose bone marrow disorders
- diagnose and monitor treatment for certain types of cancers, including leukemia, multiple myeloma, and lymphoma
- diagnose the cause of an unexplained fever, which could be from an infection in the bone marrow

WHY DO YOU NEED A BONE MARROW TEST?

Your health-care provider may order a bone marrow aspiration and a bone marrow biopsy if other blood tests show your levels of RBCs, WBCs, or platelets are not normal.

Too many or too few blood cells may mean you have a medical condition, such as cancer, that starts in your blood or bone marrow. If you are being treated for another type of cancer, these tests can find out if the cancer has spread to your bone marrow.

Bone marrow tests may also be used to see how well cancer treatment is working.

WHAT HAPPENS DURING A BONE MARROW TEST?

Bone marrow aspiration and bone marrow biopsy procedures are usually done at the same time. A health-care provider will collect the marrow samples for testing. Usually, the samples can be collected in about 10 minutes.

Before the procedure, you may be asked to put on a hospital gown. Your blood pressure, heart rate, and temperature will be checked.

You may choose to have a mild sedative, which is a medicine to help you relax. You may also have the choice to use stronger medicine that will make you sleep. Your provider can help you decide which option is best for you.

During the procedure, the following will happen:

- You will lie down on your side or your stomach, depending on which bone will be used to get the samples. Most bone marrow samples are taken from the back of the hip bone, called the "iliac crest." But other bones may also be used.
- An area of skin over the bone will be cleaned with an antiseptic.
- You will get an injection (shot) of medicine to numb the skin and the bone underneath. It may sting.
- When the area is numb, the provider will make a very small incision (cut) in your skin and insert a hollow needle. You will need to lie very still during the procedure:
  - The bone marrow aspiration is usually done first. The provider will push the needle into the bone and use a syringe attached to the needle to pull out bone marrow fluid and cells. You may feel a brief, sharp pain. The aspiration takes only a few minutes.
  - The bone marrow biopsy uses a special hollow biopsy needle inserted through the same skin opening. The provider will twist the needle into the bone to take out a small piece, or core, of bone marrow tissue. You may feel some pressure or brief pain while the sample is being taken.
- After the test, the health-care provider will cover your skin with a bandage.
- If you do not use medicine to relax or sleep, you will usually need to stay lying down for about 15 minutes to make sure that the bleeding has stopped. Afterward, you can do your usual activities as soon as you are able. If you use medicine to relax or sleep, you will need to stay longer before you can go home. You may also need to rest the next day.

591

IS THERE ANYTHING YOU NEED TO DO TO GET READY FOR THE TEST?

Your provider will tell you whether you need to fast (not eat or drink) for a few hours before the procedure.

Plan to have someone take you home after the test because you may be drowsy if you are given medicine to help you relax or sleep during the procedure.

You will receive instructions on how to prepare, but be sure to ask your provider any questions you have about the procedure.

ARE THERE ANY RISKS IN THE TEST?

After a bone marrow aspiration and bone marrow biopsy, you may feel stiff or sore where the sample was taken. This usually goes away in a few days.

Your provider may recommend or prescribe a pain reliever to help. Do not take any pain medicine your provider has not approved. Certain pain relievers, such as aspirin, could increase your risk of bleeding.

Serious symptoms are very rare but may include the following:
- increased pain or discomfort where the sample was taken
- redness, swelling, bleeding, or other fluids leaking from the site
- fever

If you have any of these symptoms, call your provider.

WHAT DO THE RESULTS MEAN?

It may take several days or even weeks to get your bone marrow test results. Your provider may have ordered many different types of tests on your marrow sample, so the results often include a lot of complex information. Your provider can explain what your results mean.

In certain cases, if your test results are not normal, you may need to have more tests to confirm a diagnosis or to decide which treatment would be best.

Bone Marrow Tests

If you have cancer that affects your bones and marrow, your test results may provide information about your cancer stage, which is how much cancer you have in your body and how fast it may be growing.

If you are already being treated for cancer, your test results may show:

- how well your treatment is working
- whether your treatment is affecting your bone marrow[1]

[1] MedlinePlus, "Bone Marrow Tests," National Institutes of Health (NIH), July 7, 2022. Available online. URL: https://medlineplus.gov/lab-tests/bone-marrow-tests. Accessed June 6, 2023.

Chapter 46 | Bleeding and Clotting Tests

Chapter Contents

WHAT ARE COAGULATION FACTOR TESTS?

Coagulation factors are proteins in your blood. They help form blood clots to stop bleeding when you have an injury. These proteins are also called "clotting factors." You have several different types of clotting factors that are all important for making blood clots.

Coagulation factor tests are blood tests that check one or more of your clotting factors to see if you:

- have too much or too little of a clotting factor
- are missing a clotting factor
- have a clotting factor that is not working properly

Your liver makes most of your clotting factors. But, normally, clotting factors are turned off, so you do not form abnormal blood clots. When you have an injury that causes bleeding, blood cells called "platelets" begin to make a soft blood clot to stop the bleeding.

The platelets release molecules into your blood that begin to turn on the clotting factors. The clotting factors work together in a chain reaction to form a harder blood clot that will stay firmly in place.

Problems with any one of your clotting factors may mean the following:

- **Your blood clots too easily, even without an injury**. This condition may lead to clots that block your blood flow and cause serious conditions, such as heart attack, stroke, or clots in the lungs.
- **Your blood does not clot enough after an injury or surgery**. If this happens, you have a bleeding disorder. Bleeding disorders can lead to serious blood loss after an injury.

Clotting factors have names, such as fibrinogen and prothrombin. Each clotting factor also has a Roman numeral name, such as "clotting factor II."

WHAT IS IT USED FOR?

A coagulation factor test is used to find out if you have a problem with any of your clotting factors that may cause too little or too much blood clotting.

Coagulation factor tests are also used to monitor people who have a known problem with clotting factors or who take medicine called "blood thinners" to lower the risk of blood clots.

You may have tests for one or more factors at a time.

WHY DO YOU NEED A COAGULATION FACTOR TEST?

You may need this test if you have the following:

- **An abnormal result on a blood test that checks how long it takes your blood to clot.** These tests include a prothrombin time and international normalized ratio (PT/INR) test and/or a partial thromboplastin time test (PTT).
- **A family health history of problems with clotting factors**. Some conditions that affect clotting factors, such as hemophilia, are inherited. It means that your parents passed the gene for the disease to you. These conditions are not common.
- **A health condition that may affect clotting factors in your blood:**
  - Conditions that may cause a bleeding disorder include:
    - severe liver disease
    - a lack of vitamin K
    - blood transfusions
    - cancer
    - immune disorders
  - Conditions that may cause a problem with blood clots include:
    - autoimmune diseases, such as lupus
    - cancer
    - obesity
    - certain infections, such as sepsis and COVID-19
    - not moving for long periods of time, such as after surgery
    - lack of vitamins B_6, B_{12}, and folate

- **Symptoms that may be from a problem with clotting factors:**
  - Symptoms of bleeding disorders may include:
    - heavy bleeding that does not stop with pressure after an injury, dental procedure, or surgery
    - frequent nosebleeds that start on their own
    - blood in the urine (pee) or stool (poop)
    - frequent, large bruises or tiny red or brown spots under the skin
    - redness, swelling, pain, or stiffness from bleeding into muscles or joints
    - heavy menstrual periods
  - Symptoms of too much blood clotting may include the following:
    - swelling, redness, warmth, and pain in your arms or legs, which may be from a clot
    - trouble breathing from a clot that is traveled to your lung
    - nausea

WHAT HAPPENS DURING A COAGULATION FACTOR TEST?

A health-care professional will take a blood sample from a vein in your arm using a small needle. After the needle is inserted, a small amount of blood will be collected into a test tube or vial. You may feel a little sting when the needle goes in or out. This usually takes less than five minutes.

WOULD YOU NEED TO DO ANYTHING TO PREPARE FOR THE TEST?

You do not need any special preparations for a coagulation factor test.

ARE THERE ANY RISKS IN THE TEST?

There is very little risk in having a blood test. You may have slight pain or bruising at the spot where the needle was put in, but most symptoms go away quickly.

WHAT DO THE RESULTS MEAN?

Your provider may need to order other tests to diagnose the cause of a problem with your clotting factors.

- Lower-than-normal levels of one or more clotting factors or a missing clotting factor may mean you have a bleeding disorder. Depending on which clotting factors were tested, your results may show the type of bleeding disorder you have and how serious it is.
  - Bleeding disorders that you inherit usually involve only one clotting factor. There is no cure for inherited bleeding disorders, but treatment can help manage your condition.
  - Bleeding disorders caused by other conditions usually involve low levels of two or more clotting factors. Treatment depends on the cause of your bleeding disorder.
- Higher-than-normal levels of one or more clotting factors may mean you have a disorder that makes your blood clot more than it should. Your provider may recommend medicine and heart-healthy lifestyle changes to help prevent clots. You may also need to avoid hormone replacement therapy (HRT) for menopause and birth control pills with estrogen because they may increase the risk of blood clots.

Talk with your provider to find out what your test results mean and what treatment is best for you.[1]

---

[1] MedlinePlus, "Coagulation Factor Tests," National Institutes of Health (NIH), August 3, 2022. Available online. URL: https://medlineplus.gov/lab-tests/coagulation-factor-tests. Accessed June 7, 2023.

Section 46.2 | **Partial Thromboplastin Time Test**

WHAT IS A PARTIAL THROMBOPLASTIN TIME TEST?

A partial thromboplastin time (PTT) test uses a blood sample to measure how long it takes for your blood to make a clot. Normally, when you get a cut or injury that causes bleeding, many different types of proteins in your blood work together to make a clot to stop the bleeding. These proteins are called "coagulation factors" or "clotting factors."

If any of your clotting factors are missing, at a low level, or not working properly, you may experience the following:

- **Your blood may clot too slowly after an injury or surgery**. If this happens, you have a bleeding disorder. Bleeding disorders can cause serious blood loss. Hemophilia is one type of bleeding disorder.
- **Your blood may clot too much and/or too quickly, even without an injury**. This condition may lead to clots that block your blood flow and cause serious conditions, such as heart attack, stroke, or clots in the lungs.

A PTT test helps check a specific group of clotting factors. It helps show how much of these clotting factors you have and how well they are working. A PTT test is often done with other tests that check clotting factors and how well they all work together.

WHAT IS IT USED FOR?

A PTT test is used to check for problems with a specific group of blood clotting factors. The test is done to:

- find the cause of too much bruising or bleeding
- find the cause of clotting problems (Causes can include certain autoimmune diseases, such as lupus and antiphospholipid syndrome (APS).)
- monitor people taking heparin, a type of medicine that is used to prevent and treat blood clots (PTT test can help make sure the dose is safe and effective.)

- check the risk of possible bleeding problems before surgery or medical procedures (A PTT test is not always used as a routine test before surgery. It may be used for certain people who may have a risk of bleeding problems.)

WHY DO YOU NEED A PARTIAL THROMBOPLASTIN TIME TEST?
You may need a PTT test if you:
- have problems with bleeding or bruising and the cause is not known
- have a blood clot in a vein or artery
- have liver disease (Your liver makes most of your clotting factors.)
- have had several miscarriages
- have been diagnosed with a bleeding or clotting disorder and do not know which clotting factors are involved
- are taking heparin (To check how this medicine is affecting you, your health-care provider may use a PTT test or another test instead.)

WHAT HAPPENS DURING A PARTIAL THROMBOPLASTIN TIME TEST?
A health-care professional will take a blood sample from a vein in your arm using a small needle. After the needle is inserted, a small amount of blood will be collected into a test tube or vial. You may feel a little sting when the needle goes in or out. This usually takes less than five minutes.

WOULD YOU NEED TO DO ANYTHING TO PREPARE FOR THE TEST?
You do not need any special preparations for a PTT test.

ARE THERE ANY RISKS IN THE TEST?
There is very little risk in having a blood test. You may have slight pain or bruising at the spot where the needle was put in, but most symptoms go away quickly.

WHAT DO THE RESULTS MEAN?

Your PTT test results will show how much time it took for your blood to clot. Results are usually given as a number of seconds. A PTT test is often ordered along with another blood test called a "prothrombin time (PT) test." A PT test measures other clotting factors that a PTT test does not check. Your provider will usually compare the results of both tests to understand how your blood is clotting. Ask your provider to explain what your test results mean for your health.

In general, if your blood takes longer than normal to clot on a PTT test, it may be a sign of:

- liver disease
- a lack of vitamin K
- certain genetic disorders that you inherit from your parents

These disorders affect certain clotting factors and increase your risk of bleeding. They include the following:

- von Willebrand disease (VWD)
- hemophilia
- too much heparin
- certain types of leukemia
- autoimmune diseases, such as antiphospholipid-antibody syndrome or lupus anticoagulant syndrome

Autoimmune diseases cause your body to make proteins called "antibodies." The antibodies related to these diseases cause too much clotting. But the results of a PTT test may show a slow clotting time. That is because the chemicals in the PTT test react with the antibodies in your blood sample. This chemical reaction makes the blood sample clot more slowly than the blood in your body. If your provider thinks that an autoimmune disease is causing a clotting problem, you will usually have other tests to make a diagnosis.

If your blood clot faster than normal on a PTT test, it may be a sign of:

- **The early stage of disseminated intravascular coagulation (DIC).** This rare but serious condition may develop if you have an infection or damage to organs or tissues that affects blood clotting. In the early stage, you have too much blood clotting. Later on, DIC starts to use up clotting factors in your blood, which leads to bleeding problems.

- **Cancer of the ovaries, colon, or pancreas that is advanced**. It means the cancer has spread to other parts of the body and is unlikely to be controlled with treatment.

Talk with your provider to learn what your test results mean.[2]

Section 46.3 | Prothrombin Time Test and International Normalized Ratio

WHAT IS A PROTHROMBIN TIME TEST WITH AN INTERNATIONAL NORMALIZED RATIO?

A prothrombin time (PT) test measures how long it takes for a clot to form in a blood sample. An international normalized ratio (INR) is a type of calculation based on PT test results.

Prothrombin is a protein made by the liver. It is one of several substances known as "clotting (coagulation) factors." When you get a cut or other injury that causes bleeding, your clotting factors work together to form a blood clot. How fast your blood clots depends on the amount of clotting factors in your blood and whether they are working correctly. If your blood clots too slowly, you may bleed too much after an injury. If your blood clots too fast, dangerous clots may form in your arteries or veins.

A PT/INR test helps diagnose the cause of bleeding or clotting disorders. It also checks to see if a medicine that prevents blood clots is working the way it should.

---

[2] MedlinePlus, "Partial Thromboplastin Time (PTT) Test," National Institutes of Health (NIH), December 15, 2022. Available online. URL: https://medlineplus.gov/lab-tests/partial-thromboplastin-time-ptt-test. Accessed June 7, 2023.

WHAT IS IT USED FOR?

A PT/INR test is most often used to:

- see how well warfarin is working (Warfarin is a blood-thinning medicine that is used to treat and prevent dangerous blood clots. Coumadin is a common brand name for warfarin.)
- find out the reason for abnormal blood clots
- find out the reason for unusual bleeding
- check clotting function before surgery
- check for liver problems

A PT/INR test is often done along with a partial thromboplastin time (PTT) test. A PTT test also checks for clotting problems.

WHY DO YOU NEED A PT/INR TEST?

You may need this test if you are taking warfarin on a regular basis. The test helps make sure you are taking the right dose.

If you are not taking warfarin, you may need this test if you have symptoms of a bleeding or clotting disorder.

Symptoms of a bleeding disorder include the following:

- unexplained heavy bleeding
- bruising easily
- unusually heavy nose bleeds
- unusually heavy menstrual periods in women

Symptoms of a clotting disorder include the following:

- leg pain or tenderness
- leg swelling
- redness or red streaks on the legs
- trouble breathing
- cough
- chest pain
- rapid heartbeat

In addition, you may need a PT/INR test if you are scheduled for surgery. It helps make sure your blood is clotting normally, so you will not lose too much blood during the procedure.

WHAT HAPPENS DURING A PT/INR TEST?

The test may be done on a blood sample from a vein or a fingertip. For a blood sample from a vein, the following will be done:

- A health-care professional will take a blood sample from a vein in your arm using a small needle. After the needle is inserted, a small amount of blood will be collected into a test tube or vial. You may feel a little sting when the needle goes in or out. This usually takes less than five minutes.

For a blood sample from a fingertip, the following will be done:

- A fingertip test may be done in a provider's office or in your home. If you are taking warfarin, your provider may recommend you test your blood regularly using an at-home PT/INR test kit. During this test, you or your provider will:
  - use a small needle to puncture your fingertip
  - collect a drop of blood and place it onto a test strip or other special instrument
  - place the instrument or test strip into a device that calculates the results (At-home devices are small and lightweight.)

If you are using an at-home test kit, you will need to review your results with your provider. Your provider will let you know how he or she would like to receive the results.

IS THERE ANYTHING YOU NEED TO DO TO GET READY FOR THE TEST?

If you are taking warfarin, you may need to delay your daily dose until after testing. Your health-care provider will let you know if there are any other special instructions to follow.

ARE THERE ANY RISKS IN THE TEST?

There is very little risk in having a blood test. You may have slight pain or bruising at the spot where the needle was put in, but most symptoms go away quickly.

WHAT DO THE RESULTS MEAN?

If you were tested because you are taking warfarin, your results will probably be in the form of INR levels. INR levels are often used because they make it easier to compare results from different labs and different test methods. If you are not taking warfarin, your results may be in the form of INR levels or the number of seconds it takes for your blood sample to clot (PT).

If you are taking warfarin, the following will be your results:

- **INR levels that are too low**. It may mean you are at risk of dangerous blood clots.
- **INR levels that are too high**. It may may mean you are at risk of dangerous bleeding.

Your health-care provider will probably change your dose of warfarin to reduce these risks.

If you are not taking warfarin and your INR or PT results are not normal, it may mean one of the following conditions:

- a bleeding disorder, a condition in which the body cannot clot blood properly, causing excessive bleeding
- a clotting disorder, a condition in which the body forms excessive clots in arteries or veins
- liver disease
- vitamin K deficiency that plays an important role in blood clotting[3]

---

[3] MedlinePlus, "Prothrombin Time Test and INR (PT/INR)," National Institutes of Health (NIH), September 21, 2022. Available online. URL: https://medlineplus.gov/lab-tests/prothrombin-time-test-and-inr-ptinr. Accessed June 7, 2023.

Chapter 47 | **Tests Used in the Assessment of Vascular Disease**

Blood tests and heart health tests can help find heart diseases or identify problems that can lead to heart diseases. There are several different types of heart health tests. Your doctor will decide which test or tests you need based on your symptoms (if any), risk factors, and medical history.[1]

CORONARY CALCIUM SCAN

A coronary calcium scan is a computed tomography (CT) scan of your heart that measures the amount of calcium in the walls of your coronary arteries. The buildup of calcium, or calcifications, is a sign of atherosclerosis or coronary heart disease (CHD).

A coronary calcium scan may be done in a medical imaging facility or hospital. The test does not use contrast dye and will take about 10–15 minutes to complete. A coronary calcium scan uses a special scanner such as an electron beam CT or a multidetector CT (MDCT) machine. An MDCT machine is a very fast CT scanner that makes high-quality pictures of the beating heart. A coronary calcium scan will determine a score that reflects the amount of calcium found in your coronary arteries, often referred to as an "Agatston score." A score of 0 is normal. In general, the higher your

[1] MedlinePlus, "Heart Health Tests," National Institutes of Health (NIH), February 28, 2017. Available online. URL: https://medlineplus.gov/hearthealthtests.html. Accessed June 21, 2023.

score, the more likely you are to have CHD. If your score is high, your doctor may recommend more tests.

A coronary calcium scan has few risks. There is a very slight risk of cancer, particularly in people younger than 40 years old who undergo multiple CT scans. However, the amount of radiation from one test is similar to the amount of radiation you are naturally exposed to over one year. Talk to your doctor and the technicians performing the test about whether you are or could be pregnant.[2]

CARDIAC CATHETERIZATION

Cardiac catheterization, also known as "cardiac cath" or "heart catheterization," is a medical procedure used to diagnose and treat some heart conditions. It lets doctors take a close look at the heart to identify problems and perform other tests or procedures.

Your health-care provider may recommend cardiac catheterization to find out the cause of symptoms such as chest pain or irregular heartbeat. Before the procedure, you may need diagnostic tests, such as blood tests, heart imaging tests, or a stress test, to determine how well your heart is working and to help guide the procedure.

During cardiac catheterization, a long, thin, flexible tube called a "catheter" is put into a blood vessel in your arm, groin or upper thigh, or neck. The catheter is then threaded through the blood vessels to your heart. It may be used to examine your heart valves or take samples of blood or heart muscle. Your doctor may also use ultrasound, a test that uses sound waves to create an image, or they may inject a dye into your coronary arteries to see whether your arteries are narrowed or blocked. Cardiac catheterization may also be used instead of some heart surgeries to repair heart defects and replace heart valves.

Cardiac catheterization is safe for most people. Problems following the procedure are rare but can include bleeding and blood clots. Your health-care provider will monitor your condition and may recommend medicines to prevent blood clots.[3]

---

[2] "Heart Tests," National Heart, Lung, and Blood Institute (NHLBI), March 24, 2022. Available online. URL: www.nhlbi.nih.gov/health/heart-tests. Accessed May 25, 2023.
[3] "Cardiac Catheterization," National Heart, Lung, and Blood Institute (NHLBI), March 24, 2022. Available online. URL: www.nhlbi.nih.gov/health/cardiac-catheterization. Accessed May 25, 2023.

CARDIAC MAGNETIC RESONANCE IMAGING

Cardiac magnetic resonance imaging (MRI) is a painless, noninvasive imaging test that uses radio waves, magnets, and a computer to create detailed pictures of your heart. No ionizing radiation is used in this type of imaging. This test can provide information on the type and seriousness of heart disease to help your doctor decide the best way to treat your condition.

Cardiac MRI can help your doctor diagnose heart diseases or problems with the blood vessels. Cardiac MRI can provide an accurate look at the heart muscle, heart chamber sizes and function, and connecting blood vessels. It is an excellent tool to look for scarring of the heart muscle like you might see in a heart attack or inflammation of the heart, as you might see with a heart infection. Cardiac MRI may be performed as a resting study or used in combination with a stress medicine or exercise to look for low blood flow to the heart muscle. Cardiac MRI is also an excellent tool for evaluating tumors or clots in the heart and to help your health-care provider monitor congenital heart disease or problems with your heart valves or aorta. Cardiac MRI may be used when images from other studies, such as an echocardiogram, are not clear. It can also help clarify results from other imaging tests such as chest x-rays and chest CT scans.

Cardiac MRI may be done in a medical imaging facility or hospital. Before your procedure, a contrast dye to highlight your heart and blood vessels may be injected into a vein in your arm. Some cardiac MRI studies do not require contrast. The MRI machine is a large, tunnel-like machine that has a table. You will lie still on the table, and the table will slide into the machine. Talk to your doctor if you are uncomfortable in tight or closed spaces to see if you need medicine to help you relax during the test. You will hear loud humming, tapping, and buzzing sounds when you are inside the machine as pictures of your heart are being taken. You will be able to hear from and talk to the technician performing the test while you are inside the machine. Your heart rhythm will be monitored by an electrocardiogram, and your pictures will be coordinated with your heartbeat. The technician may ask you to hold your breath for a few seconds multiple times during the test.

Cardiac MRI has few risks. In very rare cases, the contrast dye may cause an allergic-type reaction. Talk to your doctor and the technicians performing the test if you are or could be pregnant or are breastfeeding. If you are breastfeeding and need to receive an MRI contrast, you may be instructed to discard your breast milk for up to two days after the MRI study.

Tell your doctor if you have:

- a pacemaker or other implanted device because the MRI machine can damage these devices or cause a metallic implant to move
- had any prior surgeries, even if you do not know if metal was involved (Metal inside your body from previous surgeries (e.g., from clips or metal parts) can interfere with the MRI machine, cause the metal to move, cause artifacts in your images, or cause local heating. A lot of surgery-related metal is safe in the MRI machine, but it is important for the imaging team to carefully screen you ahead of time.)
- metal on your body from piercings, jewelry, or some transdermal skin patches because they can interfere with the MRI machine or cause skin burns (Tattoos may cause a problem because older tattoo inks may contain small amounts of metal.)

CARDIAC COMPUTED TOMOGRAPHY SCAN

A cardiac CT is a painless, noninvasive imaging test that uses x-rays to take many detailed pictures of your heart and its blood vessels. Computers can combine these pictures to create a three-dimensional (3D) model of your whole heart.

This imaging test can help doctors find heart diseases or problems with the heart or blood vessels supplying blood to the heart or the rest of the body. This test may also be used to check the results of coronary artery bypass grafting or to follow up on abnormal findings from earlier chest x-rays. You may go to a medical imaging facility or a hospital for a cardiac CT scan. The scan itself usually takes only about 15 minutes. However, it can take more than an hour to prepare for the scan, including time to take medicines such as beta blockers to slow your heart rate or nitroglycerin to help dilate your arteries. Before the test, a health-care provider will inject a contrast dye, often iodine-based, into a vein in your arm. This contrast dye highlights your blood vessels and creates clearer pictures. You may feel some discomfort from the needle, or after the contrast dye is injected, you may feel a warm flush briefly throughout your body or have a temporary metallic taste in your mouth.

The CT scanner is a large, tunnel-like machine that has a table. You will lie still on the table, and the table will slide into the scanner. Talk to your doctor if you are uncomfortable in tight or closed spaces to see if you need medicine to help you relax during the test. During the scan, the technician will monitor your heart rate with an electrocardiogram (EKG). You will hear soft buzzing, clicking, or whirring sounds when you are inside the scanner and the scanner is taking pictures. You will be able to hear from and talk to the technician performing the test while you are inside the scanner. The technician may ask you to hold your breath for a few seconds during the test.

Cardiac CT scans have some risks. In rare cases, the contrast dye may cause damage to the kidneys, particularly in people who have known chronic kidney problems. Your doctor or the imaging center may do a blood test to check your kidney function before the exam. In rare instances, some people may have an allergic reaction to the contrast dye. If you have a known allergy, you may still be able to receive contrast if you receive medicine ahead of time. There is a very slight risk of cancer, particularly in people younger than 40 years old who undergo multiple CT scans because the test uses radiation.

Talk to your doctor and the technicians performing the test about whether you are or could be pregnant or are breastfeeding.

Rarely, people with lung diseases or heart failure may have breathing problems during cardiac CT scans if they are given beta-blockers to slow their heart rates for this imaging test.[4]

---

[4] See footnote [2].

DOPPLER ULTRASOUND

A Doppler ultrasound is an imaging test that uses sound waves to show blood moving through blood vessels. A regular ultrasound also uses sound waves to create images of structures inside the body, but it cannot show blood flow.

Doppler ultrasound works by measuring sound waves that are reflected from moving objects, such as red blood cells (RBCs). This is known as the "Doppler effect."

There are different types of Doppler ultrasound tests. They include the following:

- **Color Doppler**. This type of Doppler uses a computer to change sound waves into different colors. These colors show the speed and direction of blood flow in real time.
- **Power Doppler**. A newer type of color Doppler. It can provide more detail of blood flow than standard color Doppler. But it cannot show the direction of blood flow, which can be important in some cases.
- **Spectral Doppler**. This test shows blood flow information on a graph rather than color pictures. It can help show how much of a blood vessel is blocked.
- **Duplex Doppler**. This test uses standard ultrasound to take images of blood vessels and organs. Then a computer turns the images into a graph, as in spectral Doppler.
- **Continuous wave Doppler**. In this test, sound waves are sent and received continuously. It allows for more accurate measurement of blood that flows at faster speeds.[5]

CAROTID ULTRASOUND

Carotid ultrasound is a painless imaging test that uses high-frequency sound waves to create pictures of the inside of your carotid arteries. Your carotid arteries are the major blood vessels

---

[5] MedlinePlus, "Doppler Ultrasound," National Institutes of Health (NIH), December 15, 2020. Available online. URL: https://medlineplus.gov/lab-tests/doppler-ultrasound. Accessed May 25, 2023.

that supply oxygen-rich blood to your brain. Carotid ultrasound can help detect plaque buildup in one or both of your carotid arteries. It can also see whether the buildup is blocking blood flow to the brain. If combined with Doppler ultrasound, this test can also show how blood is moving through your arteries.

Carotid ultrasound is usually done in a doctor's office or hospital. This test uses an ultrasound machine, which includes a computer, a screen, and a transducer. The transducer is a handheld device that sends and receives sound waves.

You will lie on your back on an exam table for your test. The ultrasound technician will put gel on your neck where your carotid arteries are located. The gel helps the sound waves reach your arteries. The technician will move the transducer against different areas on your neck. The transducer will detect the sound waves after they have bounced off your artery walls and blood cells. A computer will use sound waves to create and record pictures of the inside of your carotid arteries and to show how blood is flowing in your carotid arteries. Test results will help your doctor plan treatment to remove or stabilize plaque and help prevent a stroke.

Carotid ultrasound has no risks because the test uses harmless sound waves. They are the same type of sound waves that doctors use to create and record pictures of a baby inside a pregnant woman.

NUCLEAR HEART SCAN

A nuclear heart scan is an imaging test that uses special cameras and a radioactive substance called a "tracer" to create pictures of your heart. This imaging test can detect if blood is not flowing to parts of the heart and can diagnose CHD. It can also check for damaged or dead heart muscle tissue, possibly from a previous heart attack, and assess how well your heart pumps blood to your body.

You may go to a medical imaging facility or a hospital for a nuclear heart scan. Your health-care team will monitor your heart during this test with an EKG. They will take two sets of pictures, each taking 15–30 minutes. The first set of pictures is taken right after an exercise or medicine stress test because some problems happen only when the heart is working hard or beating fast. Shortly after the stress test, the health-care provider will inject the tracer into a vein in your arm. You may bruise at the injection site. You will lie still on a table that slides through a tunnel-like machine as the first set of pictures is taken. The second set of pictures will be taken on either the same day or the next day after your heartbeat has returned to normal.

Nuclear heart scans have few risks. In rare instances, some people have a treatable allergic reaction to the tracer. If you have CHD, you may have chest pain during the stress test. Medicine can help relieve your chest pain. Talk to your doctor and the technicians performing the test about whether you are or could be pregnant.

CORONARY ANGIOGRAPHY

Coronary angiography is a procedure that uses contrast dye, usually containing iodine, and x-ray pictures to detect blockages in the coronary arteries that are caused by plaque buildup. Blockages prevent your heart from getting oxygen and important nutrients.

This procedure is used to diagnose heart diseases or after abnormal results from tests such as an EKG or an exercise stress test. If you are having a heart attack, coronary angiography can help your doctors plan your treatment.

Coronary angiography is often done in a hospital. You will stay awake but receive medicine to relax during the procedure. Coronary angiography is done via a cardiac catheterization procedure. For this, your doctor will clean and numb an area on the arm, groin or upper thigh, or neck before making a small hole in the skin and a blood vessel. Your doctor will insert a catheter tube into your blood vessel. Your doctor will take x-ray pictures to help place the catheter in your coronary arteries. After the catheter is in place, your doctor will inject the contrast dye through the catheter to highlight blockages and will take x-ray pictures of your heart. If blockages are detected, your doctor may use percutaneous coronary intervention, also known as "coronary balloon angioplasty," usually with the use of a stent (a wire mesh that helps keep a blocked artery open), to improve blood flow to your heart.

After coronary angiography, your doctor will remove the catheter and close and bandage the opening on your arm, groin, or neck. You may develop a bruise and soreness where the catheter is inserted. You will stay in the hospital for a few hours or sometimes overnight. During this time, your health-care team will check your heart rate, blood pressure, and the catheter insertion site.

Coronary angiography is a common procedure that rarely causes serious problems. However, as with any invasive procedure involving the heart, there is some risk. These risks include bleeding, allergic reactions to the contrast dye, kidney problems, infection, blood vessel damage, arrhythmias, and blood clots that can trigger a heart attack or stroke. The risk of complications is higher in people who are older or who have chronic kidney disease (CKD) or diabetes.

ECHOCARDIOGRAPHY

Echocardiography, or echo, is a painless test that uses sound waves to create moving pictures of your heart. The pictures show the size and shape of your heart and how well your heart is pumping blood. A type of echo called "Doppler ultrasound" shows how well blood flows through your heart's chambers and valves.

Echo can detect blood clots inside your heart, fluid buildup in the pericardium (the sac around the heart), tumors, and problems with the aorta. The aorta is the main artery that carries oxygen-rich blood from your heart to your body. Echo can also help your doctor find the cause of abnormal heart sounds, such as heart murmurs, due to damaged heart valves. Your doctor may also use an echo to see how well your heart responds to certain treatments.

There are several types of echocardiography:

- **Transthoracic echocardiography**. This echo is the most common type of echo. It involves placing a device called a "transducer" on your chest after a gel is applied to your skin. The device sends special sound waves, called "ultrasound," through your chest wall to your heart. As the ultrasound waves bounce off the structures of your heart, a computer in the echo machine converts them into pictures on a screen.

- **Stress echocardiography**. This echo is done as part of a stress test. During a stress test, you exercise or take medicine to make your heart work hard and beat fast. A technician will use echo to create pictures of your heart before you exercise and as soon as you finish.
- **Transesophageal echocardiography**. This gives your doctor a more detailed view of your heart. During this test, the transducer is attached to the end of a flexible tube. The tube is guided down your throat and into your esophagus (the passage leading from your mouth to your stomach). Your doctor will inject medicine into a vein to help you relax during the test.
- **Fetal echocardiography**. This echo is used to look at an unborn baby's heart to check for heart problems. When recommended, the test is commonly done at about 18–22 weeks of pregnancy. For this test, the transducer is moved over the pregnant person's belly.
- **Three-dimensional (3D) echocardiography**. This 3D echo creates 3D images of your heart. This may be done as part of a transthoracic or transesophageal echo.

You may have the echocardiography in your doctor's office or at a hospital. You will not need to do anything to prepare for most types of echo. For a transesophageal echo, your doctor may ask you not to eat or drink for eight hours before the test. Echocardiography usually takes less than an hour to do. For some types of echo, your doctor will need to inject saline or a special dye into one of your veins. This makes your heart show up more clearly in the echo pictures.

For most types of echo, you will remove your clothing from the waist up. Women will be given a gown to wear during the test. You will lie on your back or left side on an exam table or stretcher. Soft, sticky patches called "electrodes" will be attached to your chest to allow an EKG to be done. An EKG is a test that records your heart's electrical activity.

For a transesophageal echo, you will be given oxygen through a tube in your nose. The back of your mouth will be numbed with gel or spray. Your doctor will gently place the tube with the transducer in your throat and guide it down until it is in place behind your heart. The pictures of your heart are then recorded as your doctor moves the transducer around in your esophagus and stomach. You should not feel any discomfort as this happens. Your throat might be sore for a few hours after the test.

If you have a transesophageal echo, you may experience some side effects from the medicine given to help you relax, such as problems breathing or nausea (feeling sick to your stomach). Rarely, the tube used causes minor throat injuries.[6]

ELECTROCARDIOGRAM

An EKG test is a simple, painless, and quick test that records your heart's electrical activity. Each time your heartbeats, an electrical signal travels through your heart. The signal triggers your heart's four chambers to contract (squeeze) in the proper rhythm so that your heart can pump blood to your body.

An EKG recording of these signals looks like wavy lines. Your provider can read these lines to look for abnormal heart activity that may be a sign of heart disease or damage.

An EKG can show:
- how fast your heart is beating
- whether the rhythm of your heartbeat is steady or irregular
- the strength and timing of the electrical signals passing through each part of your heart

Sometimes, information from an EKG can help measure the size and position of your heart's chambers.

An EKG is often the first test you will have if you have signs of a heart condition. It may be done in your provider's office, an outpatient clinic, in a hospital before surgery, or as part of another heart test called a "stress test."

---

[6] See footnote [2].

An EKG test is also called an "ECG." EKG is based on the German spelling "electrocardiogram." EKG may be preferred over ECG to avoid confusion with an EEG, a test that measures brain waves.[7]

STRESS TESTING

Stress tests show how well your heart works when it is pumping hard. Some heart diseases are easier to find when your heart is working its hardest to pump blood through your body. So stress tests check your heart while you exercise on a treadmill or stationary bicycle. If you are not able to exercise, medicine can be used to make your heart work harder, as if you were exercising.

There are different types of stress tests. They all check:
- blood flow in your heart
- your blood pressure
- the rate and rhythm of your heartbeat
- the strength of the electrical signals that control your heartbeat

Some stress tests also take pictures of your heart at rest and when it is working hard.[8]

[7] MedlinePlus, "Electrocardiogram," National Institutes of Health (NIH), February 28, 2023. Available online. URL: https://medlineplus.gov/lab-tests/electrocardiogram. Accessed May 25, 2023.
[8] MedlinePlus, "Stress Tests," National Institutes of Health (NIH), February 28, 2023. Available online. URL: https://medlineplus.gov/lab-tests/stress-tests. Accessed May 25, 2023.

Chapter 48 | Commonly Used Medications for Cardiovascular Health

Chapter Contents

For most people, aspirin is safe. But it is not right for everyone.

Ask your doctor about taking aspirin regularly if you are between the ages of 50 and 59 and you have any of the following risk factors for heart disease:

- smoking
- high blood pressure (HBP)
- high cholesterol
- diabetes

Talk with your doctor about your health history and ask if low-dose aspirin is right for you.

WHAT ARE THE BENEFITS OF TAKING ASPIRIN REGULARLY?

Taking low-dose aspirin regularly can reduce your risk of heart attack or stroke by preventing blood clots. Blood clots are clumps of thickened blood that can block blood flow to parts of the body. They can cause serious health problems or even death.

A blood clot can:

- block blood flow to your heart and cause a heart attack
- prevent blood from getting to your brain and cause a stroke

If you have already had a heart attack or stroke, aspirin can lower your risk of having another one.

Taking aspirin regularly for at least 5–10 years can also lower your risk of colorectal cancer, but experts are not sure why.

CAN TAKING ASPIRIN EVERY DAY CAUSE ANY SIDE EFFECTS?

Taking aspirin regularly is not right for everyone. For some people, it may cause side effects, such as bleeding in the stomach.

Talk with your doctor before you start taking aspirin. Be sure to tell your doctor about any health conditions you have (such as stomach problems or bleeding problems).

STEPS TO PROTECT YOUR HEALTH

Take the following steps to protect your health if you are at risk of heart attack or stroke.

Find Out If Daily Aspirin Is Right for You

Your doctor can help you decide if low-dose aspirin is the right choice for you. Talk with your doctor about:

- your risk of heart attack or stroke
- what kind of aspirin to take
- how much to take
- how often to take it
- side effects that it may cause

It is important to tell your doctor about all the other medicines you take, including vitamins, herbs, and over-the-counter (OTC) medicines (medicines you can get without a prescription). It may be dangerous to mix aspirin with other medicines.

WHAT ABOUT THE COST?

Aspirin is inexpensive and sold OTC. For some adults, aspirin is covered under the Affordable Care Act (ACA), the health-care reform law passed in 2010. Check with your insurance provider to find out what is included in your plan.

Know Your Family's Health History

Your family history affects your risk of heart attack, stroke, and colorectal cancer. Share this information with your doctor.

Use Aspirin Safely

If you and your doctor decide that regularly taking low-dose aspirin is right for you, follow these safety tips:

- Make sure you understand how much aspirin to take and how often to take it. Most people who take aspirin to prevent disease take 81 mg every day—though your doctor may recommend you take a higher dose every other day.

- Talk with your doctor before you start taking a new medicine or vitamin. Ask if it is safe to take with aspirin.
- If you drink alcohol, drink only in moderation. This means no more than one drink a day for women and no more than two drinks a day for men. Alcohol can increase some risks of taking aspirin regularly.
- Check with your doctor first if you want to stop taking aspirin regularly.

Make It Easy to Remember

Here are a few things that may help you remember to take aspirin regularly:

- Take it at the same time every day. For example, take it after you brush your teeth or when you eat breakfast.
- Put a reminder note on your bathroom mirror where you will see it each day.
- Use a weekly pillbox to keep track of the medicines you take each day.

Take Steps to Protect Your Health

Taking low-dose aspirin regularly is just one of many ways to stay healthy.

To lower your risk of heart disease, stroke, and colorectal cancer, do the following:

- Quit smoking.
- Get active.
- Watch your weight.

KEEP YOUR HEART HEALTHY

Eating healthy is another way to lower your risk of heart disease and stroke.

GET TESTED FOR COLORECTAL CANCER

If you are between the ages of 50 and 75, get screened (tested) regularly for colorectal cancer. Screening can help prevent colorectal cancer or find it early when it is easier to treat.[1]

Section 48.2 | Blood Thinner Pills

A blood thinner is a kind of drug called an "anticoagulant." "Anti" means against, and "coagulant" means to thicken into a gel or solid. Your doctor prescribes a medicine called a "blood thinner" to prevent blood clots. Blood clots can put you at risk of heart attack, stroke, and other serious medical problems.

Depending on where you receive care, you may be seen by a doctor, nurse, physician's assistant, nurse practitioner, pharmacist, or other health-care professionals.

You and your doctor will work together as a team to make sure that taking your blood thinner does not stop you from living well and safely. The information in this section will help you understand why you are taking a blood thinner and how to keep yourself healthy. There are different types of blood thinners. The most common blood thinner that doctors prescribe is warfarin (Coumadin®). Your doctor may also discuss using one of the newer blood thinners depending on your individual situation.

HOW TO TAKE YOUR BLOOD THINNER

- Always take your blood thinner as directed. For example, some blood thinners need to be taken at the same time of day every day.
- Never skip a dose, and never take a double dose.

---

[1] Office of Disease Prevention and Health Promotion (ODPHP), "Talk with Your Doctor about Taking Aspirin to Prevent Disease," U.S. Department of Health and Human Services (HHS), January 1, 2019. Available online. URL: https://health.gov/myhealthfinder/health-conditions/heart-health/talk-your-doctor-about-taking-aspirin-prevent-disease#the-basics-tab. Accessed June 7, 2023.

- If you miss a dose, take it as soon as you remember. If you do not remember until the next day, call your doctor for instructions. If this happens when your doctor is not available, skip the missed dose and start again the next day. Mark the missed dose in a diary or on a calendar.
- A pillbox with a slot for each day may help you keep track of your medicines.

CHECK YOUR MEDICINE

Check your medicine when you get it from the pharmacy.

- Does the medicine seem different from what your doctor prescribed or look different from what you expected?
- Does your pill look different from what you used before?
- Are the color, shape, and markings on the pill the same as what you were given before?

If something seems different, ask the pharmacist to double-check it. Many medication errors are found by patients.

USING OTHER MEDICINES

Tell your doctor about every medicine you take. The doctor needs to know about all of your medicines, including medicines you used before you started taking a blood thinner.

Other medicines can change the way your blood thinner works. Your blood thinner can also change how other medicines work.

It is very important to talk with your doctor about all the medicines you take, including other prescription medicines, over-the-counter (OTC) medicines, vitamins, and herbal products.

Products that contain aspirin may lessen the blood's ability to form clots and may increase your risk of bleeding when you are also taking a blood thinner. If you are taking a blood thinner, talk to your doctor before taking any medication that has aspirin in it.

Medicines you get OTC may also interact with your blood thinner. Following is a list of some common medicines that you should talk with your doctor or pharmacist about before using.

- pain relievers, cold medicines, or stomach remedies, such as:
  - Advil®
  - Aleve®
  - Alka-Seltzer®
  - Excedrin®
  - ex-lax®
  - Midol®
  - Motrin®
  - Nuprin®
  - Pamprin HB®
  - Pepto Bismol®
  - Sine-Off®
  - Tagamet HB®
  - Tylenol®
- vitamins and herbal products, such as:
  - centrum®, One A Day®, or other multivitamins
  - garlic
  - *Ginkgo biloba*
  - green tea

Talk to your doctor about every medication and OTC product that you take.

TALK TO YOUR OTHER DOCTORS

Because you take a blood thinner, you will be seen regularly by the doctor who prescribed the medicine. You may also see other doctors for different problems. When you see other doctors, it is very important that you tell them you are taking a blood thinner. You should also tell your dentist and the person who cleans your teeth.

If you use different pharmacies, make sure each pharmacist knows that you take a blood thinner.

Blood thinners can interact with medicines and treatments that other doctors might prescribe for you. If another doctor orders a new medicine for you, tell the doctor who ordered your blood thinner because dose changes for your blood thinner may be needed.

Tell Your Doctor about All Your Medicines

Always tell your doctor about all the medicines you are taking. Tell your doctor when you start taking a new medicine, when you stop taking a medicine, and if the amount of medicine you are taking changes. When you visit your doctor, bring a list of current medicines: OTC drugs, such as aspirin, and any vitamins and herbal products you take. A personal medication wallet card can help you keep track of this list.

POSSIBLE SIDE EFFECTS

When taking a blood thinner, it is important to be aware of its possible side effects. Bleeding is the most common side effect.

Call your doctor immediately if you have any of the following signs of serious bleeding:

- menstrual bleeding that is much heavier than normal
- red or brown urine
- bowel movements that are red or look like tar
- bleeding from the gums or nose that does not stop quickly
- vomit that is brown or bright red
- anything red in color that you cough up
- severe pain, such as a headache or stomach ache
- unusual bruising
- a cut that does not stop bleeding
- a serious fall or bump on the head
- dizziness or weakness

STAY SAFE WHILE TAKING YOUR BLOOD THINNER

Call your doctor and go to the hospital immediately if you have had a fall or hit your head, even if you are not bleeding. You can be bleeding but not see any blood. For example, if you fall and hit your head, bleeding can occur inside your skull. Or, if you hurt your arm during a fall and then notice a large purple bruise, this means that you are bleeding under your skin.

Because you are taking a blood thinner, you should try not to hurt yourself and cause bleeding. You need to be careful when you

629

use knives, scissors, razors, or any sharp object that can make you bleed.

You also need to avoid activities and sports that could cause injury. Swimming and walking are safe activities. If you would like to start a new activity that will increase the amount of exercise you get every day, talk to your doctor.

You can still do many things that you enjoy. If you like to work in the yard, you still can. Just be sure to wear sturdy shoes and gloves to protect yourself. If you like to ride your bike, be sure you wear a helmet.

Tell Others

Keep a current list of all the medicines you take. Ask your doctor about whether you should wear a medical alert bracelet or necklace. If you are badly injured and unable to speak, the bracelet lets health-care workers know that you are taking a blood thinner.

To prevent injury indoors, do the following:
- Be very careful using knives and scissors.
- Use an electric razor.
- Use a soft toothbrush.
- Use waxed dental floss.
- Do not use toothpicks.
- Wear shoes or nonskid slippers in the house.
- Be careful when you trim your toenails.
- Do not trim corns or calluses yourself.

To prevent injury outdoors, do the following:
- Always wear shoes.
- Wear gloves when using sharp tools.
- Avoid activities and sports that can easily hurt you.
- Wear gardening gloves when doing yard work.

FOOD AND YOUR BLOOD THINNER

If your doctor has prescribed warfarin, the foods you eat can affect how well your blood thinner works for you. High amounts of vitamin K can work against warfarin. Other blood thinners are not affected by vitamin K. Ask your doctor if your diet can affect how well your blood thinner works.

If you are taking a blood thinner, you should avoid drinking alcohol.

Call your doctor if you are unable to eat for several days for whatever reason. Also, call if you have stomach problems, vomiting, or diarrhea that lasts longer than one day. These problems could affect your blood thinner dose.

Keep Your Diet the Same
Do not make any major changes in your diet or start a weight loss plan unless you talk to your doctor first.

BLOOD TESTS
You will have to have your blood tested often if you are taking warfarin. The blood test helps your doctor decide how much medicine you need.

The international normalized ratio (INR) blood test measures how fast your blood clots and lets the doctor know if your dose needs to be changed. Testing your blood helps your doctor keep you in a safe range. If there is too much blood thinner in your body, you could bleed too much. If there is not enough, you could get a blood clot.

Regular blood tests are not needed for some of the newer blood thinners.

POINTS TO REMEMBER
- Take your blood thinner as directed by your doctor.
- Go for blood tests as directed.
- Never skip a dose.
- Never take a double dose.[2]

---

[2] Agency for Healthcare Research and Quality (AHRQ), "Blood Thinner Pills: Your Guide to Using Them Safely," U.S. Department of Health and Human Services (HHS), November 2018. Available online. URL: www.ahrq.gov/patients-consumers/diagnosis-treatment/treatments/btpills/btpills.html. Accessed June 7, 2023.

Section 48.3 | **Statins**

Statins are drugs used to lower cholesterol. Your body needs some cholesterol to work properly. But, if you have too much in your blood, it can stick to the walls of your arteries and narrow or even block them.

If diet and exercise do not reduce your cholesterol levels, you may need to take cholesterol medicine. Often, this medicine is a statin. Statins interfere with the production of cholesterol in your liver. They lower low-density lipoprotein (LDL; bad) cholesterol levels and raise high-density Lipoprotein (HDL; good) cholesterol levels. This can slow the formation of plaques in your arteries.

Statins are relatively safe for most people. But they are not recommended for pregnant patients or those with active or chronic liver disease. They can also cause serious muscle problems. Some statins also interact adversely with other drugs. You may have fewer side effects with one statin drug than with another.[3]

HOW DO STATINS WORK IN CONTROLLING CHOLESTEROL?

Statins are a class of medicines used to lower cholesterol in the blood. Most of the cholesterol in your blood is made by the liver. Statins work by reducing the amount of cholesterol made by the liver and by helping the liver remove cholesterol that is already in the blood.

According to James P. Smith, M.D., M.S., deputy director of the Division of Metabolism and Endocrinology at the U.S. Food and Drug Administration (FDA), "An important first step is to have a discussion with your health-care provider about your risk of having heart disease or a stroke, how a statin would reduce that risk, and any side effects that you should consider."

WHY IS IT IMPORTANT TO KEEP CHOLESTEROL LEVELS IN THE BLOOD LOW?

Your body needs cholesterol, but too much of it in your blood can lead to buildup on the walls of your arteries (this buildup is called

---

[3] MedlinePlus, "Statins," National Institutes of Health (NIH), April 27, 2016. Available online. URL: https://medlineplus.gov/statins.html. Accessed May 30, 2023.

"plaque"), putting you at higher risk of heart disease and stroke. According to the Centers for Disease Control and Prevention (CDC), heart disease is the leading cause of death for both men and women in the United States.

YOU HAVE HEARD ABOUT "GOOD" AND "BAD" CHOLESTEROL. WHAT IS THE DIFFERENCE?

Cholesterol is carried in the bloodstream by different types of particles called "lipoproteins." The majority is carried on LDL particles and is sometimes referred to as "bad cholesterol" because high levels of LDL particles can lead to heart disease and stroke. HDL particles, on the other hand, carry cholesterol back to the liver for removal from the body. Since people with higher levels of HDL cholesterol tend to have a lower risk of heart disease, this is sometimes referred to as "good cholesterol." Your health-care provider should help you interpret what your numbers mean for your cardiovascular health.

YOU THOUGHT A HEALTHY DIET AND REGULAR EXERCISE WOULD KEEP YOUR CHOLESTEROL IN CHECK. NOT SO?

"A heart-healthy diet, regular physical activity, and maintaining a healthy weight are all very important components of a lifestyle that can help lower cholesterol and reduce the risk of heart disease and stroke," says Dr. Smith. "But other factors that are out of our control, such as genetics, also play a role. For many people, cholesterol simply cannot be lowered enough by lifestyle changes alone."

For people who are at increased risk of having a heart attack or stroke, statins may be recommended even when cholesterol levels might not seem too high. "Statins have a well-established track record for reducing the risk for heart attacks and strokes," Dr. Smith says. "Whether or not a statin is appropriate for a specific patient should involve a conversation between the patient and his or her healthcare provider."

YOU HAVE HEARD THAT THERE ARE SOME RISKS TO TAKING STATINS. SHOULD YOU BE WORRIED?

Statins are typically very well tolerated. Two risks that patients may be aware of are muscle-related complaints and an increased risk of developing type 2 diabetes. "Muscle complaints are quite common even among people not taking statins, so it is important to have your health-care provider evaluate any symptoms before stopping your medication," Dr. Smith explains. "It is rare for statins to cause serious muscle problems."

Similarly, the risk of developing diabetes as a result of a statin is small. "The benefits of statins in reducing heart attacks and strokes should generally outweigh this small increased risk," Dr. Smith says.

YOU HAVE HEARD YOU SHOULD NOT DRINK GRAPEFRUIT JUICE IF YOU ARE TAKING A STATIN. IS THAT TRUE?

Grapefruit juice and fresh grapefruit can affect the way some medicines work. That is true with certain statins, too—but only some of them. In addition, other medications can also interact with statins. Dr. Smith advises patients to ensure that their health-care provider and pharmacist know about all the prescription and nonprescription medications they take.[4]

SIDE EFFECTS OF STATINS

Statin labels have been updated to outline the potential for nonserious and reversible side effects, which include:
- memory loss and confusion
- increased blood sugar
- increased hemoglobin A1c levels

DRUG INTERACTIONS WITH STATINS

There is an increased risk of muscle injury when statins are used with:
- cholesterol-lowering drugs known as "fibrates"
- large doses of niacin
- RANEXA® (ranolazine), a medication used to treat angina
- colchicine, a medication primarily used to treat gout

[4] "Controlling Cholesterol with Statins," U.S. Food and Drug Administration (FDA), February 16, 2017. Available online. URL: www.fda.gov/consumers/consumer-updates/controlling-cholesterol-statins. Accessed May 30, 2023.

The Lovastatin label has been extensively updated with drugs that should not be used with the medication and dose limitations.

Before starting a statin, patients should inform their healthcare professional about all medicines that they are taking or plan to take. Some medicines may interact with statins, increasing the risk of side effects.[5]

---

[5] "Cholesterol-Lowering Drugs Get Labeling Changes," U.S. Food and Drug Administration (FDA), May 22, 2015. Available online. URL: www.fda.gov/drugs/special-features/cholesterol-lowering-drugs-get-labeling-changes. Accessed May 30, 2023.

Chapter 49 | Iron Supplements for Anemia: Recommendations and Dosages

Chapter Contents

Iron is a mineral that has many functions. Iron helps red blood cells (RBCs) carry oxygen through the body and supports a child's ability to learn. Having enough iron in the body can help prevent iron deficiency and iron deficiency anemia.

WHAT HAPPENS IF YOUR CHILD DOES NOT GET ENOUGH IRON?

If your child does not get enough iron, your child may develop anemia. Anemia is when there are not enough RBCs in the body or your child's ability to carry oxygen throughout the body is lowered. There are many causes of anemia. In young children, one common cause is not enough iron. Children who do not receive enough iron, either from iron-rich foods or from supplements, are at greater risk of developing anemia.

WHEN DOES YOUR CHILD NEED IRON? AND HOW MUCH?

All children need iron. It is important at all stages of your child's development. Babies fed only breast milk, only formula, or a mix of breast milk and formula have different needs when it comes to iron.

Talk to your child's doctor or nurse about your child's iron needs at his or her next checkup.

Breast Milk
- Talk with your child's nurse or doctor about if your child needs iron supplements before six months old.
- Once your child starts to eat foods, it is important to give foods with iron to meet nutritional needs.

Formula
- Your child's iron needs can be met by standard infant formulas for the first 12 months of life.
- Choose a formula that is fortified with iron. Most commercial infant formulas sold in the United States contain iron.

- Standard iron-fortified infant formulas contain enough iron (12 mg/dL) to support your growing child's needs.
- Once your child starts to eat foods, introduce your child to foods that contain iron.

ONCE YOUR CHILD STARTS TO EAT SOLID FOODS, HOW CAN YOU MAKE SURE YOUR CHILD GETS ENOUGH IRON?

When your child is about six months old, you can start giving solid foods to your child. Make sure to choose foods that contain iron. Iron found in foods comes in two forms: heme and nonheme iron.

- Heme iron is commonly found in animal products and is more easily absorbed by the body. Sources of heme iron include the following:
  - red meat (e.g., beef, pork, lamb, goat, or venison)
  - seafood (e.g., fatty fish)
  - poultry (e.g., chicken or turkey)
  - eggs
- Nonheme iron can be found in plants and iron-fortified products. This type of iron is less easily absorbed by the body and will require careful planning to get enough iron for your baby. Sources of nonheme iron include the following:
  - iron-fortified infant cereals
  - tofu
  - beans and lentils
  - dark green leafy vegetables

  Pairing nonheme iron sources with foods high in vitamin C can help your baby absorb the iron he or she needs to support development. Vitamin C-rich fruits and vegetables include the following:
  - citrus fruits (e.g., oranges)
  - berries
  - papaya
  - tomatoes
  - sweet potatoes
  - broccoli

- cabbage
- dark green leafy vegetables

Making sure your child is getting enough iron is important. Some children may need more iron than others. Talk to your child's doctor or nurse about iron at your child's next checkup.[1]

Section 49.2 | Intake Recommendations for Iron in Adults

Iron is a mineral that is naturally present in many foods, added to some food products, and available as a dietary supplement. Iron is an essential component of hemoglobin, an erythrocyte (red blood cell (RBC)) protein that transfers oxygen from the lungs to the tissues. As a component of myoglobin, another protein that provides oxygen, iron supports muscle metabolism and healthy connective tissue. Iron is also necessary for physical growth, neurological development, cellular functioning, and the synthesis of some hormones.

Dietary iron has two main forms: heme and nonheme. Plants and iron-fortified foods contain nonheme iron only, whereas meat, seafood, and poultry contain both heme and nonheme iron. Heme iron, which is formed when iron combines with protoporphyrin IX, contributes about 10–15 percent of total iron intakes in Western populations.

Most of the 3–4 grams of elemental iron in adults is in hemoglobin. Much of the remaining iron is stored in the form of ferritin or hemosiderin (a degradation product of ferritin) in the liver, spleen, and bone marrow or is located in myoglobin in muscle tissue. Transferrin is the main protein in blood that binds to iron and transports it throughout the body. Humans typically lose only small amounts of iron in the urine, feces, gastrointestinal (GI) tract, and

---

[1] "Iron," Centers for Disease Control and Prevention (CDC), November 16, 2021. Available online. URL: www.cdc.gov/nutrition/infantandtoddlernutrition/vitamins-minerals/iron.html. Accessed May 25, 2023.

skin. Losses are greater in menstruating women because of blood loss. Hepcidin, a circulating peptide hormone, is the key regulator of both iron absorption and the distribution of iron throughout the body, including in plasma.

The assessment of iron status depends almost entirely on hematological indicators. However, these indicators are not sensitive or specific enough to adequately describe the full spectrum of iron status, and this can complicate the diagnosis of iron deficiency. A complementary approach is to consider how iron intakes from the diet and dietary supplements compare with recommended intakes.

Iron deficiency progresses from the depletion of iron stores (mild iron deficiency) to iron deficiency erythropoiesis (erythrocyte production) and finally to iron deficiency anemia (IDA). With iron deficiency erythropoiesis (also known as "marginal iron deficiency"), iron stores are depleted, and transferrin saturation declines, but hemoglobin levels are usually within the normal range. IDA is characterized by low hemoglobin concentrations and decreases in hematocrit (the proportion of RBCs in blood by volume) and mean corpuscular volume (a measure of erythrocyte size).

Serum ferritin concentration, a measure of the body's iron stores, is currently the most efficient and cost-effective test for diagnosing iron deficiency. Because serum ferritin decreases during the first stage of iron depletion, it can identify low iron status before the onset of IDA. A serum ferritin concentration lower than 30 mcg/L suggests iron deficiency, and a value lower than 10 mcg/L suggests IDA. However, serum ferritin is subject to influence by inflammation (e.g., due to infectious disease), which elevates serum ferritin concentrations.

Hemoglobin and hematocrit tests are the most commonly used measures to screen patients for iron deficiency, even though they are neither sensitive nor specific. Often, hemoglobin concentrations are combined with serum ferritin measurements to identify IDA. Hemoglobin concentrations lower than 11 g/dL in children under 10 years of age or lower than 12 g/dL in individuals aged 10 years or older suggest IDA. Normal hematocrit values are approximately 41–50 percent in males and 36–44 percent in females.

SOURCES OF IRON
Food

The richest sources of heme iron in the diet include lean meat and seafood. Dietary sources of nonheme iron include nuts, beans, vegetables, and fortified grain products. In the United States, about half of dietary iron comes from bread, cereal, and other grain products. Breast milk contains highly bioavailable iron but in amounts that are not sufficient to meet the needs of infants older than four to six months.

In the United States, Canada, and many other countries, wheat and other flour are fortified with iron. Infant formulas are fortified with 12 mg of iron per liter.

Heme iron has higher bioavailability than nonheme iron, and other dietary components have less effect on the bioavailability of heme than nonheme iron. The bioavailability of iron is approximately 14–18 percent from mixed diets that include substantial amounts of meat, seafood, and vitamin C (ascorbic acid, which enhances the bioavailability of nonheme iron) and 5–12 percent from vegetarian diets. In addition to ascorbic acid, meat, poultry, and seafood can enhance nonheme iron absorption, whereas phytate (present in grains and beans) and certain polyphenols in some nonanimal foods (such as cereals and legumes) have the opposite effect. Unlike other inhibitors of iron absorption, calcium might reduce the bioavailability of both nonheme and heme iron. However, the effects of enhancers and inhibitors of iron absorption are attenuated by a typical mixed Western diet, so they have little effect on most people's iron status.

Several food sources of iron are listed in Table 49.1. Some plant-based foods that are good sources of iron, such as spinach, have low iron bioavailability because they contain iron absorption inhibitors, such as polyphenols.

The U.S. Department of Agriculture (USDA) lists the nutrient content of many foods and provides a comprehensive list of foods containing iron arranged by nutrient content and by food name.

Table 49.1. The Iron Content of Selected Foods

Food	Milligrams per Serving	% DV*
Breakfast cereals, fortified with 100% of the DV for iron, 1 serving	18	100
Oysters, eastern, cooked with moist heat, 3 ounces	8	44
White beans, canned, 1 cup	8	44
Beef liver, pan-fried, 3 ounces	5	28
Lentils, boiled and drained, ½ cup	3	17
Spinach, boiled and drained, ½ cup	3	17
Tofu, firm, ½ cup	3	17
Chocolate, dark, 45–69% cacao solids, 1 ounce	2	11
Kidney beans, canned, ½ cup	2	11
Sardines, Atlantic, canned in oil, drained solids with bone, 3 ounces	2	11
Chickpeas, boiled and drained, ½ cup	2	11
Tomatoes, canned, stewed, ½ cup	2	11
Beef, braised bottom round, trimmed to ⅛" fat, 3 ounces	2	11
Potato, baked, flesh and skin, 1 medium potato	2	11
Cashew nuts, oil roasted, 1 ounce (18 nuts)	2	11
Green peas, boiled, ½ cup	1	6
Chicken, roasted, meat and skin, 3 ounces	1	6
Rice, white, long grain, enriched, parboiled, drained, ½ cup	1	6
Bread, whole wheat, 1 slice	1	6
Bread, white, 1 slice	1	6
Raisins, seedless, ¼ cup	1	6
Spaghetti, whole wheat, cooked, 1 cup	1	6

Iron Supplements for Anemia: Recommendations and Dosages

Table 49.1. Continued

Food	Milligrams per Serving	% DV*
Tuna, light, canned in water, 3 ounces	1	6
Turkey, roasted, breast meat and skin, 3 ounces	1	6
Nuts, pistachio, dry roasted, 1 ounce (49 nuts)	1	6
Broccoli, boiled and drained, ½ cup	1	6
Egg, hard-boiled, 1 large	1	6
Rice, brown, long or medium grain, cooked, 1 cup	1	6
Cheese, cheddar, 1.5 ounces	0	0
Cantaloupe, diced, ½ cup	0	0
Mushrooms, white, sliced and stir-fried, ½ cup	0	0
Cheese, cottage, 2% milk fat, ½ cup	0	0
Milk, 1 cup	0	0

DV = daily value. The U.S. Food and Drug Administration (FDA) developed DVs to help consumers compare the nutrient contents of foods and dietary supplements within the context of a total diet. The DV for iron is 18 mg for adults and children aged four and older. The FDA requires food labels to list iron content. Foods providing 20 percent or more of the DV are considered to be high sources of a nutrient, but foods providing lower percentages of the DV also contribute to a healthful diet.

Dietary Supplements

Iron is available in many dietary supplements. Multivitamin/multimineral supplements with iron, especially those designed for women, typically provide 18 mg of iron (100% of the daily value (DV)). Multivitamin/multimineral supplements for men or seniors frequently contain less or no iron. Iron-only supplements usually deliver more than the DV, with many providing 65 mg of iron (360% of the DV).

Frequently used forms of iron in supplements include ferrous and ferric iron salts, such as ferrous sulfate, ferrous gluconate, ferric citrate, and ferric sulfate. Because of its higher solubility, ferrous iron in dietary supplements is more bioavailable than ferric iron. High doses of supplemental iron (45 mg/day or more) may cause GI side effects, such as nausea and constipation. Other forms of supplemental iron, such as heme iron polypeptides, carbonyl iron, iron amino-acid chelates, and polysaccharide-iron complexes, might have fewer GI side effects than ferrous or ferric salts.

The different forms of iron in supplements contain varying amounts of elemental iron. For example, ferrous fumarate is 33 percent elemental iron by weight, whereas ferrous sulfate is 20 percent and ferrous gluconate is 12 percent elemental iron. Fortunately, elemental iron is listed in the Supplement Facts panel, so consumers do not need to calculate the amount of iron supplied by various forms of iron supplements.

Approximately 14–18 percent of Americans use a supplement containing iron. Rates of use of supplements containing iron vary by age and gender, ranging from 6 percent of children aged 12–19 years to 60 percent of women who are lactating and 72 percent of pregnant women.

Calcium might interfere with the absorption of iron although this effect has not been definitively established. For this reason, some experts suggest that people take individual calcium and iron supplements at different times of the day.

RECOMMENDED INTAKES

Intake recommendations for iron and other nutrients are provided in the Dietary Reference Intakes (DRIs) developed by the Food and Nutrition Board (FNB) at the Institute of Medicine (IOM) of the National Academies (formerly National Academy of Sciences (NAS)). DRI is the general term for a set of reference values used for planning and assessing nutrient intakes of healthy people. These values, which vary by age and gender, include the following:

- **Recommended dietary allowance (RDA)**. RDA is the average daily level of intake sufficient to meet the nutrient requirements of nearly all (97–98%) healthy individuals, often used to plan nutritionally adequate diets for individuals.
- **Adequate intake (AI)**. Intake at this level is assumed to ensure nutritional adequacy, established when evidence is insufficient to develop an RDA.

Iron Supplements for Anemia: Recommendations and Dosages

- **Estimated average requirement (EAR).** The average daily level of intake estimated to meet the requirements of 50 percent of healthy individuals, usually used to assess the nutrient intakes of groups of people and to plan nutritionally adequate diets for them, can also be used to assess the nutrient intakes of individuals.
- **Tolerable upper intake level (UL).** Maximum daily intake is unlikely to cause adverse health effects.

Table 49.2 lists the current iron RDAs for nonvegetarians. The RDAs for vegetarians are 1.8 times higher than for people who eat meat. This is because heme iron from meat is more bioavailable than nonheme iron from plant-based foods, and meat, poultry, and seafood increase the absorption of nonheme iron.

For infants from birth to six months, the FNB established an AI for iron that is equivalent to the mean intake of iron in healthy, breastfed infants.

Table 49.2. Recommended Dietary Allowances (RDAs) for Iron

Age	Male (mg)	Female (mg)	Pregnancy (mg)	Lactation (mg)
Birth to 6 months	0.27*	0.27*	—	—
7–12 months	11	11	—	—
1–3 years	7	7	—	—
4–8 years	10	10	—	—
9–13 years	8	8	—	—
14–18 years	11	15	27	10
19–50 years	8	18	27	9
>51 years	8	8	—	—

* Adequate intake (AI).

IRON INTAKES AND STATUS

People in the United States usually obtain adequate amounts of iron from their diets, but infants, young children, teenage girls,

647

pregnant women, and premenopausal women are at risk of obtaining insufficient amounts. The average daily iron intake from foods is 11.5–13.7 mg/day in children aged 2–11 years, 15.1 mg/day in children and teens aged 12–19 years, and 16.3–18.2 mg/day in men and 12.6–13.5 mg/day in women older than 19. The average daily iron intake from foods and supplements is 13.7–15.1 mg/day in children aged 2–11 years, 16.3 mg/day in children and teens aged 12–19 years, and 19.3–20.5 mg/day in men and 17.0–18.9 mg/day in women older than 19. The median dietary iron intake in pregnant women is 14.7 mg/day.

Rates of iron deficiency vary by race and other sociodemographic factors. Almost 6 percent of White and Black toddlers aged one to three years in the United States are iron-deficient (defined as at least two abnormal results for the child's age and gender on transferrin saturation, free erythrocyte protoporphyrin, and/or serum ferritin tests), compared with 12 percent of Hispanic toddlers. Deficiency (including IDA) is more common among children and adolescents in food-insecure households than in food-secure households. Among pregnant women, deficiency based on depleted iron stores is more common in Mexican American (23.6%) and non-Hispanic Black women (29.6%) than in non-Hispanic White women (13.9%).

Some groups are at risk of obtaining excess iron. Individuals with hereditary hemochromatosis, which predisposes them to absorb excessive amounts of dietary iron, have an increased risk of iron overload. One study suggests that elderly people are more likely to have chronic positive iron balance and elevated total body iron than iron deficiency. Among 1,106 elderly White adults aged 67–96 years in the Framingham Heart Study, 13 percent had high iron stores (serum ferritin levels higher than 300 mcg/L in men and 200 mcg/L in women), of which only 1 percent was due to chronic disease. The authors did not assess genotypes, so they could not determine whether these results were due to hemochromatosis.

HEALTH RISKS FROM EXCESSIVE IRON
Adults with normal intestinal function have very little risk of iron overload from dietary sources of iron. However, supplements

containing 25 mg of iron or more can reduce zinc absorption and plasma zinc concentrations. High-dose iron supplements can also cause GI effects, including gastric upset, constipation, nausea, abdominal pain, vomiting, and diarrhea. Taking iron supplements with food can help minimize these adverse effects. Case reports, some involving doses of 130 mg iron, suggest that some people develop even more serious GI effects, including gastritis and gastric lesions (along with iron deposits in the gastric mucosa in some cases).

Acute intakes of more than 20 mg/kg iron (about 1,365 mg iron for a person weighing 150 lb) from supplements or medicines can lead to corrosive necrosis of the intestine, which might lead to fluid and blood loss, shock, tissue damage, and organ failure, especially if food is not taken at the same time as the iron. In severe cases (e.g., one-time ingestions of 60 mg/kg, or about 4,090 mg iron for a 150-lb person), overdoses of iron can lead to multisystem organ failure, coma, convulsions, and even death.

Hemochromatosis, a disease caused by a mutation in the hemochromatosis (*HFE*) gene, is associated with an excessive buildup of iron in the body. About 1 in 10 Whites carry the most common *HFE* mutation (C282Y), but only 4.4 Whites per 1,000 are homozygous for the mutation and have hemochromatosis. The condition is much less common in other ethnic groups. Without treatment by periodic chelation or phlebotomy, people with hereditary hemochromatosis typically develop signs of iron toxicity by their 30s. These effects can include liver cirrhosis, hepatocellular carcinoma, heart disease, and impaired pancreatic function. The American Association for the Study of Liver Diseases recommends that treatment of hemochromatosis include the avoidance of iron and vitamin C supplements.

The FNB has established ULs for iron from food and supplements based on the amounts of iron that are associated with GI effects following supplemental intakes of iron salts (see Table 49.3). The ULs apply to healthy infants, children, and adults. Physicians sometimes prescribe intakes higher than the UL, such as when people with IDA need higher doses to replenish their iron stores.

Table 49.3. Tolerable Upper Intake Levels (ULs) for Iron

Age	Male (mg)	Female (mg)	Pregnancy (mg)	Lactation (mg)
Birth to 6 months	40	40	—	—
7–12 months	40	40	—	—
1–3 years	40	40	—	—
4–8 years	40	40	—	—
9–13 years	40	40	—	—
14–18 years	45	45	45	45
19+ years	45	45	45	45

INTERACTIONS WITH MEDICATIONS

Iron can interact with certain medications, and some medications can have an adverse effect on iron levels. A few examples are provided below. Individuals taking these and other medications on a regular basis should discuss their iron status with their health-care providers.

Levodopa

Some evidence indicates that in healthy people, iron supplements reduce the absorption of levodopa (found in Sinemet® and Stalevo®), used to treat Parkinson disease (PD) and restless leg syndrome (RLS), possibly through chelation. In the United States, the labels for levodopa warn that iron-containing dietary supplements might reduce the amount of levodopa available to the body and, thus, diminish its clinical effectiveness.

Levothyroxine

Levothyroxine (Levothroid®, Levoxyl®, Synthroid®, Tirosint®, and Unithroid®) is used to treat hypothyroidism, goiter, and thyroid cancer. The simultaneous ingestion of iron and levothyroxine can result in clinically significant reductions in levothyroxine efficacy in some patients. The labels for some of these products warn that iron supplements can reduce the absorption of levothyroxine tablets and advise against administering levothyroxine within four hours of iron supplements.

Proton Pump Inhibitors

Gastric acid plays an important role in the absorption of nonheme iron from the diet. Because proton pump inhibitors, such as lansoprazole (Prevacid®) and omeprazole (Prilosec®), reduce the acidity of stomach contents, they can reduce iron absorption. Treatment with proton pump inhibitors for up to 10 years is not associated with iron depletion or anemia in people with normal iron stores. But patients with iron deficiency taking proton pump inhibitors can have suboptimal responses to iron supplementation.

Iron and Healthful Diets

The federal government's 2020–2025 *Dietary Guidelines for Americans* (*DGA*) notes that "Because foods provide an array of nutrients and other components that have benefits for health, nutritional needs should be met primarily through foods…. In some cases, fortified foods and dietary supplements are useful when it is not possible otherwise to meet needs for one or more nutrients (e.g., during specific life stages such as pregnancy)."

The *DGA* describes a healthy dietary pattern as one that:
- includes a variety of vegetables; fruits; grains (at least half whole grains); fat-free and low-fat milk, yogurt, and cheese; and oils
  - Many ready-to-eat breakfast cereals are fortified with iron, and some fruits and vegetables contain iron.
- includes a variety of protein foods such as lean meats; poultry; eggs; seafood; beans, peas, and lentils; nuts and seeds; and soy products
  - Oysters and beef liver have high amounts of iron. Beef, cashews, chickpeas, and sardines are good sources of iron. Chicken, tuna, and eggs contain iron.

- limits foods and beverages higher in added sugars, saturated fat, and sodium
- limits alcoholic beverages
- stays within your daily calorie needs[2]

[2] Office of Dietary Supplements (ODS), "Iron," National Institutes of Health (NIH), April 5, 2022. Available online. URL: https://ods.od.nih.gov/factsheets/Iron-HealthProfessional. Accessed May 25, 2023.

Chapter 50 | **Blood Transfusion**

A blood transfusion is a common, safe medical procedure in which healthy donor blood is given to you through an intravenous (IV) line inserted in one of your blood vessels. Blood transfusions replace the blood that is lost through surgery or injury. This treatment also provides blood if your body is not making blood properly on its own.

Four types of blood products may be given through blood transfusions:

- whole blood
- red blood cells (RBCs), the blood cells that carry oxygen throughout the body
- platelets, blood cell fragments that help your blood clot
- plasma, the fluid part of the blood

Most of the blood used for transfusions comes from whole blood donations given by volunteer blood donors.

Sometimes, people have their own blood collected and stored a few weeks before an elective surgery in case it is needed.

After a doctor determines that you need a blood transfusion, your blood will be tested to make sure that the blood you are given is a good match. Blood transfusions usually take one to four hours to complete. You will be monitored during and after the procedure.

Blood transfusions are usually very safe because donated blood is carefully tested, handled, and stored. However, there is a small chance that your body may have a mild or even a severe reaction to the donor blood.

Other complications of blood transfusions may include the following:

- fever
- heart or lung problems
- alloimmunization when the body's natural defense system attacks donor blood cells
- rare but serious reactions where donated white blood cells (WBCs) attack your body's healthy tissues

Some people also have health problems from getting too much iron after frequent transfusions. There is also a very small chance of getting an infectious disease, such as hepatitis B or C or human immunodeficiency virus (HIV), through a blood transfusion. For HIV, that chance is less than 1 in 1 million. Scientific research and careful medical controls make the supply of donated blood very safe.

Blood transfusions are needed for the following conditions:

- anemia
- bleeding disorders
- iron deficiency anemia
- sickle cell disease (SCD)
- thalassemia[1]

[1] "Treatments for Blood Disorders," National Heart, Lung, and Blood Institute (NHLBI), March 24, 2022. Available online. URL: www.nhlbi.nih.gov/health/blood-bone-marrow-treatments. Accessed May 29, 2023.

Part 7 | **Additional Help and Information**

Chapter 51 | **Glossary of Terms Related to Blood and Circulatory Disorders**

ablation: The removal or destruction of a body part or tissue or its function.

addiction: A chronic, relapsing disease characterized by compulsive drug seeking and use accompanied by neurochemical and molecular changes in the brain.

allergy: An abnormally high sensitivity to certain substances, such as pollens or foods.

alopecia: The lack or loss of hair from areas of the body where hair is usually found.

anemia: A condition in which the number of red blood cells is less than normal, resulting in less oxygen carried to the body's cells.

aneurysm: A weak or thin spot on an artery wall that has stretched or ballooned out from the wall and filled with blood, or damage to an artery leading to pooling of blood between the layers of the blood vessel walls.

antibiotic: A drug that can destroy or prevent the growth of bacteria.

artery: Any of the thick-walled blood vessels that carry blood away from the heart to other parts of the body.

atherosclerosis: A blood vessel disease characterized by deposits of lipid material on the inside of the walls of large to medium-sized arteries, which make the artery walls thick, hard, brittle, and prone to breaking.

biopsy: To remove cells or tissues from the body for testing and examination under a microscope.

This glossary contains terms excerpted from documents produced by several sources deemed reliable.

calories: The energy provided by food/nutrients.

carcinoma: Cancer that begins in the skin or in tissues that line or cover internal organs.

chlamydia: A common sexually transmitted disease caused by the bacterium *Chlamydia trachomatis*.

cholesterol: A waxy substance, produced naturally by the liver and also found in foods, that circulates in the blood and helps maintain tissues and cell membranes.

cocaine: A highly addictive stimulant drug derived from the coca plant that produces profound feelings of pleasure.

depression: A disorder marked by sadness, inactivity, difficulty with thinking and concentration, significant increase or decrease in appetite and time spent sleeping, feelings of dejection and hopelessness, and, sometimes, suicidal thoughts or an attempt to commit suicide.

diabetes: A condition characterized by high blood glucose, resulting from the body's inability to use blood glucose for energy.

dialysis: The process of filtering wastes from the blood artificially.

diuretic: A chemical that stimulates the production of urine.

edema: The swelling of a cell that results from the influx of large amounts of water or fluid into the cell.

emphysema: A disease that affects the tiny air sacs in the lungs.

gallstone: Solid material that forms in the gallbladder or common bile duct. Gallstones are made of cholesterol or other substances found in the gallbladder.

gene: The basic unit of heredity. Genes play a role in how high a person's risk is for certain diseases.

germ cell tumor: A type of tumor that begins in the cells that give rise to sperm or eggs.

hemorrhagic stroke: Sudden bleeding into or around the brain.

hormone: A substance that stimulates the function of a gland.

human immunodeficiency virus (HIV): The virus that causes acquired immunodeficiency syndrome (AIDS), which is the most advanced stage of HIV infection.

hypertension: Characterized by persistently high arterial blood pressure defined as a measurement greater than or equal to 140 mm Hg systolic pressure over 90 mm Hg diastolic pressure.

Glossary of Terms Related to Blood and Circulatory Disorders

imaging: In medicine, a process that makes pictures of areas inside the body.

immune system: The complex group of organs and cells that defends the body against infections and other diseases.

immunosuppressant: A drug given to stop the natural responses of the body's immune system.

injection drug use: A method of illicit drug use. The drugs are injected directly into the body into a vein, into a muscle, or under the skin with a needle and syringe.

intracerebral hemorrhage: This occurs when a vessel within the brain leaks blood into the brain.

invasive cancer: Cancer that has spread beyond the layer of tissue in which it developed and is growing into surrounding healthy tissues.

jaundice: A condition in which the skin and the whites of the eyes become yellow, urine darkens, and the color of stool becomes lighter than normal.

lipoprotein: Small globules of cholesterol covered by a layer of protein, produced by the liver.

lobe: A portion of an organ, such as the liver, lung, breast, thyroid, or brain.

lupus: A chronic inflammatory disease that occurs when the body's immune system attacks its own tissues and organs.

lymph nodes: Small glands that help the body fight infection and disease. They filter a fluid called "lymph" and contain white blood cells.

magnetic resonance imaging (MRI): A type of imaging involving the use of magnetic fields to detect subtle changes in the water content of tissues.

medical test: Tests designed to rule out or avoid disease.

metabolism: Metabolism refers to all of the processes in the body that make and use energy, such as digesting food and nutrients and removing waste through urine and feces.

monoclonal antibody: A type of protein made in the laboratory that can bind to substances in the body, including tumor cells.

mutation: Any change in the deoxyribonucleic acid (DNA) of a cell. Mutations may be caused by mistakes during cell division, or they may be caused by exposure to DNA-damaging agents in the environment.

neoplasm: An abnormal mass of tissue that results when cells divide more than they should or do not die when they should.

obstruction: A clog or blockage that prevents liquid from flowing easily.

oncologist: A doctor who specializes in treating cancer. Some oncologists specialize in a particular type of cancer treatment.

pancreas: A large gland that helps digest food and also makes some important hormones.

positron emission tomography (PET) scan: In a PET scan, the patient is given radioactive glucose (sugar) through a vein. A scanner then tracks the glucose in the body.

plaque: Fatty cholesterol deposits found along the inside of artery walls that lead to atherosclerosis and stenosis of the arteries.

prognosis: A prediction of the probable outcome of a disease.

radiation: The emission of energy in waves or particles. Often used to treat cancer cells.

recurrence: When cancer comes back after a period when no cancer can be found.

relapse: Return of the manifestations of disease after an interval of improvement.

resection: Surgery to remove tissue, an organ, or part of an organ.

scrotum: The sac of skin that contains the testes.

sexually transmitted disease (STD): An infectious disease that spreads from person to person during sexual contact.

stage: How much cancer is in the body and how far it has spread.

stroke: A stroke occurs when blood flow to your brain stops.

subarachnoid hemorrhage: Bleeding within the meninges, or outer membranes, of the brain into the clear fluid that surrounds the brain.

transient ischemic attack (TIA): A short-lived stroke that lasts from a few minutes up to 24 hours, often called a "ministroke."

transmission: The spread of disease from one person to another.

triglycerides: A type of fat in your blood, triglycerides can contribute to the hardening and narrowing of your arteries if levels are too high.

ulcer: An open lesion on the surface of the skin or a mucosal surface caused by superficial loss of tissue, usually with inflammation.

ultrasound: A type of test in which sound waves too high to hear are aimed at a structure to produce an image of it.

urinalysis: A test of a urine sample that can reveal many problems of the urinary tract and other body systems.

urinary tract: The path that urine takes as it leaves the body. It includes the kidneys, ureters, bladder, and urethra.

vaccine: A substance meant to help the immune system respond to and resist disease.

virus: A microscopic infectious agent that requires a living host cell in order to replicate.

x-ray: A type of high-energy radiation. In low doses, x-rays are used to diagnose diseases by making pictures of the inside of the body.

Chapter 52 | **Directory of Resources Related to Blood and Circulatory Disorders**

GENERAL

American Society of Hematology (ASH)
2021 L St., N.W., Ste. 900
Washington, DC 20036
Phone: 202-776-0544
Toll-Free: 866-828-1231
Fax: 202-776-0545
Website: www.hematology.org

Iron Disorders Institute (IDI)
P.O. Box 4891
Greenville, SC 29608
Website: www.irondisorders.org
Email: info@irondisorders.org

National Heart, Lung, and Blood Institute (NHLBI)
31 Center Dr.
Bldg. 31
Bethesda, MD 20892
Toll-Free: 877-NHLBI4U
(877-645-2448)
Website: www.nhlbi.nih.gov
Email: nhlbiinfo@nhlbi.nih.gov

National Institute of Arthritis and Musculoskeletal and Skin Diseases (NIAMS)
One AMS Cir.
Bethesda, MD 20892-3675
Phone: 301-495-4484
Toll-Free: 877-22-NIAMS
(877-226-4267)
Fax: 301-718-6366
Website: www.niams.nih.gov
Email: NIAMSinfo@mail.nih.gov

Resources in this chapter were compiled from several sources deemed reliable; all contact information was verified and updated in July 2023.

National Institute of Diabetes and Digestive and Kidney Diseases (NIDDK)
9000 Rockville Pike
Bethesda, MD 20892
Toll-Free: 800-860-8747
Website: www.niddk.nih.gov
Email: healthinfo@niddk.nih.gov

National Organization for Rare Disorders (NORD)
1900 Crown Colony Dr., Ste. 310
Quincy, MA 02169
Phone: 617-249-7300
Website: https://rarediseases.org

The Nemours Foundation/ KidsHealth®
Website: https://kidshealth.org

ANEMIA

American Sickle Cell Anemia Association (ASCAA)
2390 E. 79th St.
Langston Hughes Cleveland Clinic Center
Cleveland, OH 44104
Phone: 216-229-8600
Fax: 216-229-4500
Website: www.ascaa.org
Email: irabragg@ascaa.org

The Aplastic Anemia and MDS International Foundation (AAMDSIF)
4330 East-West Hwy., Ste. 230
Bethesda, MD 20814
Phone: 301-279-7202
Toll-Free: 800-747-2820
Website: www.aamds.org
Email: help@aamds.org

Diamond Blackfan Anemia Foundation, Inc. (DBAF)
P.O. Box 1092
West Seneca, NY 14224
Phone: 716-674-2818
Website: https://dbafoundation.org
Email: DBAF@dbafoundation.org

Fanconi Anemia (FA) Research Fund
360 E. 10th Ave., Ste. 201
Eugene, OR 97401
Phone: 541-687-4658
Toll-Free: 888-FANCONI
(888-326-2664)
Fax: 541-687-0548
Website: www.fanconi.org
Email: info@fanconi.org

ANEURYSMS

American Association of Neurological Surgeons (AANS)

5550 Meadowbrook Industrial Ct.
Rolling Meadows, IL 60008-3852
Phone: 847-378-0500
Toll-Free: 888-566-AANS
(888-566-2267)
Fax: 847-378-0600
Website: www.aans.org
Email: info@aans.org

American Stroke Association (ASA)

7272 Greenville Ave.
Dallas, TX 75231
Toll-Free: 888-4-STROKE
(888-478-7653)
Website: www.strokeassociation.org

Brain Aneurysm Foundation (BAF)

269 Hanover St.
Hanover, MA 02339
Phone: 781-826-5556
Toll-Free: 888-BRAIN-02
(888-272-4602)
Fax: 781-826-5566
Website: www.bafound.org
Email: office@bafound.org

Brain Resources and Information Network (BRAIN)

P.O. Box 5801
Bethesda, MD 20824
Toll-Free: 800-352-9424
Fax: 301-402-2186
Website: www.ninds.nih.gov
Email: braininfo@ninds.nih.gov

ANTIPHOSPHOLIPID ANTIBODY SYNDROME

APS Foundation of America, Inc. (APSFA)

P.O. Box 801
LaCrosse, WI 54602-0801
Website: https://apsfa.org

BLEEDING AND CLOTTING DISORDERS

Cure HHT

P.O. Box 329
Monkton, MD 21111
Phone: 410-357-9932
Fax: 410-472-5559
Website: https://curehht.org
Email: hhtinfo@curehht.org

Foundation for Women & Girls with Blood Disorders (FWGBD)

P.O. Box 1358
Montclair, NJ 07042
Website: www.fwgbd.org

National Blood Clot Alliance (NBCA)

P.O. Box 825687
Philadelphia, PA 19182-5687
Phone: 703-935-8845
Toll-Free: 877-4-NO-CLOT
(877-466-2568)
Website: www.stoptheclot.org
Email: info@stoptheclot.org

Preeclampsia Foundation

3840 W. Eau Gallie Blvd., Ste. 104
Melbourne, FL 32934
Phone: 321-421-6957
Toll-Free: 800-665-9341
Website: www.preeclampsia.org
Email: info@preeclampsia.org

BLOOD DONATION

American Association of Blood Banks (AABB)

4550 Montgomery Ave., Ste. 700
N. Twr.
Bethesda, MD 20814
Phone: 301-907-6977
Fax: 301-907-6895
Website: www.aabb.org
Email: publicrelations@aabb.org

America's Blood Centers

1717 K St., N.W., Ste. 900
Washington, DC 20006
Phone: 202-393-5725
Fax: 202-899-2621
Website: www.americasblood.org

The American National Red Cross

431 18th St., N.W.
Washington, DC 20006
Phone: 202-303-5214
Toll-Free: 800-RED-CROSS
(800-733-2767)
Website: www.redcross.org
Email: customercare@redcross.org

BONE MARROW DONATION AND STEM CELL TRANSPLANTATION

Center for International Blood and Marrow Transplant Research (CIBMTR)

9200 W. Wisconsin Ave., Ste.
C5500
Milwaukee, WI 53226
Phone: 414-805-0700
Fax: 414-805-0714
Website: www.cibmtr.org
Email: contactus@cibmtr.org

INDEX

INDEX

Page numbers followed by "n" refer to citation information; by "t" indicate tables; and by "f" indicate figures.

A

AAA *see* abdominal aortic aneurysm

abdominal aortic aneurysm (AAA), smoking 551

ABI *see* ankle-brachial index

ABO test, blood typing 10

ACE *see* angiotensin-converting enzyme

acetaminophen, stroke 480

acquired immunodeficiency syndrome (AIDS)
adult non-Hodgkin lymphoma (NHL) 203
anemia 138
hemophilia 313

activated protein C (APC), factor V Leiden thrombophilia 340

acute chest syndrome, sickle cell disease (SCD) 105

acute lymphocytic leukemia (ALL), children 147

acute myeloid leukemia (AML)
Diamond-Blackfan anemia 59
leukemia 148
myelodysplastic syndrome (MDS) 226

see also childhood acute myeloid leukemia (AML)

acute nonlymphocytic leukemia, lymphoid stem cell 158

acute promyelocytic leukemia (APL) *see* adult acute myeloid leukemia (AML)

ADHD *see* attention deficit hyperactivity disorder

adult acute myeloid leukemia (AML), overview 165–169

Advil®, blood thinner 628

AF *see* atrial fibrillation

afibrinogenemia
factor I deficiency 333
fibrinogen levels 583

Agency for Healthcare Research and Quality (AHRQ)
publication
blood thinner pills 631n

agranulocytes, leukocytes 6

AIDS *see* acquired immunodeficiency syndrome

AIDS-related lymphoma, overview 207–212

albumin
childhood Hodgkin lymphoma (HL) 187
immunoglobulin A (IgA) vasculitis 321
plasma cell neoplasms 267

Index

671

C

Index

Index

Index

Index

O

obesity
  atherosclerosis 443
  blood clotting disorders 289
  chronic venous insufficiency
    (CVI) 544
  coagulation factor tests 598
  excessive blood clots 376
  factor V Leiden thrombophilia 340
  food and alcohol 44
  heart attack 465
  renal artery stenosis (RAS) 498
  thrombotic thrombocytopenic
    purpura (TTP) 397
Office of Dietary Supplements (ODS)
  publication
    iron 652n
Office of Disease Prevention and
  Health Promotion (ODPHP)
  publications
    blood thinner pills 626n
    healthy heart 45n
Office on Women's Health (OWH)
  publications
    iron deficiency anemia 84n
    varicose veins and spider
      veins 548n
One a Day®, blood thinner pills 628
ophthalmoscopy, primary CNS
  lymphoma 216
oral contraceptives, factor V Leiden
  thrombophilia 340
orthostatic hypotension *see*
  hypotension
osmotic pressure
  blood function and composition 4
  capillaries 35
osteosarcoma, Diamond-Blackfan
  anemia 59
OTC *see* over-the-counter
over-the-counter (OTC)
  aspirin 624

blood clotting disorders 290
bruises 362
hypertension 407
hypotension 425
vasculitis 513
overweight
  childhood acute myeloid leukemia
    (AML) 163
  chronic venous insufficiency
    (CVI) 540
  coronary artery disease
    (CAD) 451
  excessive blood clots 376
  food and alcohol 44
  hypertension 408
  preeclampsia 421
  renal artery stenosis (RAS) 498
  stroke 474
oxygen, depicted 35f

P

packed cell volume (PCV), blood
  function and composition 4
PAD *see* peripheral artery disease
PAH *see* pulmonary arterial
  hypertension
pale tongue, anemia 51
pallor
  autoimmune hemolytic anemia
    (AIHA) 114
  Diamond-Blackfan anemia 57
  pyruvate kinase deficiency 100
palpitations
  platelet count 243
  Takayasu arteritis 521
PAN *see* polyarteritis nodosa
pancytopenia
  Langerhans cell histiocytosis
    (LCH) 274
  Waldenström
    macroglobulinemia 221

Index

Index

701

Index

Index

Index

X

X-inactivation
  glucose-6-phosphate
    dehydrogenase deficiency 93
  paroxysmal nocturnal
    hemoglobinuria (PNH) 124
x-ray
  arteriovenous malformations
    (AVMs) 537
  childhood acute lymphoblastic
    leukemia (ALL) 150

childhood acute myeloid leukemia
  (AML) 161
childhood Hodgkin lymphoma
  (HL) 187
coronary angiography 616
coronary artery disease (CAD) 453
excessive blood clots 377
plasma cell neoplasms 266
pulmonary hypertension 416
renal artery stenosis (RAS) 500